Neuroradiology Test and Syllabus
Part 1

Peter E. Weinberg, M.D.
Section Editor

Solomon Batnitzky, M.D.
John R. Bentson, M.D.
R. Nick Bryan, M.D., Ph.D.
Thomas P. Naidich, M.D.
Joseph F. Sackett, M.D.
Robert A. Zimmerman, M.D.

 American College of Radiology
Reston, Virginia   1990

Sets Published
- Chest Disease
- Bone Disease
- Genitourinary Tract Disease
- Gastrointestinal Disease
- Head and Neck Disorders
- Pediatric Disease
- Nuclear Radiology
- Radiation Pathology and Radiation Biology
- Chest Disease II
- Bone Disease II
- Genitourinary Tract Disease II
- Gastrointestinal Disease II
- Head and Neck Disorders II
- Nuclear Radiology II
- Cardiovascular Disease
- Emergency Radiology
- Bone Disease III
- Gastrointestinal Disease III
- Chest Disease III
- Pediatric Disease II
- Nuclear Radiology III
- Head and Neck Disorders III
- Genitourinary Tract Disease III
- Diagnostic Ultrasound
- Breast Disease
- Bone Disease IV
- Pediatric Disease III
- Chest Disease IV
- Neuroradiology

Sets in Preparation
- Gastrointestinal Disease IV
- Nuclear Radiology IV
- Magnetic Resonance
- Biological Effects of Diagnostic and Other Low-Level Radiation
- Cardiovascular Disease II
- Emergency Radiology II
- Genitourinary Tract Disease IV
- Head and Neck Disorders IV
- Bone Disease V
- Pediatric Disease IV
- Diagnostic Ultrasound II

Note: The American College of Radiology and the Editors of the Professional Self-Evaluation and Continuing Education Program, in developing new and revised material for this volume, sought to include the most current and accurate data. However, it is possible that some errors may have been printed. Radiopharmaceutical, contrast agent, and other drug dosages are, we believe, accurate and in accordance with standards current with the publication date. It is recommended, however, *that readers carefully review the manufacturer's package insert to ensure that recommended dosages and interventions are in accordance with any recommendations of this volume.*

AMERICAN COLLEGE OF RADIOLOGY
PROFESSIONAL SELF-EVALUATION AND CONTINUING EDUCATION
PROGRAM

BARRY A. SIEGEL, M.D., *Editor in Chief*
> Professor of Radiology and Medicine and Director, Division of Nuclear Medicine, Edward Mallinckrodt Institute of Radiology, Washington University School of Medicine, St. Louis, Missouri

ANTHONY V. PROTO, M.D., *Associate Editor*
> Professor of Radiology and Interim Chairman, Department of Radiology, Medical College of Virginia, Virginia Commonwealth University, Richmond, Virginia

ELIAS G. THEROS, M.D., *Editor Emeritus*
> Isadore Meschan Distinguished Professor of Radiology, Bowman Gray School of Medicine of Wake Forest University, Winston-Salem, North Carolina

SET 28:

Neuroradiology Test and Syllabus
Part 1

Editor

PETER E. WEINBERG, M.D., Attending Physician, Scripps Memorial Hospital, La Jolla, California; formerly Professor of Radiology and Director of Neuroradiology, Northwestern Memorial Hospital and Northwestern University, Chicago, Illinois

Co-Authors

SOLOMON BATNITZKY, M.D., Professor of Diagnostic Radiology and Chief of Section of Neuroradiology, University of Kansas Medical Center, Kansas City, Kansas

JOHN R. BENTSON, M.D., Professor of Radiology and Chief of Neuroradiology, University of California School of Medicine, Los Angeles, California

R. NICK BRYAN, M.D., PH.D., Director of Neuroradiology, Johns Hopkins Hospital, Baltimore, Maryland

THOMAS P. NAIDICH, M.D., Director of Neuroradiology, Baptist Hospital of Miami, Miami, Florida

JOSEPH F. SACKETT, M.D., Professor and Chairman, Department of Radiology, Clinical Science Center, University of Wisconsin, Madison, Wisconsin

ROBERT A. ZIMMERMAN, M.D., Section Chief of Pediatric Neuroradiology and Section Chief of Pediatric MRI, Children's Hospital, and Staff Neuroradiologist, Hospital of the University of Pennsylvania, Philadelphia, Pennsylvania

Publishing Coordinators:	*G. Rebecca Haines and Thomas M. Rogers*
Publishing Consultant:	*Earle V. Hart*
Administrative Assistant:	*Janice Cameron*
Copy Editor:	*John N. Bell*
Text Processing:	*Fusako T. Nowak*
Composition:	*Karen Finkle and Barbara Ginsburg*
Index:	*Camille Joslyn*
Lithography:	*Lanman Progressive, Washington, D.C.*
Typesetting:	*Publication Technology Corp., Burke, Va.*
Printing:	*John D. Lucas Printing, Baltimore, Md.*

Library of Congress Cataloging-in-Publication Data

Neuroradiology test and syllabus / Peter E. Weinberg, section editor ; Solomon Batnitzky ... [et al.].
    p. cm. — (Professional Self-Evaluation and Continuing Education Program ; set 28)
On cover: Committee on Professional Self-Evaluation and Continuing Education, Commission on Education, American College of Radiology.
    Includes bibliographical references.
    Includes index.
    ISBN 1-55903-028-3 : $230.00. — ISBN 1-55903-000-3 (series)
    1. Nervous system—Radiography—Examinations, questions, etc. I. Weinberg, Peter E., 1935– . II. Batnitzky, Solomon. III. American College of Radiology. Commission on Education. Committee on Professional Self-Evaluation and Continuing Education. IV. Series.
    [DNLM: W1 PR606 set 28 / WL 18 N4943]
RC349.R3N484 1990
616.8′047572′076—dc20
DNLM/DLC   90-714
for Library of Congress   CIP

ACR COMMITTEE ON PROFESSIONAL SELF-EVALUATION AND CONTINUING EDUCATION, COMMISSION ON EDUCATION

Additional Contributors

SCOTT W. ATLAS, M.D., Associate Professor of Radiology, Neuroradiology Section, University of Pennsylvania School of Medicine, Philadelphia, Pennsylvania

BRUCE BAUER, M.D., Head of Division of Plastic Surgery, Children's Memorial Hospital, and Assistant Professor of Surgery, Northwestern University Medical School, Chicago, Illinois

DEAN A. ELIAS, M.D., Director of Neuroradiology, Chicago Neurosurgical Center, Columbus Hospital, Chicago, Illinois

MICHAEL T. GOREY, M.D., Assistant Professor of Radiology, Cornell University Medical College, New York, and Attending Neuroradiologist, North Shore University Hospital, Manhasset, New York

MICHELE H. JOHNSON, M.D., Assistant Professor, Section of Neuroradiology, Departments of Diagnostic Imaging and Neurosurgery, Temple University Hospital, Philadelphia, Pennsylvania

ANDREW J. KURMAN, M.D., Assistant Professor of Radiology, Northeastern Ohio Universities College of Medicine, and Director of Neuroradiology, Akron General Medical Center, Akron, Ohio

DAVID G. McLONE, M.D., PH.D., Professor of Surgery (Neurosurgery), Northwestern University Medical School, and Division Head of Pediatric Neurosurgery, Children's Memorial Hospital, Chicago, Illinois

ERIC J. RUSSELL, M.D., Director of Neuroradiology, Northwestern Memorial Hospital, and Associate Professor of Radiology, Northwestern University Medical School, Chicago, Illinois

SUSAN W. WEATHERS, M.D., Assistant Professor of Radiology, Baylor College of Medicine and the Veterans Administration Medical Center, Houston, Texas

DAVID YOUSEFZADEH, M.D., Professor of Radiology and Pediatrics and Director of Pediatric Radiology, University of Chicago and Wyler Children's Hospital, Chicago, Illinois

Author's Preface

This is the first *Neuroradiology Test and Syllabus* in the College's Professional Self-Evaluation and Continuing Education Program. Prior to this syllabus, neuroradiology was included in those syllabi covering disorders of the head and neck. The third *Disorders of the Head and Neck Syllabus*, which was published in 1985, included case material involving the brain and spinal cord, as well as diseases of the orbits, paranasal sinuses, larynx, salivary glands, mandible, ears, and neck. However, with the advent of magnetic resonance imaging (MRI) and the increasing utilization of computed tomography, it is no longer practical to include neuroradiology and the radiology of other head and neck lesions in one syllabus.

Because of the large amount of material covered, this syllabus is being published in two separate volumes. In this syllabus, we have included both adult neuroradiological case material, which is likely to be commonly encountered in the daily practice of radiology, and also several pediatric neuroradiology cases, which have not been presented in previous syllabi. Many of the chapters include examples of MRI. However, we have not attempted to cover this subject comprehensively, since it will be presented in a separated syllabus to be published in the near future.

As chairman of the Committee for the *Neuroradiology Test and Syllabus*, I would like to express my gratitude to my principal co-authors and Committee members: Drs. Solomon Batnitzky, John R. Bentson, R. Nick Bryan, Thomas P. Naidich, Joseph F. Sackett, and Robert A. Zimmerman. I would also like to thank each of the other contributing authors for their important additions to this syllabus. Most of the case material in this syllabus was written shortly after the advent of MRI, and therefore, the original manuscripts did not include material on this subject. Nevertheless, we believed that it was necessary to include MRI illustrations to demonstrate the importance of this imaging technique in the diagnosis of many neurological disorders. I greatly appreciate the willingness of the authors to add pertinent illustrations and additional text to their already completed manuscripts. Their effort has resulted in a more comprehensive and meaningful presentation of modern neuroradiological imaging.

On behalf of the members of the Neuroradiology Committee I would like to express special thanks to the co-editors of this syllabus: Barry A. Siegel, M.D., Editor in Chief, and Elias G. Theros, M.D., Editor Emeritus. They are deserving of the highest praise for their tireless efforts and expert guidance. Their critical review of every chapter led to many suggestions and revisions, which immeasurably improved the quality of this syllabus.

Special tribute is also due to the staff of the American College of Radiology who are responsible for the publication of this syllabus. Earle Hart was involved in the development and organization of the test and syllabus. We are grateful to him and to his successor as Director of Publications, G. Rebecca Haines, for their enthusiastic support and guidance. Tom Rogers has been involved in all aspects of the production of this syllabus. Tom did a masterful job of editing the manuscripts and assuring the highest quality of the extensive illustrations. I would also like to thank Susan DeBusk, my former secretary, who was helpful in the early phases of development of this syllabus.

Peter E. Weinberg, M.D.
Section Chairman

Editor's Preface

The Professional Self-Evaluation and Continuing Education Program of the American College of Radiology has now reached the 18th anniversary since publication of the inaugural volume in the series. These years have witnessed many important improvements and changes in the program, and this current volume represents one such change. In recognition of the increasing complexity of both neuroradiology and the now distinct subspecialty of head and neck radiology, the educational packages in these areas have been separated. Hence, this volume, which is the 28th in the series, is the first to be devoted entirely to the radiology of the central nervous system.

Despite its evolution over many years, the fundamental concept of the Self-Evaluation Program remains unaltered. In each section of the self-evaluation examination, the participant must first carefully analyze one or more images of an individual patient, then integrate the radiologic findings with pertinent clinical data, and finally select the most likely diagnosis from a carefully chosen list of alternatives. The primary questions in each case are designed to reproduce the diagnostic problems that challenge radiologists daily in their own reading rooms. The primary question of each case is accompanied by one or more satellite questions, which are carefully crafted to probe the reader's cognitive knowledge, primarily in relation to the disorders that constitute the case's differential diagnosis. The syllabus provides the answers to the test questions but, more importantly, is also intended to guide the participant step-by-step through the differential diagnosis by showing how the experts "weigh the evidence" in reaching a diagnosis. The syllabus discussions of the satellite questions are designed to serve as brief reviews of their respective topics to help participants keep abreast of rapid advances in radiologic knowledge.

The process by which a self-evaluation test and its accompanying syllabus are developed is an arduous one. It involves several intensive but lively meetings of the authors at which cases are selected and the questions fine-tuned. Although each of the syllabus discussions represents the individual labor of one or two principal authors, the whole package is subjected to rigorous and critical review by both the section chairman and the series editors. The goal is to ensure that program participants are provided with a syllabus that contains the latest information and so will derive maximal educational benefit.

All radiologists are indebted to Dr. Peter E. Weinberg and his colleagues, Drs. Solomon Batnitzky, John R. Bentson, R. Nick Bryan,

Thomas P. Naidich, Joseph F. Sackett, and Robert A. Zimmerman, for the preparation of the *Neuroradiology Test and Syllabus*. This *opus magnus* provides coverage of a wide variety of diseases of the brain and spinal cord. Although the emphasis is on computed tomography, reflecting the fact that work on this project began several years ago before the general availability of magnetic resonance imaging, the anatomic, physiologic, and pathologic principles encompassed in these discussions freely cross the boundaries between CT and MRI. Moreover, as Dr. Weinberg notes in his preface, the authors have given of their time extraordinarily to provide the relevant MRI updates to their respective discussions. Our readers will surely recognize that the *Neuroradiology Test and Syllabus* is a large package, comprising two volumes. This also reflects the outstandingly thorough job done by Dr. Weinberg and his co-authors and their liberal use of excellent illustrative material throughout the syllabus. Because of the larger size of this package (and the necessarily greater cost), the Committee on Continuing Education in Postgraduate Education of the College's Commission on Education has determined that program participants are eligible to earn a larger number of continuing medical education credits (up to 25 hours) for this set than for past installments in the series.

As always, special thanks are due to the dedicated publications staff of the American College of Radiology, under the highly competent and professional direction of G. Rebecca Haines. Principal editorial kudos go to Thomas M. Rogers, whose patience, attention to detail, and unswerving standards for excellence make the complex production process work so smoothly. The work of this Committee was initiated with the guidance of Mr. Earle V. Harte, Jr. His keen editorial eye and helpful advice in his continuing role as a consultant to the Self-Evaluation Program remain invaluable.

Finally, thanks are due from me and my colleagues—Drs. Anthony V. Proto, Associate Editor and Chairman of the Committee on Professional Self-Evaluation and Continuing Education, and Elias G. Theros, Editor Emeritus—to all the radiologists whose continued enthusiastic support for the Self-Evaluation Program is its *raison d'etre*. Since the inception of this program, nearly 170,000 subscriptions have been recorded in aggregate. Knowledge of this is suitable compensation for all those who have donated their expertise (and many long hours) to ensure the success of this educational venture.

Barry A. Siegel, M.D.
Editor in Chief

Neuroradiology Test

For you to derive the maximum benefit from this program, you should complete the following test, and send your answer sheet to the ACR for scoring, before you proceed to the syllabus.

If for any reason you refer to the syllabus material, or any other references, in answering the questions, please be sure to so indicate when answering Question 155, the first demographic data question. Your score will then *not* be used in developing the norm tables.

NOTE: You must return your answer sheet for scoring, whether or not you use reference materials, in order to claim the 25 hours of Category I credit.

CASE 1: Questions 1 through 5

This 44-year-old man presented with a 1-year history of intermittent severe headaches and dizziness. You are shown pre- and postcontrast infusion computed tomographic (CT) scans (Figures 1-1 and 1-2).

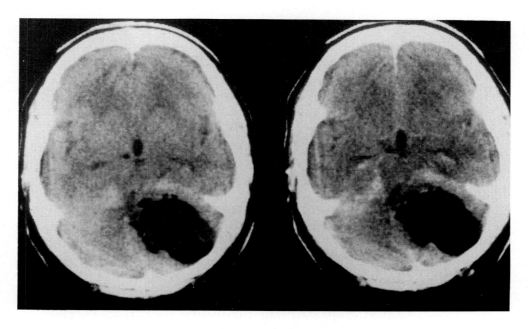

Figure 1-1

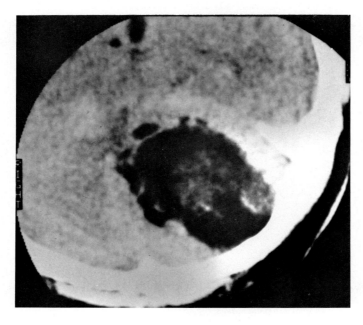

Figure 1-2

CASE 1 (Cont'd)

1. Which *one* of the following is the MOST likely diagnosis?

   (A) Arachnoid cyst
   (B) Dermoid tumor
   (C) Hemangioblastoma
   (D) Cystic metastatic tumor
   (E) Cerebellar astrocytoma

QUESTIONS 2 THROUGH 5: MARK YOUR ANSWER SHEET TRUE (T) OR FALSE (F) FOR EACH OF THE RESPONSE CHOICES.

2. Concerning arachnoid cysts,

   (A) in a minority of cases, they are differentiated from epidermoid tumors by analysis of their CT attenuation values
   (B) the most common site of occurrence in the posterior fossa is the cerebellopontine angle cistern
   (C) the presence of hydrocephalus is an important factor to be considered in distinguishing them from developmentally large cisternae magnae
   (D) those occurring in the cerebellopontine angle cistern do not extend above the tentorium
   (E) the demonstration of contrast within the cysts on delayed positive-contrast cisternography excludes the diagnosis

CASE 1 (Cont'd)

3. Concerning dermoid tumors,

   (A) they are usually distinguishable from arachnoid cysts on contrast-enhanced CT because their capsules are enhanced
   (B) calcification of the lesions is frequently observed on CT scans
   (C) they are composed of elements of one germ layer, the ectoderm
   (D) they are differentiated from arachnoid cysts on magnetic resonance imaging
   (E) CT demonstration of fat in the ventricular system is an indication of rupture of the lesions

4. Concerning hemangioblastomas,

   (A) calcification of the mural nodules is seen in approximately 25% of cases
   (B) they are the most common primary cerebellar tumors in adults
   (C) the mural nodules usually abut a pial surface
   (D) they usually demonstrate ring blush on contrast-enhanced CT
   (E) CT is more accurate than is angiography in demonstrating multiple small solid lesions

5. Concerning cerebellar astrocytomas,

   (A) most cystic tumors with mural nodules are smaller than hemangioblastomas
   (B) hydrocephalus is usually not seen with laterally located cystic astrocytomas
   (C) solid astrocytomas are usually hyperdense on noncontrast CT
   (D) CT demonstrates calcification in approximately one-half of cases
   (E) angiography commonly demonstrates intense tumor blush of the mural nodules

This 64-year-old man presented with a 3-week history of intermittent states of confusion. You are shown pre- and postcontrast computed tomographic (CT) scans (Figure 2-1).

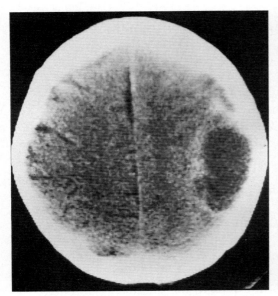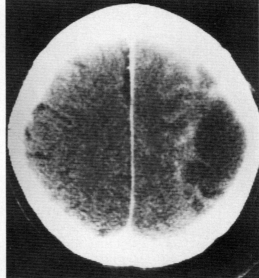

Figure 2-1

6. Which *one* of the following is the MOST likely diagnosis?

    (A) Infiltrating glioma
    (B) Subdural hematoma
    (C) Hemorrhagic infarct
    (D) Cortical vein thrombosis
    (E) Meningioma

QUESTIONS 7 THROUGH 10: MARK YOUR ANSWER SHEET TRUE (T) OR FALSE (F) FOR EACH OF THE RESPONSE CHOICES.

7. Concerning gliomatous tumors,

    T (A) magnetic resonance imaging (MRI) with paramagnetic contrast agents more reliably differentiates tumor growth from associated edema than does noncontrast MRI in cases of malignant glioma

    T (B) gliomas spread along white matter tracts

    T (C) hemorrhage occurs in 20% of all intracranial gliomas

    F (D) low-grade gliomas exhibit moderate contrast enhancement

    F (E) angiography demonstrates tumor vascularity in approximately 80% of malignant gliomas

8. Concerning CT findings of subdural hematoma (SDH),

    F (A) the density of the hematoma is an accurate indicator of its age

    T (B) unilateral obliteration of cortical sulci is a reliable finding for differentiation between isodense SDH and acute infarction

    F (C) buckling of the gray matter-white matter interface is seen with both SDH and meningioma

    T (D) MRI is more sensitive than CT for the detection of subacute SDH

    T (E) rebleeding into a chronic SDH simulates a hemorrhagic infarct

CASE 2 (Cont'd)

9. Concerning cerebral infarcts,

    (A) mass effect on CT is seen in approximately 60% of all infarcts during the first week
    (B) the combination of mass effect and associated contrast enhancement on CT virtually excludes the diagnosis
    (C) approximately 20% are demonstrated only on the contrast-enhanced scan
    (D) ring enhancement on CT is uncommon unless there is associated hemorrhage
    (E) those secondary to occlusion of a superficial cortical vein involve the white matter

10. Concerning meningiomas,

    (A) a low-density area adjacent to the tumor is most frequently caused by atrophy
    (B) nonenhancing low-density areas can be seen in 15% of benign meningiomas
    (C) tumor vessels usually arise only from internal carotid artery branches
    (D) extensive white matter edema occurs
    (E) intratumoral hemorrhage is highly specific for malignant meningioma

CASE 3: Questions 11 through 14

This 66-year-old man presented with severe headaches. You are shown pre- and postcontrast computed tomographic (CT) scans (Figures 3-1 and 3-2).

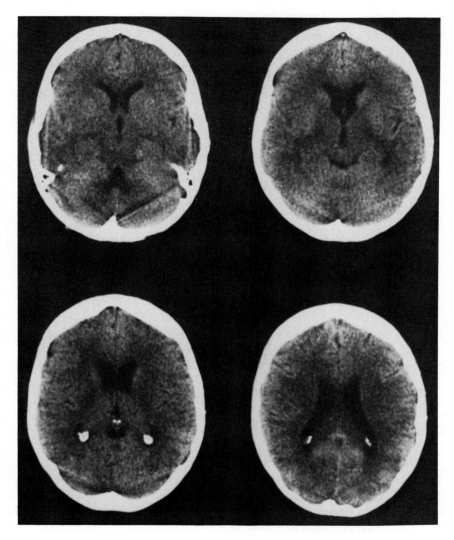

Figure 3-1

CASE 3 (Cont'd)

11. Which *one* of the following is the MOST likely diagnosis?

   (A) Subarachnoid hemorrhage
   (B) Cerebellar infarction
   (C) Diffuse leptomeningeal metastatic neoplasm
   (D) Arteriovenous malformation
   (E) Metastatic parenchymal tumors

QUESTIONS 12 THROUGH 14: MARK YOUR ANSWER SHEET TRUE (T) OR FALSE (F) FOR EACH OF THE RESPONSE CHOICES.

12. Concerning cerebellar infarction,

   (A) cerebellar arteries do not freely communicate over the surface of the cerebellum
   (B) a common presenting symptom is vertigo
   (C) the superior cerebellar artery is the most common vessel involved
   (D) absent filling of the posterior inferior cerebellar artery on angiography confirms the diagnosis
   (E) nodular and ring-like enhancement on CT makes differentiation from neoplasm difficult
   (F) obliteration of posterior fossa cisterns on CT suggests poor prognosis

13. Concerning leptomeningeal spread of neoplasm,

   (A) leptomeningeal metastases are usually not diagnosed on CT unless they produce hydrocephalus and obliteration of the cisterns
   (B) squamous cell carcinoma commonly invades the leptomeninges
   (C) most lymphomas demonstrate involvement of both the leptomeninges and deep-brain structures on contrast-enhanced CT
   (D) in the majority of cases, leptomeningeal carcinomatosis cannot be differentiated from bacterial meningitis by CT

T-8 / *Neuroradiology*

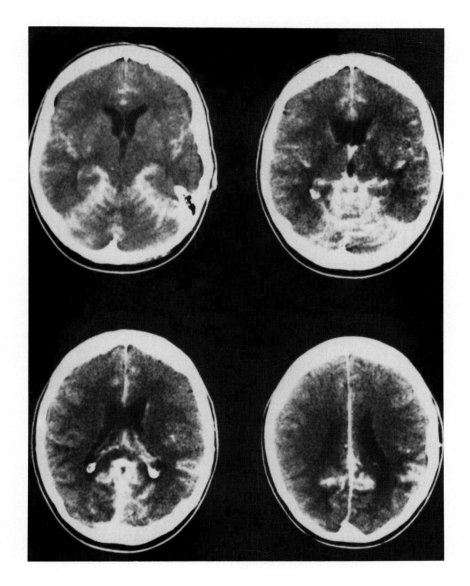

Figure 3-2

CASE 3 (Cont'd)

14. Concerning arteriovenous malformations,

   (A) in the absence of hemorrhage, mass effect is not seen on CT
   (B) noncontrast CT demonstrates mixed increased and decreased densities only when hemorrhage is present
   (C) on CT, low-density areas in the parenchyma adjacent to an arteriovenous malformation most commonly represent edema
   (D) CT evidence of calcification is seen in less than one-third of cases
   (E) the predominant site of hemorrhage is the subarachnoid space

CASE 4: Questions 15 through 19

For each numbered image (Questions 15 through 19) select the *one* lettered diagnosis (A, B, C, D, or E) that is MOST likely. Each lettered diagnosis may be used once, more than once, or not at all.

15. Figure 4-1
16. Figure 4-2
17. Figure 4-3
18. Figure 4-4
19. Figure 4-5

    (A) Tuberous sclerosis
    (B) Lipoma of the corpus callosum
    (C) Agenesis of the corpus callosum
    (D) Sturge-Weber syndrome
    (E) Colloid cyst

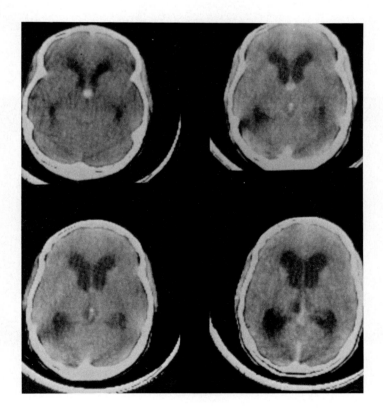

Figure 4-1

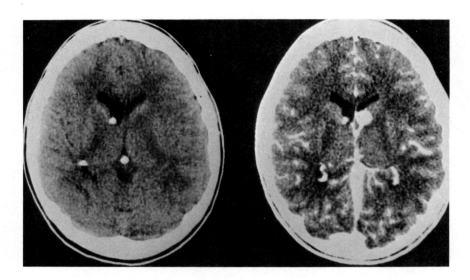

Figure 4-2

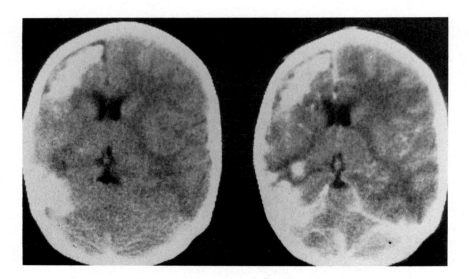

Figure 4-3

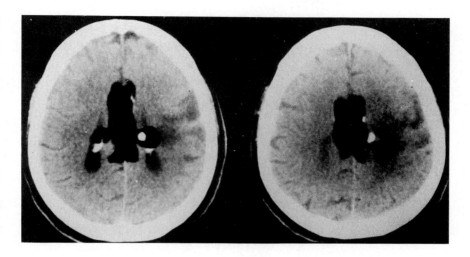

Figure 4-4

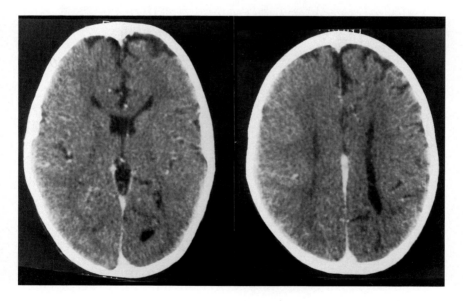

Figure 4-5

This 33-year-old man had a left sixth cranial nerve palsy. You are shown postcontrast CT sections of the sellar and parasellar regions obtained by using both soft tissue (Figure 5-1) and bone (Figures 5-2 and 5-3) window settings.

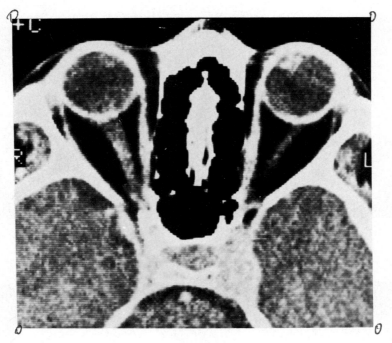

Figure 5-1

20. Which *one* of the following is the MOST likely diagnosis?

    (A) Aneurysm
    (B) Pituitary adenoma
    (C) Parasellar meningioma
    (D) Trigeminal neuroma
    (E) Dural arteriovenous malformation

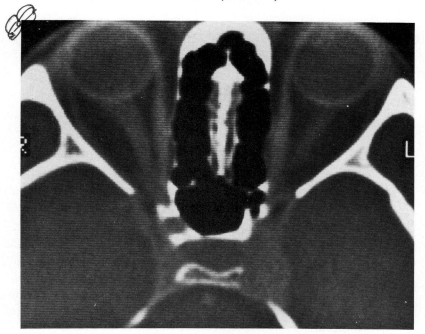

Figure 5-2

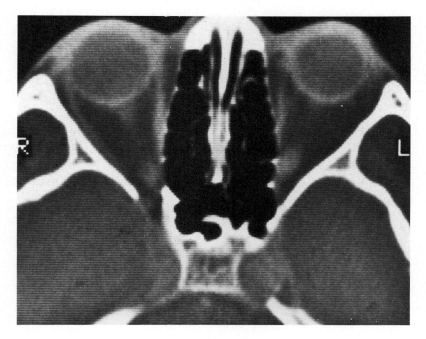

Figure 5-3

CASE 5 (Cont'd)

QUESTIONS 21 THROUGH 24: MARK YOUR ANSWER SHEET TRUE (T) OR FALSE (F) FOR EACH OF THE RESPONSE CHOICES.

21. Concerning CT of the sellar and parasellar areas,

    (A) the cavernous sinuses are normally symmetrical
    (B) the pituitary stalk lies anterior to the optic chiasm
    (C) contrast infusion is necessary to demonstrate the internal carotid artery within the cavernous sinus by CT scanning
    (D) on contrast-enhanced CT performed by drip infusion, the density of the pituitary gland is nearly the same as that of the cavernous sinus
    (E) on CT, disease processes within the cavernous sinus are more often recognized by change in form than by change in density

22. Concerning parasellar meningiomas involving the cavernous sinus,

    (A) bone erosion is more common than sclerosis
    (B) calcification of the tumor is usually evident on CT scans
    (C) the tumor usually extends into the anterior part of the middle fossa
    (D) the most specific diagnostic sign of this tumor on angiography is blood supply from the middle meningeal artery
    (E) encasement of the internal carotid artery favors the diagnosis of meningioma

23. Concerning trigeminal neuromas,

    T (A) they are usually confined to the cavernous sinus region and middle fossa
    T (B) the pattern of bone erosion is similar to that with other tumors of the cavernous sinus region and middle fossa
    F (C) they frequently exhibit an intense tumor blush on angiography
    T (D) the incidence is higher in patients with neurofibroma-tosis
    T (E) calcification is rarely seen in them

24. Concerning parasellar vascular lesions,

    T (A) aneurysms of the cavernous portions of the carotid arteries are bilateral in about 5% of patients
    F (B) dural arteriovenous malformations (AVMs) usually cause enlargement of the cavernous sinus
    F (C) aneurysms of the cavernous portions of the carotid arteries are more readily treatable than dural AVMs of the cavernous sinus
    F (D) patients with aneurysms of the cavernous portions of the carotid artery usually present with symptoms caused by rupture
    T (E) in patients with cavernous sinus AVMs, bilateral eye signs usually indicate bilateral AVMs

This 46-year-old woman presented with a 1-month history of headaches and mild hemiparesis. You are shown pre- and postcontrast computed tomographic scans (Figure 6-1).

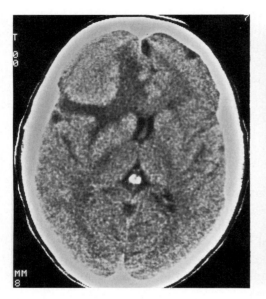
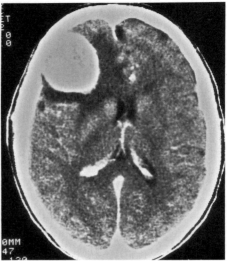

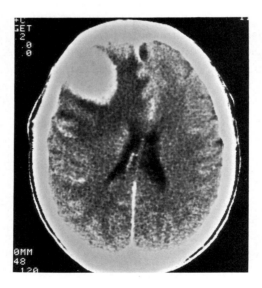

Figure 6-1

CASE 6 (Cont'd)

25. Which *one* of the following is the MOST likely diagnosis?

    (A) Cerebral hematoma
    (B) Glioma
    (C) Meningioma
    (D) Metastasis
    (E) Abscess

QUESTIONS 26 THROUGH 29: MARK YOUR ANSWER SHEET TRUE (T) OR FALSE (F) FOR EACH OF THE RESPONSE CHOICES.

26. Concerning gliomas,

    (A) calcification of gliomas tends to be diffuse rather than focal
    (B) bilateral cerebral hypodensity on computed tomography (CT) suggests infiltration of the corpus callosum
    (C) the presence of multiple cavities within a cerebral mass lesion is a reliable sign favoring glioma or other neoplasm over cerebral abscess
    (D) an enhancing cerebral mass without surrounding edema seen on CT scanning is more likely to be a glioma than a metastasis
    (E) they are less likely than metastases to occur at the corticomedullary junction

27. Concerning cerebral edema,

    (A) the amount of edema around a tumor is usually proportional to the tumor's degree of malignancy
    (B) the pattern of edema reliably differentiates cerebral abscesses from neoplasms
    (C) the direction of white matter fiber tracts strongly influences the pattern of edema, as demonstrated by CT or magnetic resonance imaging (MRI)
    (D) it is less likely to spread along the fiber tracts of the corpus callosum than along the fiber tracts of the ipsilateral cerebral hemisphere

Case 6—Test / T-19

28. Regarding meningiomas,

   (A) the base of the skull is the most common site of origin of intracranial meningiomas
   (B) the amount of associated cerebral edema predicts the histologic type
   (C) less than 10% are cystic
   (D) erosion of bone is more commonly seen with meningiomas of the skull vault than with those of the skull base
   (E) when multiple they may be of the same histological type or belong to different tumor types in the same patient

29. Concerning cerebral hematomas,

   (A) contrast enhancement is usually of the ring type
   (B) the edema adjacent to them is usually maximal on the day of the bleed
   (C) the hematocrit has little effect on their CT density
   (D) in the absence of trauma, the presence of multiple high-density lesions on CT suggests bleeding diathesis
   (E) in the absence of hypertension, the cause of most hemorrhages will be apparent on CT provided that both pre- and postcontrast scans are performed

This 35-year-old man presented with recent onset of left hemiparesis. You are shown pre- and postcontrast computed tomographic scans (Figure 7-1).

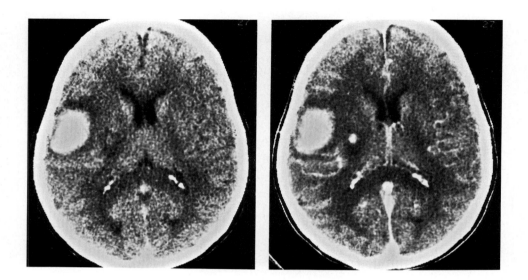

Figure 7-1

30. Which *one* of the following is the MOST likely diagnosis?

    (A) Hypertensive hemorrhage
    (B) Arteriovenous malformation
    (C) Metastatic disease
    (D) Mycotic aneurysm
    (E) Cavernous hemangioma

CASE 7 (Cont'd)

QUESTIONS 31 THROUGH 33: MARK YOUR ANSWER SHEET TRUE (T) OR FALSE (F) FOR EACH OF THE RESPONSE CHOICES.

31. Concerning cerebral arteriovenous malformations (AVMs),

   (A) their likelihood of rupture increases with increasing lesion size
   (B) they usually derive their blood supply from only one major artery
   (C) large AVMs and neoplasms of similar size produce similar degrees of ventricular shift
   (D) a single draining vein is more typically associated with venous angiomas than with AVMs
   (E) aneurysms associated with them rarely bleed

32. Concerning cerebral metastases,

   (A) they can involve all intracranial structures, including the pituitary and pineal glands
   (B) those most likely to bleed are melanoma and chorio-carcinoma
   (C) hemorrhage from metastases is less likely to spread to the subarachnoid or ventricular spaces than hemorrhage related to hypertension or AVMs
   (D) when there is associated hemorrhage, the tumor itself is usually recognizable on CT by performing postcontrast scans

CASE 7 (Cont'd)

33. Concerning mycotic aneurysms,

    (A) the territory of the middle cerebral artery is most commonly involved
    (B) they are usually larger than congenital aneurysms when first detected
    (C) medical treatment is frequently successful, obviating surgical therapy
    (D) an unusual location is generally the main CT or angiographic finding suggesting that an aneurysm may be mycotic
    (E) cerebrovascular accidents due to fungal diseases, such as aspergillosis and mucormycosis, are usually due to rupture of mycotic aneurysms

CASE 8: Questions 34 through 38

This 16-year-old boy presented with a 1-week history of headache, vomiting, dysarthria, and seizures. You are shown pre- and postcontrast computed tomographic (CT) scans (Figures 8-1 and 8-2).

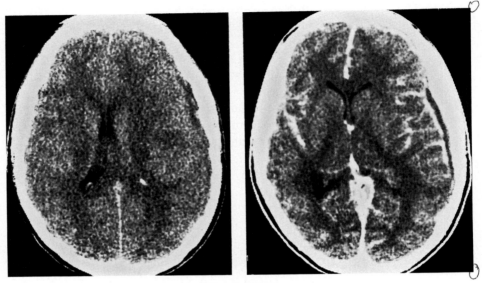

Figure 8-1

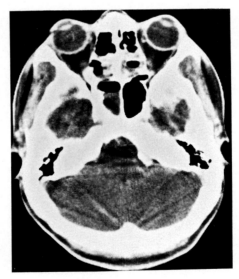

Figure 8-2

CASE 8 (Cont'd)

34. Which *one* of the following is the MOST likely diagnosis?

    (A) Subdural hematoma
    (B) Subdural hygroma
    (C) Subdural empyema
    (D) Epidural abscess
    (E) Malignant subdural effusion

QUESTIONS 35 THROUGH 38: MARK YOUR ANSWER SHEET TRUE (T) OR FALSE (F) FOR EACH OF THE RESPONSE CHOICES.

35. Concerning subdural hematomas,

    (A) less than 50% are associated with skull fractures
    (B) when acute they are similar in shape to chronic epidural hematomas
    (C) they are more often bilateral in young children than in adults
    (D) contrast enhancement around their margins indicates a superimposed infection
    (E) different densities within them are usually due to either settling or rebleeding

36. Concerning subdural hygromas,

    (A) most are considered sequelae of subdural hematomas
    (B) they show marginal contrast enhancement less often than do subdural hematomas
    (C) they are more common in children than in adults
    (D) they infrequently form immediately after head trauma
    (E) when associated with meningitis, the most common organism responsible is *Hemophilus influenzae*

37. Concerning subdural empyemas,

(A) most cases are related to acute sinusitis
(B) CT usually shows marginal contrast enhancement
(C) no angiographically recognizable abnormalities are seen in adjacent cerebral vessels
(D) surgical drainage is usually not necessary if the responsible organism is known
(E) clinical signs and symptoms are usually much more marked than those associated with subdural hematomas of similar size

38. Concerning epidural abscesses,

(A) they have the same shape on CT scans as subdural empyemas
(B) they are more common than subdural infections following neurosurgical procedures
(C) they are more commonly associated with abnormalities of the cranial vault than are subdural empyemas
(D) their presence is indicated by the separation of a dural venous sinus from the skull
(E) separation of the dura from the skull is readily apparent on CT scans, especially after contrast infusion

This 31-year-old man presented with progressive visual field defect. You are shown pre- and postcontrast computed tomographic (CT) sections (Figures 9-1 to 9-4).

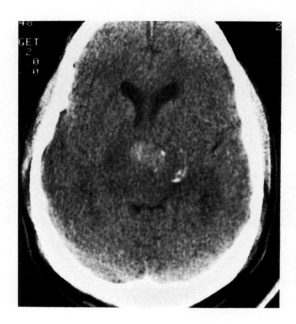

Figure 9-1

39. Which *one* of the following is the MOST likely diagnosis?

    (A) Hypothalamic glioma
    (B) Tuberculum meningioma
    (C) Craniopharyngioma
    (D) Giant aneurysm
    (E) Pituitary tumor with hemorrhage

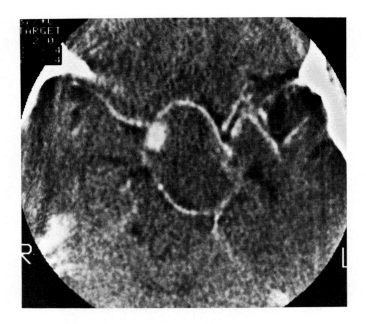

Figure 9-2

QUESTIONS 40 THROUGH 43: MARK YOUR ANSWER SHEET
TRUE (T) OR FALSE (F) FOR EACH OF THE RESPONSE
CHOICES.

40. Concerning suprasellar masses,

(A) they all produce similar changes in the sella
(B) craniopharyngiomas and giant aneurysms are the two
     suprasellar masses most likely to be calcified
(C) a tuberculum meningioma is less likely to present with
     visual field changes than are other suprasellar tumors
(D) hypothalamic gliomas are more likely to receive major
     arterial feeders from the ophthalmic arteries than are
     other suprasellar tumors
(E) bleeding from a pituitary tumor may mimic curvilinear
     calcification

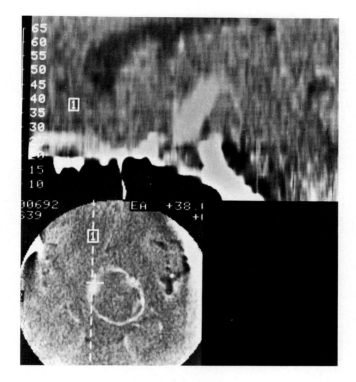

Figure 9-3

41. Concerning tuberculum meningiomas,

   (A) calcification is less common than in craniopharyngiomas

   (B) blood supply is mainly from the middle meningeal artery

   (C) the adjacent planum sphenoidale is commonly eroded

   (D) the pattern of displacement of the internal carotid and anterior cerebral arteries is different from that seen with suprasellar pituitary tumors

   (E) when erosion of the dorsum sellae is seen with this tumor, it usually reflects increased intracranial pressure rather than the effect of adjacent mass

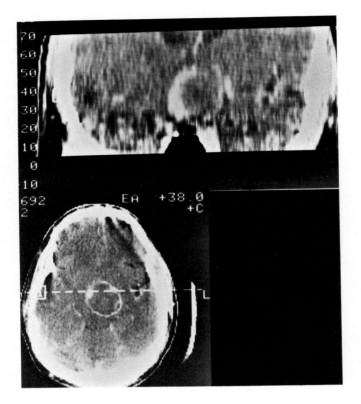

Figure 9-4

42. Concerning craniopharyngiomas,

    (A) calcification is usually peripheral and curvilinear
    (B) they are more often calcified in adults than in children
    (C) they are more likely than other suprasellar masses to grow into the posterior fossa
    (D) visual changes are less common than endocrine changes
    (E) if the solid portion of a partly cystic tumor can be removed, the tumor will rarely recur

CASE 9 (Cont'd)

43. Concerning giant aneurysms,

T (A) most suprasellar giant aneurysms arise from the internal carotid artery
T (B) their CT pattern is most specific when the aneurysm is partially thrombosed
F (C) they are usually found in elderly patients with generalized arteriosclerotic disease
F (D) following contrast infusion, CT usually shows intense uniform contrast enhancement
T (E) when CT shows no calcification within a suprasellar mass, aneurysm is very unlikely

This 2-year-old girl presented with weakness of the lower extremities. You are shown a midsagittal magnetic resonance (MR) image of the craniovertebral junction (0.5 T; TR, 500 msec; TE, 30 msec) (Figure 10-1).

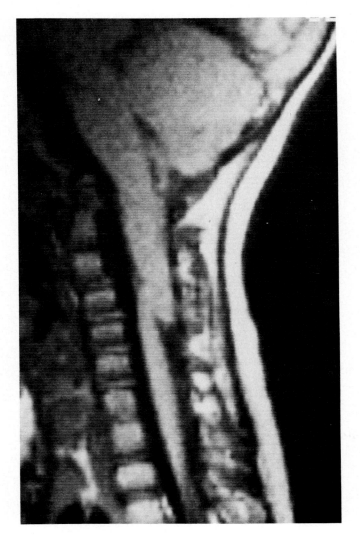

Figure 10-1

CASE 10 (Cont'd)

44. Which *one* of the following is the MOST likely diagnosis?

   (A) Cerebellar tumor with tonsillar herniation
   (B) Inferior extraventricular extension of fourth ventricular ependymoma
   (C) Chiari II malformation
   (D) Spinal cord astrocytoma
   (E) Foramen magnum-upper cervical neurinoma

QUESTIONS 45 THROUGH 49: MARK YOUR ANSWER SHEET TRUE (T) OR FALSE (F) FOR EACH OF THE RESPONSE CHOICES.

45. Tonsillar herniation:

   (A) may be diagnosed confidently when the lower poles of the tonsils lie inferior to the lower lip of the foramen magnum
   (B) is the most common mass displacement caused by space-occupying intracranial lesions
   (C) is more common with occipital glioma than with anterior falcine meningioma
   (D) is more common with external obstructive hydrocephalus than with aqueductal stenosis
   (E) is associated with a positive Lhermitte's sign

46. Tumors that grow downward through the foramen magnum into the posterior cervical subarachnoid space include:

   (A) ependymoma
   (B) medulloblastoma
   (C) cerebellar astrocytoma
   (D) epidermoid tumor of the fourth ventricle
   (E) meningioma

47. Concerning the Chiari malformations,

T (A) clinically evident myelomeningocele signifies Type II

T (B) cervical "spur" and "kink" signify Type I

F (C) segmentation anomalies of the cervical spine and skull base are more commonly associated with Type I than with Type II

F (D) hydrocephalus occurs more frequently with Type I than with Type II

T (E) downbeat nystagmus suggests the presence of Type I

48. Spinal cord astrocytomas:

F (A) represent hematogenous dissemination of cerebral astrocytomas

T (B) extend over several cord segments

T (C) remain buried within the substance of the cord and displace relatively normal but compressed cord tissue circumferentially

T (D) are associated with intramedullary cysts in more than 25% of cases

T (E) generally present clinically with both hydrocephalus and papilledema

49. A "dumbbell" neurinoma:

T (A) implies underlying neurofibromatosis

F (B) is commonly calcified

T (C) usually causes foraminal enlargement

F (D) is characteristically hyperdense on noncontrast computed tomography

T (E) exhibits enhancement on infusion computed tomography

This 16-month-old boy presented with painful swelling at the glabella. You are shown a photograph of the patient's face (Figure 11-1), direct coronal noncontrast computed tomographic (CT) scans through the glabella (Figure 11-2; soft tissue window) and the nasofrontal junction (Figure 11-3; bone window image), and axial noncontrast CT scans through the nasofrontal junction and glabella (Figure 11-4).

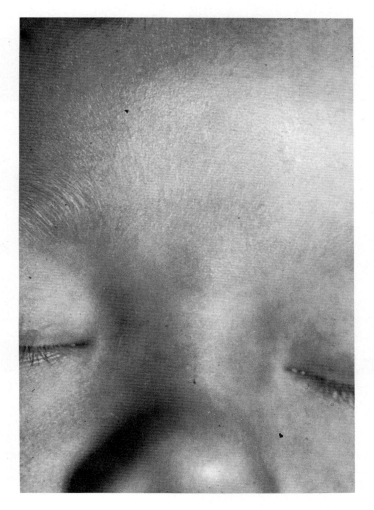

Figure 11-1

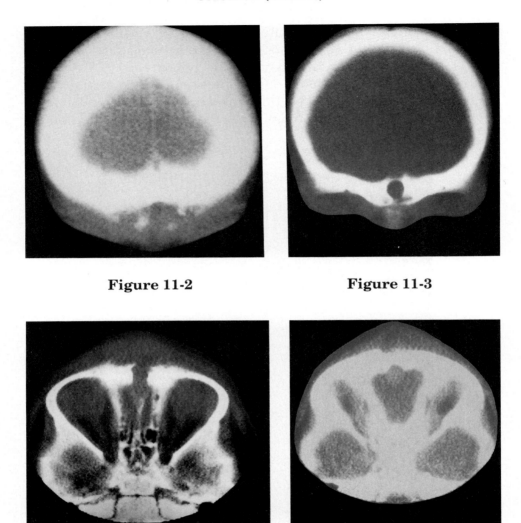

Figure 11-2   Figure 11-3

Figure 11-4

50. Which *one* of the following is the MOST likely diagnosis?

   (A) Infected dermal sinus/epidermoid cyst
   (B) Nasal glioma
   (C) Nasofrontal cephalocele
   (D) Histiocytosis X
   (E) Sinus pericranii

QUESTIONS 51 THROUGH 55: MARK YOUR ANSWER SHEET TRUE (T) OR FALSE (F) FOR EACH OF THE RESPONSE CHOICES.

51. Nasal dermal sinuses:

   (A) lie in the true midline of the body
   (B) present as sinus ostia or as cysts with nearly equal frequency
   (C) extend intracranially in 80% of cases
   (D) progress to squamous cell carcinoma in approximately 2% of cases
   (E) are associated with a widened foramen cecum and distorted crista galli only when the dermoid elements enter the cranial cavity

52. Concerning nasal gliomas and cephaloceles,

   (A) an intranasal mass that is connected directly to the brain is a nasal cephalocele, not a nasal glioma
   (B) extranasal gliomas typically present as midline lesions at the nasal root
   (C) in infants, nasal gliomas are more common than inflammatory nasal polyps
   (D) nasal gliomas are very low-grade neoplasms
   (E) nasal gliomas are easily identified by their characteristically increased attenuation on computed tomography

53. Concerning cephaloceles,

   (A) the size of the fluid space within the sac determines patient prognosis
   (B) sincipital cephaloceles are closely linked with other neural tube defects
   (C) in nasofrontal cephaloceles, the ethmoid bone is displaced inferiorly

54. Concerning histiocytosis X,

   (A) calvarial lesions are more commonly parietal than temporal
   (B) involvement of the posterior pituitary gland most commonly accounts for concurrent diabetes insipidus
   (C) calvarial lesions frequently erode the outer table to present as tender soft tissue masses
   (D) calvarial lesions commonly erode through dura into the underlying cortex
   (E) computed tomographic demonstration of a central density within the calvarial lesion rules out this diagnosis

55. Concerning sinus pericranii,

   (A) it signifies chronic elevation of intracranial pressure
   (B) it most commonly involves the frontal region
   (C) it lies within 2 cm of the true midline, to either side of the superior sagittal sinus
   (D) it is usually associated with well-defined calvarial defects
   (E) it communicates with the dural venous sinuses via emissary and diploic veins

CASE 12: Questions 56 through 61

This full-term infant girl was born with the umbilical cord wound once about the neck and had Apgar scores of 9 and 9 at 1 and 5 minutes, respectively. On day 13 she developed cyanosis, apnea, and seizures. Gram stain and cultures and titers of virus in blood and in cerebrospinal fluid were all negative. Physical examination showed a lethargic girl with weak grasp, increased extensor tone, posturing, and weakly up-going toes bilaterally. You are shown four sections of a noncontrast computed tomographic (CT) scan obtained at 8 weeks of age (Figure 12-1).

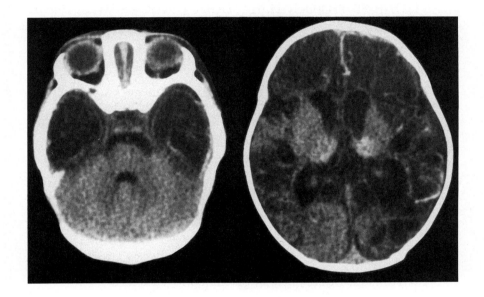

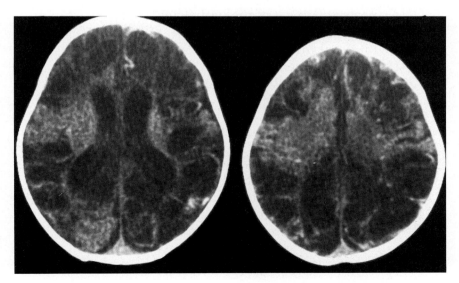

Figure 12-1

CASE 12 (Cont'd)

56. Which *one* of the following is the MOST likely diagnosis?

   (A) Multicystic encephalomalacia
   (B) Porencephaly
   (C) Schizencephaly
   (D) Hydranencephaly
   (E) Middle cerebral artery emboli

QUESTIONS 57 THROUGH 61: MARK YOUR ANSWER SHEET TRUE (T) OR FALSE (F) FOR EACH OF THE RESPONSE CHOICES.

57. Features characteristic of multicystic encephalomalacia include:

   (A) origin of cysts prior to the third month of gestation
   (B) bilateral involvement
   (C) direct continuity between the lesion cavities and the ventricles
   (D) uniform size of individual cysts
   (E) smooth lesion walls

58. Features characteristic of porencephaly include:

   (A) postnatal onset of the pathology
   (B) smooth lesion walls
   (C) bilateral involvement
   (D) multiloculated cysts
   (E) continuity between lesions and ventricles

59. Features characteristic of schizencephaly include:

   (A) heterotopias of gray matter
   (B) concurrent zones of polymicrogyria
   (C) thrombosis of multiple middle cerebral artery branches
   (D) absence of the interhemispheric fissure
   (E) bilateral, paramedian hemorrhages

This 1-month-old boy presented with a palpable skin-covered lumbosacral mass and spina bifida. You are shown 5.0-MHz sonograms taken through the lesion (Figure 14-1). (A and B) Longitudinal (sagittal) sonograms oriented like a myelogram, with cephalic toward the top, caudal toward the bottom, and anterior toward the reader's left. (C through F) Axial sonograms oriented like CT scans, with ventral toward the top of each image (panel C is the most cephalic and panel F is the most caudal of these axial images).

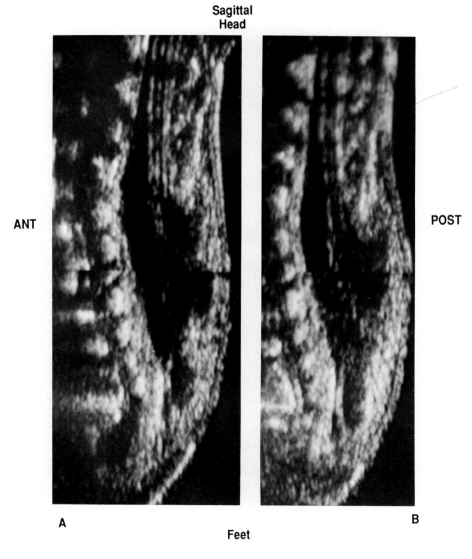

Figure 14-1

CASE 14 (Cont'd)

68. Which *one* of the following is the MOST likely diagnosis?

    (A) Lipomyelomeningocele
    (B) Simple meningocele
    (C) Myelocystocele
    (D) Sacrococcygeal teratoma
    (E) Dermal sinus with dermoid/epidermoid tumor

Transverse
Ventral

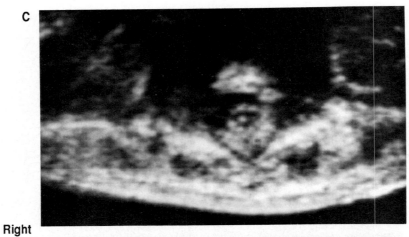

Dorsal

Transverse
Ventral

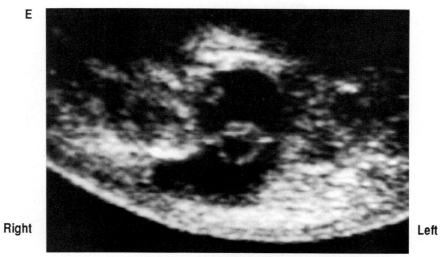

E

Right   Left

F

Dorsal

QUESTIONS 69 THROUGH 73: MARK YOUR ANSWER SHEET TRUE (T) OR FALSE (F) FOR EACH OF THE RESPONSE CHOICES.

69. Lipomyelomeningoceles are commonly associated with:

T (A) Chiari I malformation
T (B) Chiari II malformation
T (C) clinical progression to paraparesis and urinary incontinence despite initial normal neurological examination
T (D) partial dorsal myeloschisis
T (E) extracanalicular protrusion of the spinal cord

70. Simple meningoceles contain:

F (A) dura
T (B) arachnoid
F (C) dermoid/epidermoid tumors
F (D) herniated spinal cord
F (E) intrinsic nerve roots

71. Myelocystoceles commonly:

T (A) are associated with meningoceles
T (B) are associated with hydromyelia
T (C) contain an ependyma-lined cyst
T (D) are associated with cloacal exstrophy
F (E) indicate concurrent Dandy-Walker malformation

72. Sacrococcygeal teratomas commonly:

T (A) lie within or below the intergluteal crease
T (B) extend into the pelvis below a normal sacrum
F (C) are associated with myelomeningocele
F (D) are associated with concurrent pineal teratomas
T (E) contain fibroadipose tissue

73. Dermal sinuses of the back:

F (A) usually appear at sites of prior spinal taps because of implantation of dermal elements along the needle tract

T (B) nearly always extend to and stop at the coccyx

T (C) suggest the likelihood of concurrent dermoid/epidermoid tumors

T (D) rarely become infected

T (E) typically pass progressively more cephalically from their origin at the skin to their deep termination

This 40-year-old woman had slowly progressive lower extremity weakness and hyper-reflexia. You are shown scans from a CT-myelogram, including reformatted sagittal and coronal images (Figures 15-1 through 15-3).

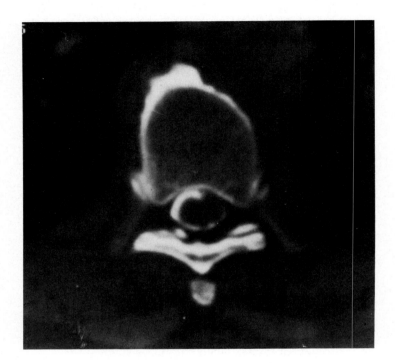

Figure 15-1

74. Which *one* of the following is the MOST likely diagnosis?

    (A) Neurofibroma
    (B) Astrocytoma
    (C) Meningioma
    (D) Ependymoma
    (E) Herniated thoracic disc

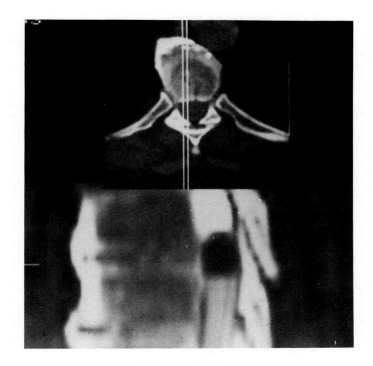

Figure 15-2

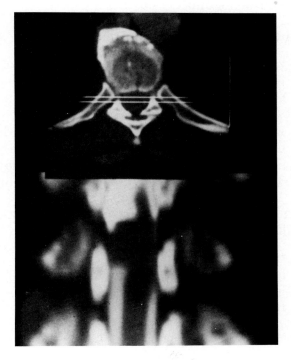

Figure 15-3

QUESTIONS 75 THROUGH 78: MARK YOUR ANSWER SHEET TRUE (T) OR FALSE (F) FOR EACH OF THE RESPONSE CHOICES.

75. Concerning spinal neoplasms,

    T (A) expanded neural foramina in patients with von Recklinghausen's disease are indicative of neurofibromas
    F (B) astrocytoma of the spinal cord in childhood is a rapidly progressive neoplasm
    F (C) the most common calcified lesion impinging upon the thoracic spinal canal is a meningioma
    T (D) ependymoma is the most common tumor found at or below the conus medullaris
    T (E) lipoma is usually associated with dysraphism

76. Spinal lesions that are typically intradural and extramedullary include:

    T (A) epidermoid tumor
    F (B) meningioma
    T (C) neurofibroma
    F (D) astrocytoma
    T (E) neuroblastoma

77. Regarding intradural spinal tumors,

    F (A) use of gadolinium-DTPA during magnetic resonance imaging (MRI) is inappropriate
    T (B) C1-C2 spinal puncture is safer than lumbar puncture when performing myelography
    F (C) noncontrast CT scanning is accurate for diagnosis
    F (D) CSF cytology is a highly sensitive means of diagnosis
    F (E) seeding of the spinal subarachnoid space occurs only with tumors arising in the central nervous system

78. Disorders of the spinal cord frequently associated with cystic medullary changes include:

    T (A) trauma
    T (B) astrocytoma
    F (C) multiple sclerosis
    T (D) hemangioblastoma

CASE 16: Questions 79 and 80

This 58-year-old man presented with progressive myelopathy. You are shown frontal and lateral views from a myelogram produced with a water-soluble contrast agent (Figures 16-1 and 16-2).

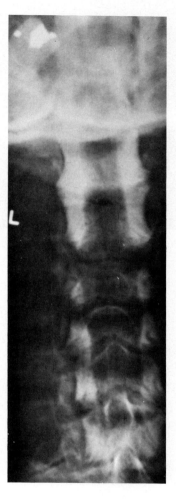

Figure 16-1

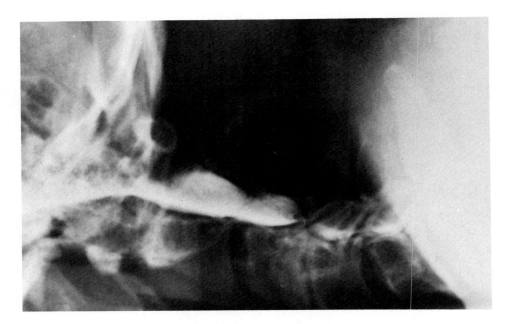

Figure 16-2

79. Which *one* of the following is the MOST likely diagnosis?

    (A) Disc herniation
    (B) Cervical spondylosis
    (C) Congenital cervical spinal stenosis
    (D) Ossified posterior longitudinal ligament
    (E) Cervical astrocytoma

CASE 16 (Cont'd)

QUESTION 80: MARK YOUR ANSWER SHEET TRUE (T) OR
FALSE (F) FOR EACH OF THE RESPONSE CHOICES.

80. Concerning cervical myelography with water-soluble contrast agents,

   (A) fluids should be restricted to avoid contrast medium-
   induced emesis and aspiration
   (B) in patients with kyphosis, the prone position is
   preferred to bring contrast agent upward from the
   lumbar region to the cervical region
   (C) lateral cervical spinal puncture is best accomplished
   by aligning the needle with the posterior aspect of the
   dens
   (D) flexion and extension views are required for accurate
   diagnosis of cord compression
   (E) postmyelography headache is minimized if the patient
   lies prone for 12 hours after the procedure

This 35-year-old man was involved in a motorcycle accident. He was not wearing a helmet. You are shown a noncontrast computed tomographic (CT) scan (Figure 17-1).

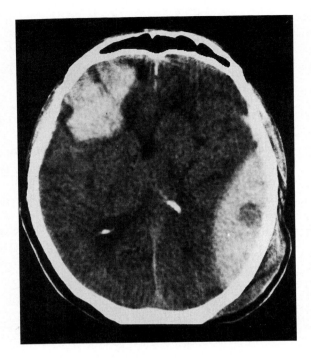

Figure 17-1

81. Which *one* of the following CT features is MOST indicative of an unusual degree of urgency in the treatment of this patient?

    (A) Degree of midline shift of the ventricles
    (B) Location of the epidural hematoma
    (C) Lucency within the epidural hematoma
    (D) Size of the intracerebral hematoma
    (E) Degree of ventricular compression

QUESTIONS 82 AND 83: MARK YOUR ANSWER SHEET TRUE (T) OR FALSE (F) FOR EACH OF THE RESPONSE CHOICES.

82. Concerning head trauma,

F (A) skull radiography is the most valuable initial radiologic study to exclude basilar skull fracture

F (B) in the "battered child" syndrome, intracerebral hematoma is more common than extracerebral hematoma

T (C) current neurosurgical management of patients with intracranial hematoma includes both CT scanning and epidural pressure monitoring

T (D) the recovery rate in acute subdural hematoma is high

T (E) venous epidural hematoma results from tearing of dural bridging veins

83. Concerning basilar skull fractures,

T (A) early diagnosis is of primary importance in a patient with acute head injury

T (B) meningitis is often associated

T (C) CT findings include pneumocephalus and an air-fluid level in the sphenoid sinus

F (D) surgical management is usually necessary

F (E) the site of CSF leak is best demonstrated by CT scanning after intrathecal injection of a water-soluble contrast agent

CASE 18: Questions 84 through 87

This adult patient presents with low back and radicular pain. You are shown a CT-myelogram (Figure 18-1).

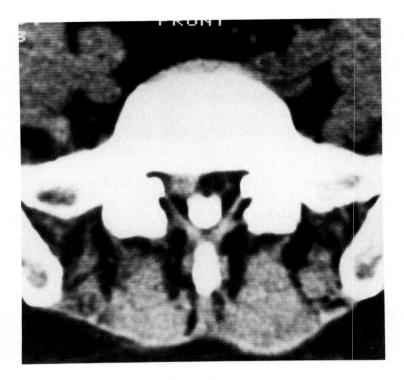

Figure 18-1

84. Which *one* of the following is the MOST likely diagnosis?

    (A) Conjoined nerve root
    (B) Perineural cyst
    (C) Neurinoma
    (D) Extruded disc fragment
    (E) Arachnoid cyst

CASE 18 (Cont'd)

QUESTIONS 85 THROUGH 87: MARK YOUR ANSWER SHEET TRUE (T) OR FALSE (F) FOR EACH OF THE RESPONSE CHOICES.

85. A conjoined lumbar nerve root:

  (A) often resembles a herniated disc on axial CT
  (B) has a higher attenuation value on CT than a spinal neoplasm or disc fragment
  (C) is best differentiated from disc herniation by CT-myelography
  (D) is a normal anatomic variant
  (E) is of minimal clinical importance

86. Concerning spinal neurinomas,

  (A) most have an extradural component
  (B) when found in neurofibromatosis, they are usually malignant
  (C) when intradural, myelography or CT-myelography is required for radiologic diagnosis
  (D) when extradural, they have higher attenuation values on CT than does disc material
  (E) they can be diagnosed from the radiographic finding of expanded neural foramen

87. Regarding herniated discs,

  (A) they can be routinely differentiated from postoperative scar on CT when epidural fat is absent
  (B) they are associated with destruction of adjacent bone
  (C) midline location causes a monoradiculopathy
  (D) intraforaminal migration is best diagnosed by myelography

This 29-year-old man presented with bilateral lower extremity weakness and upper extremity dysesthesias. You are shown selected images from a computed tomographic (CT) study (Figure 19-1) of the cervical spine. Figure 19-1A was obtained without contrast administration. Figures 19-1B and C were obtained 4 and 24 hours, respectively, after intrathecal metrizamide injection. Figure 19-1D was obtained at the level of C1 4 hours after intrathecal metrizamide injection.

Pre-metrizamide

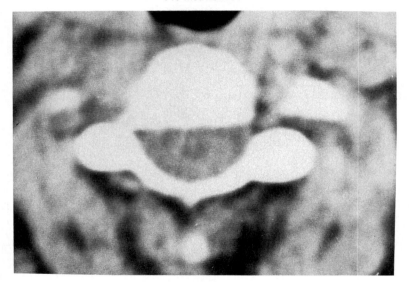

A

4 hr post-metrizamide

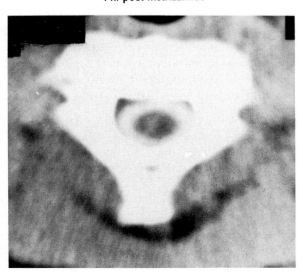

B

Figure 19-1

24 hr post-metrizamide

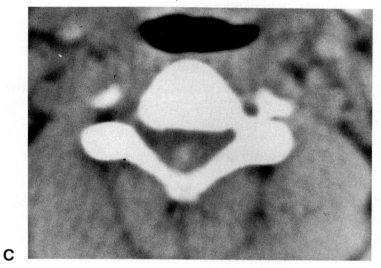

C

4 hr post-metrizamide

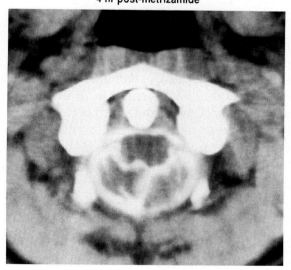

D

88. Which *one* of the following is the MOST likely diagnosis?

(A) Neurofibromatosis
(B) Hematomyelia
(C) Hemangioblastoma
(D) Post-traumatic spinal cord cyst
(E) Syringohydromyelia

QUESTIONS 89 THROUGH 92: MARK YOUR ANSWER SHEET TRUE (T) OR FALSE (F) FOR EACH OF THE RESPONSE CHOICES.

89. Concerning von Recklinghausen's neurofibromatosis,

(A) it is associated with neoplasms of endocrine origin
(B) it is transmitted as an autosomal recessive trait
(C) it is associated with hypertension
(D) it is associated with aqueductal stenosis and hydro-cephalus
(E) there is an increased incidence of astrocytomas

90. Spinal cord hemangioblastomas:

(A) usually exhibit early venous drainage by angiography
(B) are associated with retinal lesions
(C) are associated with renal hamartomas
(D) most often present with hemorrhage
(E) usually occur as solitary lesions

CASE 19 (Cont'd)

91. Post-traumatic spinal cord cysts:

 (A) are the most common cause of progression of symptoma-
     tology after spinal cord injury
 (B) typically produce ascending levels of neurological dys-
     function as they enlarge
 (C) are associated with cord atrophy
 (D) do not accumulate metrizamide on delayed CT scans
 (E) are readily distinguished from myelomalacia by ultra-
     sonography

92. Concerning syringohydromyelia,

 (A) the most common plain film finding is scoliosis
 (B) dissociated sensory loss is a common presentation
 (C) myelographic demonstration of a normal-size cord
     excludes the diagnosis
 (D) the foramen of Magendie is partially blocked in most
     cases
 (E) the cyst extends into the brain stem in approximately
     one-third of cases

CASE 20: Questions 93 through 97

This 16-year-old boy presented with seizures. You are shown pre- and postcontrast computed tomographic (CT) scans (Figure 20-1).

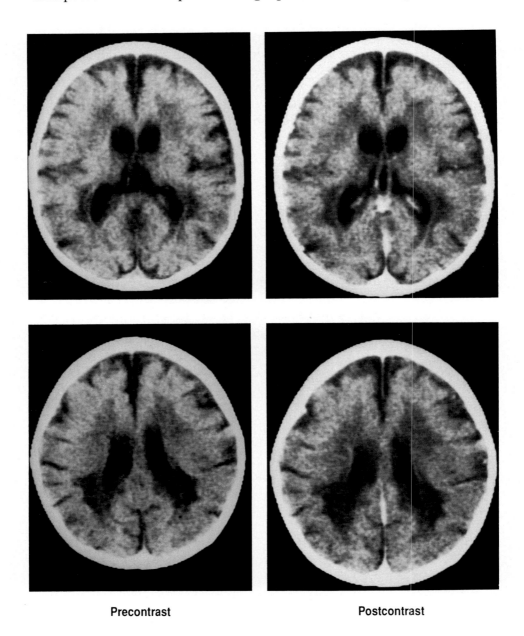

Precontrast   Postcontrast

Figure 20-1

CASE 20 (Cont'd)

93. Which *one* of the following is the MOST likely diagnosis?

    (A) Multiple sclerosis
    (B) Progressive multifocal leukoencephalopathy
    (C) Adrenoleukodystrophy
    (D) Acute obstructive hydrocephalus
    (E) Venous infarction

QUESTIONS 94 THROUGH 96: MARK YOUR ANSWER SHEET TRUE (T) OR FALSE (F) FOR EACH OF THE RESPONSE CHOICES.

94. Conditions that predispose to progressive multifocal leukoencephalopathy include:

    T (A) leukemia
    T (B) intrathecal methotrexate therapy
    T (C) exposure to measles
    T (D) immunosuppressive therapy
    T (E) acquired immunodeficiency syndrome

95. Concerning adrenoleukodystrophy,

    T (A) contrast enhancement is usually bifrontal
    T (B) lateral ventricular enlargement is usually symmetrical
    F (C) it typically occurs in young male patients
    T (D) definitive diagnosis requires brain biopsy
    T (E) adrenal cortical hyperplasia is common

96. On CT, enlargement of the lateral ventricles and periventricular hypodensity are characteristic of:

    T (A) treatment with intrathecal methotrexate
    T (B) obstructive hydrocephalus
    T (C) subcortical arteriosclerotic encephalopathy (Binswanger's disease)
    T (D) nonspecific leukoencephalopathy related to advanced age
    F (E) steroid therapy

97. Cerebral venous infarction is MOST commonly associated with which *one* of the following?

    (A) Dehydration
    (B) Pregnancy
    (C) Meningitis
    (D) Vein of Galen aneurysm
    (E) Meningioma

CASE 21: Questions 98 through 102

This 42-year-old woman was evaluated for headaches. You are shown a postcontrast computed tomographic (CT) scan (Figure 21-1) and a subsequent vertebral angiogram (Figure 21-2).

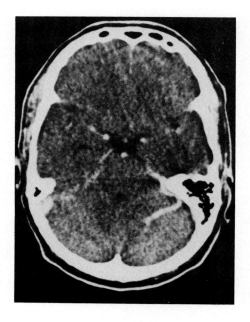

Figure 21-1

98. Which *one* of the following is the MOST likely diagnosis?

    (A) Glioblastoma multiforme
    (B) Hemangioblastoma
    (C) Arteriovenous malformation
    (D) Cavernous hemangioma
    (E) Venous angioma

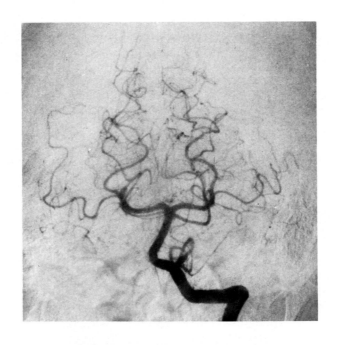

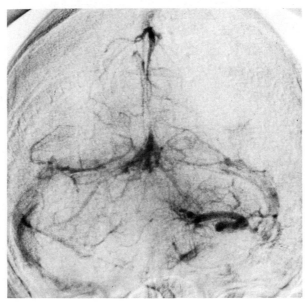

Figure 21-2

CASE 21 (Cont'd)

QUESTIONS 99 THROUGH 102: MARK YOUR ANSWER SHEET TRUE (T) OR FALSE (F) FOR EACH OF THE RESPONSE CHOICES.

99. Angiographic features that suggest glioblastoma multiforme include:

   (A) tumor stain that persists late into the venous phase
   (B) encasement of larger intracranial vessels
   (C) calcification on scout film
   (D) arteriovenous shunting
   (E) hypervascularity

100. Concerning intracranial arteriovenous malformations,

   (A) calcification is visible on plain radiographs in the majority of cases
   (B) they rarely involve the dura
   (C) they frequently extend across the corpus callosum
   (D) they commonly produce arterial spasm
   (E) they are associated with lückenschädel

101. Angiograms of intracerebral cavernous hemangiomas typically show:

   (A) enlarged feeding arteries
   (B) early draining veins
   (C) mass effect
   (D) calcification on scout film
   (E) associated aneurysms

102. Concerning venous angiomas,

    (A) they are benign neoplasms
    (B) they are often incidental findings
    (C) they are characterized by early draining veins
    (D) they are frequently associated with vascular malforma-
           tions of the skin and mucous membranes
    (E) they occur predominantly in the white matter

CASE 22: Questions 103 through 107

This 32-year-old woman presented with diplopia, gait disturbance, slurred speech, and right leg weakness. You are shown postcontrast computed tomographic (CT) scans (Figure 22-1). The precontrast CT scans were normal.

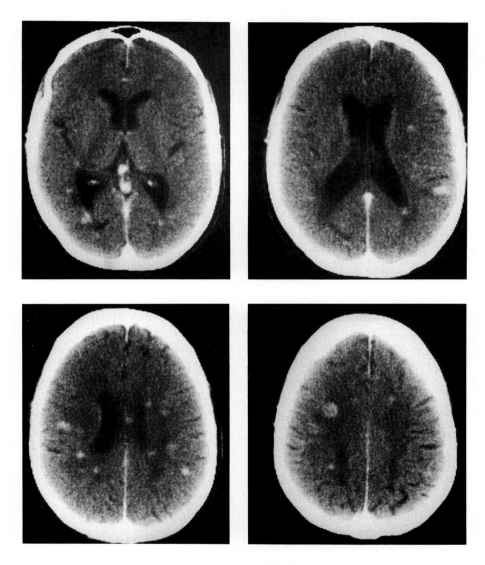

Figure 22-1

CASE 22 (Cont'd)

103. Which *one* of the following is the MOST likely diagnosis?

    (A) Metastases
    (B) Cysticercosis
    (C) Cerebral infarcts
    (D) Lymphoma
    (E) Multiple sclerosis

QUESTION 104: MARK YOUR ANSWER SHEET TRUE (T) OR FALSE (F) FOR EACH OF THE RESPONSE CHOICES.

104. Concerning cysticercosis,

    (A) humans acquire the infection by ingesting ova of the pork tapeworm
    (B) living cysticerci produce little inflammatory reaction in the brain
    (C) serologic tests are positive in 80% of patients
    (D) the most common neurological symptom is seizure
    (E) encysted larvae can be killed by anthelmintic drugs

105. On noncontrast CT scans, hyperdense brain metastases are MOST commonly due to which *one* of the following?

    (A) Malignant melanoma
    (B) Breast carcinoma
    (C) Lung carcinoma
    (D) Choriocarcinoma
    (E) Colon carcinoma

106. Cerebral infarction manifested on CT as multiple contrast-enhancing lesions is MOST likely due to which *one* of the following?

    (A) Embolism
    (B) Moya Moya disease
    (C) Anoxia
    (D) Venous thrombosis
    (E) Atherosclerotic occlusion (large artery thrombosis)

CASE 24: Questions 113 through 116

This 13-year-old boy presented with severe headaches and new onset of seizures. You are shown contrast-enhanced computed tomographic (CT) images in three planes: axial (Figure 24-1), coronal (Figure 24-2), and sagittal (Figure 24-3).

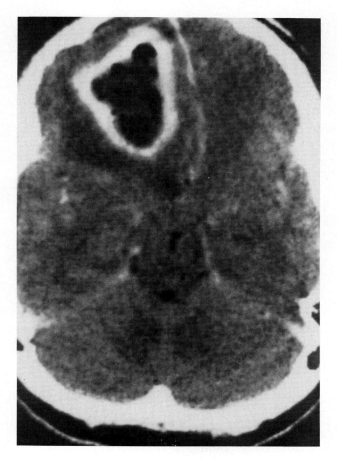

Figure 24-1

CASE 24 (Cont'd)

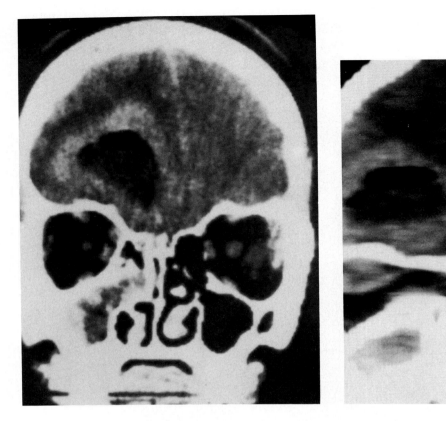

Figure 24-2   Figure 24-3

113. Which *one* of the following is the MOST likely diagnosis?

    (A) Pneumatocele
    (B) Ruptured dermoid
    (C) Necrotic glioma
    (D) Mucocele with extension
    (E) Brain abscess

CASE 24 (Cont'd)

QUESTIONS 114 THROUGH 116: MARK YOUR ANSWER SHEET TRUE (T) OR FALSE (F) FOR EACH OF THE RESPONSE CHOICES.

114. Concerning intracranial pneumatoceles,

   F (A) the occipital lobe is the most common site of occurrence after closed head injury
   T (B) most are accompanied by rhinorrhea or otorrhea
   T (C) they commonly present weeks to months following head injury
   T (D) they usually resolve spontaneously

115. Concerning spontaneous or surgical rupture of a dermoid,

   T (A) sudanophilic material enters the cerebrospinal fluid
   T (B) multiple "implantation dermoids" commonly occur along the ependyma and meninges
   F (C) intraventricular fat-cerebrospinal fluid levels are seen on CT
   T (D) hydrocephalus is a common complication
   T (E) abnormal contrast enhancement of the meninges is commonly seen on CT

116. Tumors that exhibit regions of low (fat-density) attenuation on CT include:

   T (A) teratomas
   T (B) epidermoids
   T (C) dermoids
   T (D) lipomatous meningiomas
   F (E) cysticercomas

This 57-year-old man presented with a 3-month history of interscapular pain and had decreased sensation below the T6 level. You are shown anteroposterior and lateral radiographs of the midthoracic spine (Figures 25-1 and 25-2), a lateral tomogram (Figure 25-3), a computed tomographic (CT) scan at the level of T6 (Figure 25-4), and a CT scan at the level of T7 obtained following intrathecal injection of metrizamide (Figure 25-5).

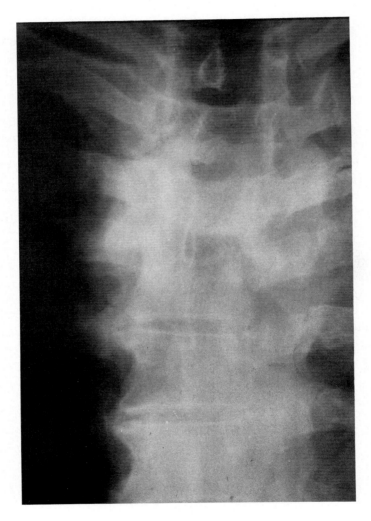

Figure 25-1

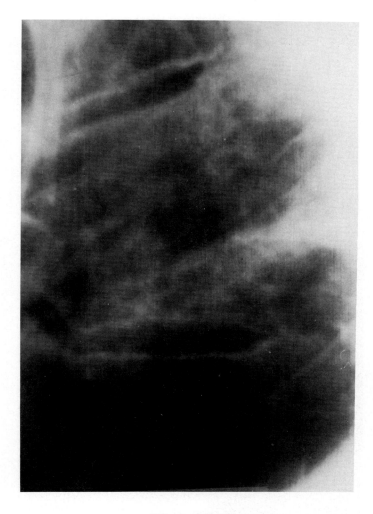

Figure 25-2

117. Which *one* of the following is the MOST likely diagnosis?

    (A) Metastases
    (B) Chordoma
    (C) Plasmacytoma
    (D) Tuberculosis
    (E) Lymphoma

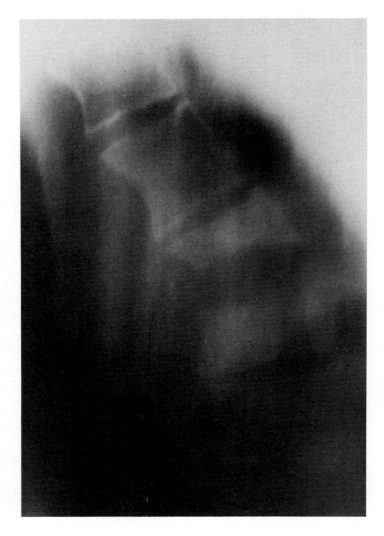

Figure 25-3

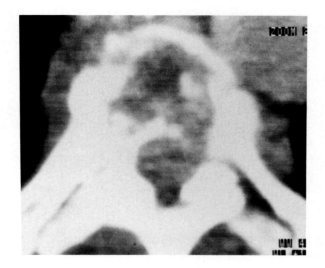

Figure 25-4

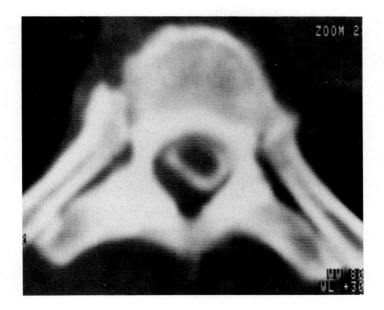

Figure 25-5

QUESTIONS 118 AND 119: MARK YOUR ANSWER SHEET
TRUE (T) OR FALSE (F) FOR EACH OF THE RESPONSE
CHOICES.

118. Concerning chordomas,

T (A) approximately 20% are located in the thoracic spine
T (B) calcified prevertebral masses simulate those seen with
tuberculosis
F (C) they affect the vertebral bodies more often than the
posterior elements
T (D) distant metastases are rare

119. Frequent radiographic features of solitary plasmacytoma
include:

F (A) involvement of the intervertebral disc space
T (B) lytic destruction of the neural arch early in the
destructive phase
T (C) replacement of the trabecular pattern of the vertebral
body
F (D) intensely increased activity on bone scintigraphy

This 5-month-old girl was examined because of an increased head circumference. You are shown precontrast (Figure 26-1A) and postcontrast (Figure 26-1B) computed tomographic (CT) scans.

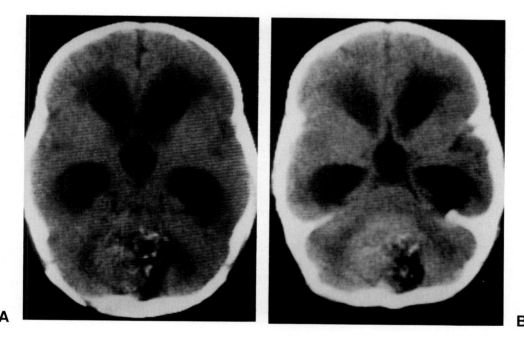

A   B

Figure 26-1

120. Which *one* of the following is the MOST likely diagnosis?

    (A) Medulloblastoma
    (B) Astrocytoma
    (C) Choroid plexus papilloma
    (D) Ependymoma
    (E) Neuroblastoma

CASE 26 (Cont'd)

QUESTIONS 121 THROUGH 123: MARK YOUR ANSWER SHEET TRUE (T) OR FALSE (F) FOR EACH OF THE RESPONSE CHOICES.

121. Concerning medulloblastoma,

   T (A) metastatic spread outside of the central nervous system is usually to the lungs
   T (B) the frequency of calcification as seen on CT is between 25 and 35%
   T (C) it typically is a hypodense mass on noncontrast CT
   F (D) it is generally curable even when subarachnoidal and ventricular spread has occurred

122. Concerning cerebellar astrocytoma of childhood,

   T (A) it is usually a low-grade neoplasm
   F (B) it usually shows contrast enhancement on CT
   T (C) it is cystic more often than other pediatric posterior fossa neoplasms
   F (D) the tumor exhibits calcification on CT in over 50% of cases
   F (E) it commonly seeds the subarachnoid space

123. Concerning tumors of the fourth ventricular choroid plexus,

   F (A) they are usually carcinomatous in patients under 5 years of age
   T (B) with papillomas, hydrocephalus results almost exclusively from overproduction of cerebrospinal fluid
   T (C) choroid plexus meningiomas arise in the fourth ventricle less frequently than in the lateral ventricle

This 48-year-old woman presented with a 1-year history of confusion and progressive left hemiparesis. You are shown skull radiographs in lateral (Figure 27-1) and Towne's projections (Figure 27-2), pre- and postcontrast axial computed tomographic (CT) scans (Figures 27-3 and 27-4, respectively), and a postcontrast coronal CT scan (Figure 27-5).

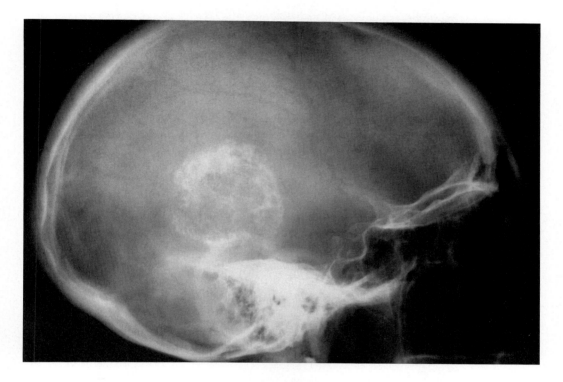

Figure 27-1

124. Which *one* of the following is the MOST likely diagnosis?

    (A) Choroid plexus papilloma
    (B) Tuberous sclerosis
    (C) Pineal tumor
    (D) Ependymoma
    (E) Intraventricular meningioma

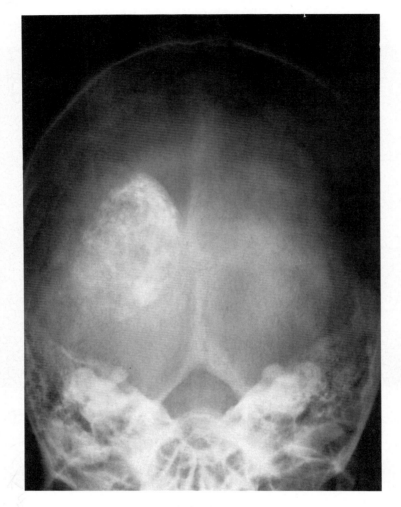

Figure 27-2

CASE 27 (Cont'd)

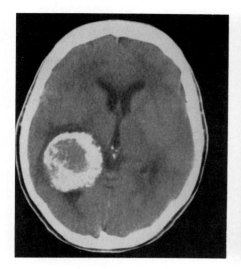 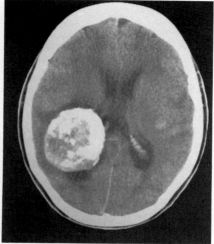

Figure 27-3

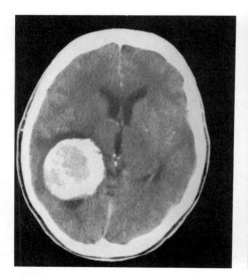 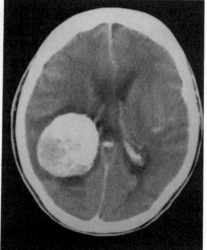

Figure 27-4

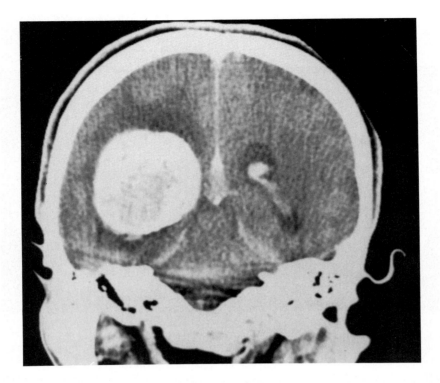

Figure 27-5

QUESTIONS 125 THROUGH 129: MARK YOUR ANSWER
SHEET TRUE (T) OR FALSE (F) FOR EACH OF THE RESPONSE
CHOICES.

125. Concerning choroid plexus papillomas,

   (A) the usual site in adults is the fourth ventricle
   (B) they are multiple in less than 10% of cases
   (C) calcification is seen on skull radiographs in most cases
   (D) transependymal extension into the cerebral paren-
       chyma suggests malignancy

CASE 27 (Cont'd)

126. Concerning tuberous sclerosis,

  T (A) the frequency of calcification in the intracranial tubers increases with age

  T (B) cerebral heterotopia occasionally mimics its appearance on CT

  T (C) neoplastic degeneration is more common with subependymal tubers in the region of the foramen of Monro than with tubers located elsewhere

  F (D) on CT, contrast enhancement of tubers generally occurs only in those that have undergone neoplastic transformation

  T (E) scattered areas of cranial vault sclerosis are more common in children than in adults

127. Concerning pineal tumors,

  T (A) loss of upward conjugate eye movement is a common finding

  T (B) tumors of germ cell origin (germinomas) are the most common types

  F (C) pineoblastoma and medulloblastoma cannot be distinguished histologically

  T (D) pineocytoma is the type most likely to seed via the cerebrospinal fluid (CSF)

  T (E) calcification within or surrounding a pineoblastoma is common

128. Concerning ependymomas,

  F (A) the trigone of the lateral ventricle is the most common supratentorial site of origin

  T (B) seeding into the subarachnoid space of the spine or cerebrum is common

  T (C) in most cases, seeding into the spinal subarachnoid space is not apparent clinically

  T (D) angiographically, they have a characteristic, highly vascular angio-architecture

129. Concerning intraventricular meningiomas,

F (A) most are the result of CSF seeding from spinal meningiomas

T (B) the foramen of Monro is the most common site

T (C) they occur more often in the left lateral ventricle than in the right

T (D) the angiographic features are specific

T (E) when multiple and calcified, they suggest neurofibromatosis

This 59-year-old man presented with persistent headaches. You are shown a lateral skull radiograph (Figure 28-1) and two computed tomographic (CT) images at the same level, with soft tissue and bone window settings (Figure 28-2).

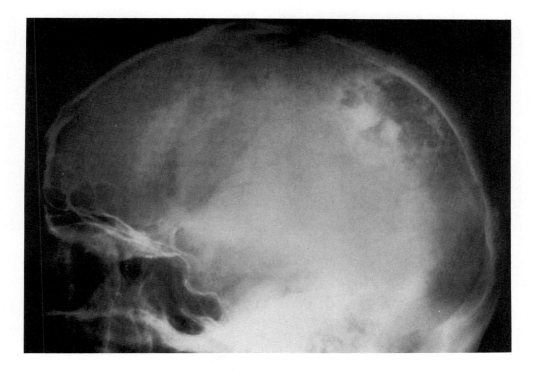

Figure 28-1

130. Which *one* of the following is the MOST likely diagnosis?

    (A) Hemangioma
    (B) Epidermoid tumor
    (C) Paget's disease of bone
    (D) Meningioma
    (E) Fibrous dysplasia

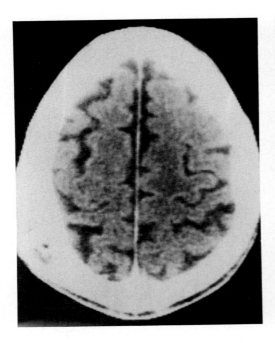 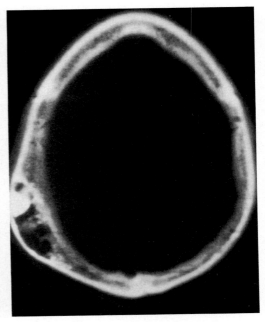

Figure 28-2

QUESTIONS 131 THROUGH 133: MARK YOUR ANSWER SHEET TRUE (T) OR FALSE (F) FOR EACH OF THE RESPONSE CHOICES.

131. Concerning epidermoid tumors,

   (A) they arise in either the intradiploic or the subarachnoid spaces

   (B) in the suprasellar region they mimic craniopharyngioma on intrathecally enhanced CT

   (C) they contain only keratin

   (D) a hyperdense lesion is an uncommon presentation on noncontrast CT

   (E) they are more common than meningiomas in the cerebellopontine angle in adults

132. Concerning sarcomatous change in Paget's disease of the calvarium,

   T (A) it occurs in one-third of affected patients
   T (B) it often occurs within 10 years of initial diagnosis
   T (C) cortical destruction is a reliable sign on CT scanning
   F (D) fibrosarcoma is the most common tumor

133. Convexity meningiomas are associated with:

   T (A) hyperostosis
   T (B) enlarged vascular channels
   F (C) demineralization of the floor of the sella
   T (D) blistering of bone
   F (E) displacement of the calcified pineal gland

CASE 29: Questions 134 through 138

This 42-year-old woman had nine episodes of transient ischemic attacks, consisting of parathesias and weakness in both hands and arms, during the 6 weeks prior to admission. She has been treated for hypertension for the past year. You are shown frontal views of right and left carotid angiograms (Figures 29-1 and 29-2).

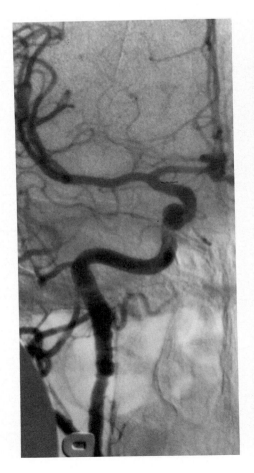

Figure 29-1

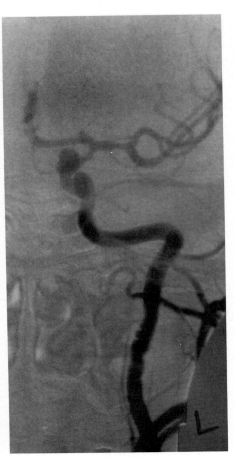

Figure 29-2

CASE 29 (Cont'd)

134. Which *one* of the following is the MOST likely diagnosis?

    (A) Fibromuscular dysplasia
    (B) Dissecting aneurysm (dissecting hematoma)
    (C) Atherosclerosis
    (D) Spasm or arterial waves
    (E) Takayasu's arteritis

QUESTIONS 135 THROUGH 138: MARK YOUR ANSWER SHEET TRUE (T) OR FALSE (F) FOR EACH OF THE RESPONSE CHOICES.

135. Concerning cervical fibromuscular dysplasia,

    (A) it is bilateral in approximately 10% of cases
    (B) it spares the common carotid bifurcation and origin of the internal carotid artery in nearly all cases
    (C) it rarely involves the petrous portion of the internal carotid artery
    (D) histologically, it is usually subadventitial hyperplasia
    (E) it is associated with intracranial aneurysms in nearly one-third of cases

136. Concerning dissecting hematoma (dissecting aneurysm),

    (A) when traumatic, its level of origin is usually C1-2
    (B) when spontaneous, it is frequently associated with ptosis of the eyelid
    (C) hypertension is present in most patients
    (D) it rarely extends into the petrous portion of the internal carotid artery
    (E) the angiographic appearance of alternating areas of widening and narrowing ("string of beads") is more typical of dissecting hematoma than of fibromuscular dysplasia

CASE 29 (Cont'd)

137. Concerning atherosclerosis,

(A) lesions of the internal carotid artery usually involve the proximal 1 to 2 cm or the bifurcation
(B) the main trunk of the middle cerebral artery proximal to its bifurcation is a common intracranial site of involvement
(C) ulcerations, when present, are usually located on the anterior wall of the internal carotid artery at its origin
(D) ulcerations are not usually found at the origins of the vertebral arteries

138. Concerning Takayasu's arteritis,

(A) it is found exclusively in young Japanese women
(B) two or more aortic arch branches are involved in over 80% of cases
(C) the right subclavian artery is the most commonly involved vessel
(D) the intracranial vessels are spared
(E) it usually does not affect the origins of the brachio-cephalic vessels from the aortic arch

CASE 30: Questions 139 through 143

This 14-year-old boy presented with headaches and paralysis of upward gaze. You are shown precontrast (Figure 30-1) and postcontrast (Figure 30-2) computed tomographic (CT) scans.

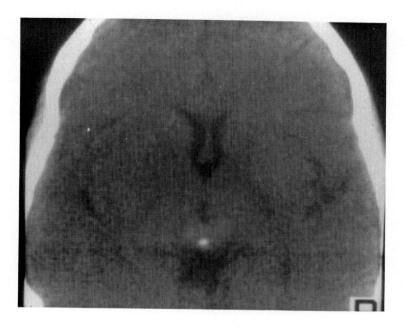

Figure 30-1

139. Which *one* of the following is the MOST likely diagnosis?

    (A) Astrocytoma
    (B) Germinoma
    (C) Arteriovenous malformation
    (D) Teratoma
    (E) Meningioma

CASE 30 (Cont'd)

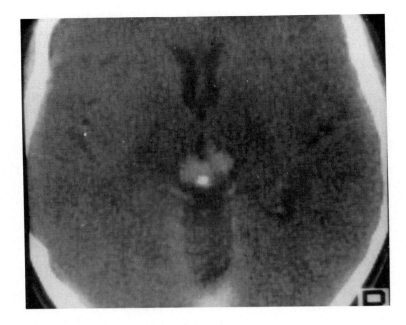

Figure 30-2

QUESTION 140: MARK YOUR ANSWER SHEET TRUE (T) OR
FALSE (F) FOR EACH OF THE RESPONSE CHOICES.

140. CT findings that suggest the presence of a pineal tumor
include:

T (A) calcification exceeding 1×1 cm in size
T (B) calcification in a patient under 6 years of age
T (C) calcification surrounded by contrast-enhancing tissue
T (D) calcification and fat
T (E) a small ring-like calcification with a cerebrospinal fluid
central density

CASE 30 (Cont'd)

141. Arteriographic signs of pineal mass include *all* of the following EXCEPT:

 (A) neovascularity
 (B) elevation of the internal cerebral vein
 (C) posterior displacement of the posterior medial choroidal arteries
 (D) caudal displacement of the precentral cerebellar veins
 (E) medial displacement of the basal vein of Rosenthal

QUESTIONS 142 AND 143: MARK YOUR ANSWER SHEET TRUE (T) OR FALSE (F) FOR EACH OF THE RESPONSE CHOICES.

142. Concerning pineoblastomas,

 (A) CT occasionally demonstrates subarachnoid spread of tumor before the primary site is identified
 (B) there is an increased incidence in patients with congenital retinoblastoma
 (C) they have an appearance on CT similar to that of pineal astrocytomas
 (D) they occur more commonly in men

143. Arterial blood supply to tentorial meningiomas originates in the:

 (A) internal carotid artery
 (B) vertebral artery
 (C) external carotid artery
 (D) posterior cerebral artery

This 20-year-old woman with a history of drug abuse presented with right-sided headache. She was admitted in a confused state with right hemiparesis and fever. You are shown two noncontrast computed tomographic (CT) scans (Figure 31-1), the lateral arterial phase of the left carotid angiogram (Figure 31-2), the lateral arterial phase of the left vertebral angiogram (Figure 31-3), and the frontal early and late arterial phases of the left vertebral angiogram (Figures 31-4 and 31-5).

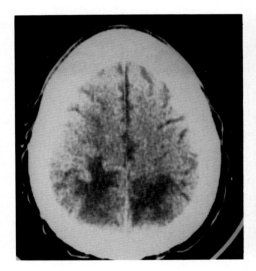 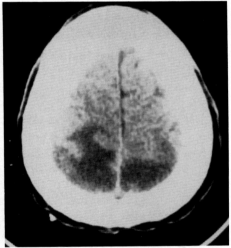

Figure 31-1

144. Which *one* of the following is the MOST likely diagnosis?

  (A) Drug-induced vasculitis
  (B) Tuberculous meningitis
  (C) Systemic lupus erythematosus
  (D) Subarachnoid hemorrhage due to ruptured aneurysm
  (E) Temporal arteritis

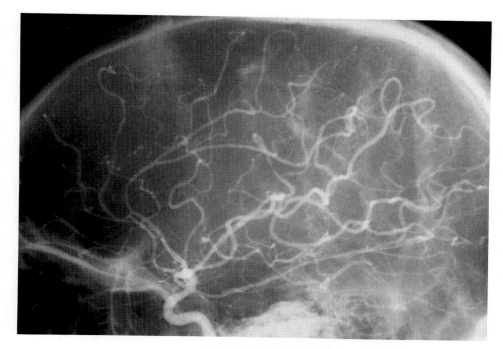

Figure 31-2

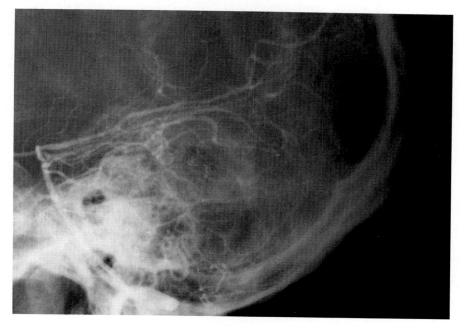

Figure 31-3

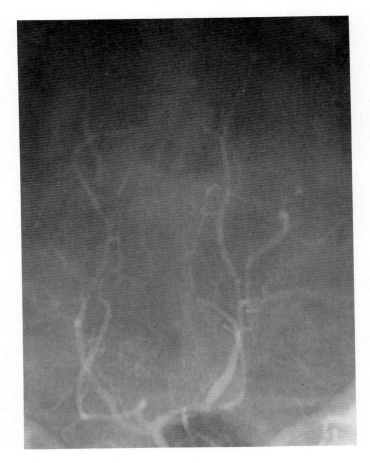

Figure 31-4

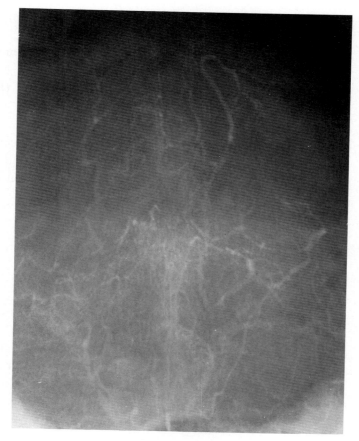

Figure 31-5

QUESTIONS 145 THROUGH 149: MARK YOUR ANSWER SHEET TRUE (T) OR FALSE (F) FOR EACH OF THE RESPONSE CHOICES.

145. Concerning drug-induced vasculitis,

   (A) heroin is the most frequently incriminated drug

   (B) it occurs after oral as well as intravenous use of the offending drugs

   (C) segmental narrowing of the medium-sized and small arteries is angiographically demonstrable

   (D) the vascular changes are reversible

   (E) steroids are very effective treatment

CASE 31 (Cont'd)

146. Concerning tuberculous meningitis,

   (A) invasion of arterial walls by mycobacteria commonly produces aneurysm
   (B) it characteristically affects the large vessels at the base of the brain
   (C) the thick basilar exudate narrows the arteries
   (D) small-vessel changes in the absence of vascular changes at the base are common findings
   (E) basilar enhancement on CT is a more common finding than in the other meningitides

147. Concerning systemic lupus erythematosus,

   (A) involvement of the central nervous system is rare
   (B) it typically involves small vessels
   (C) occlusion of large and medium-sized arteries is frequently demonstrable by angiography
   (D) verrucous endocarditis with or without associated bacterial endocarditis occurs in approximately one-third of patients
   (E) anti-native DNA antibodies are the most specific indicator of the disease

148. Concerning spasm due to subarachnoid hemorrhage,

   (A) it occurs in less than one-third of patients
   (B) it usually begins within the first 12 hours
   (C) it is maximal 6 to 12 days following onset
   (D) the segmental narrowing typically involves the proximal arteries more than the distal ones
   (E) it does not involve the extradural portion of the internal carotid artery

149. Concerning temporal arteritis,

    F (A) it is a disease of adolescents and young adults
    T (B) occlusion of branches of the ophthalmic artery results
        in blindness in one or both eyes in 25% of patients
    T (C) it characteristically affects the internal carotid and
        vertebral arteries where they pierce the dura
    F (D) arteries on the surface of the brain are commonly
        involved
    T (E) false-negative biopsy of the superficial temporal artery
        is more common early in the course of the disease

This 36-year-old woman presented with a 2-year history of progressive weakness in both lower extremities, with associated bladder and bowel dysfunction. You are shown two frontal views from a myelogram with nonionic water-soluble contrast agent (Figure 32-1) and four sections from a computed tomographic (CT) study of the spine performed after the myelogram (Figure 32-2).

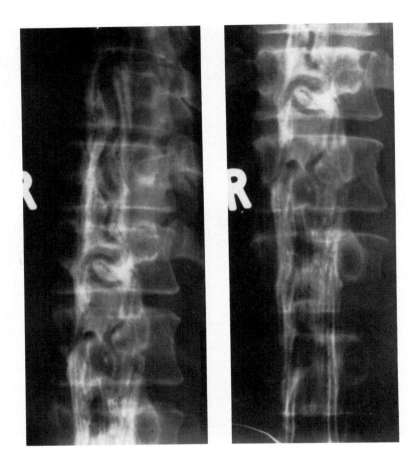

Figure 32-1

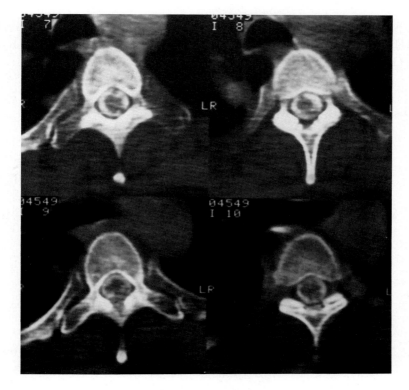

Figure 32-2

150. Which *one* of the following is the MOST likely diagnosis?

    (A) Drop metastases
    (B) Arachnoiditis
    (C) Hemangioblastoma
    (D) Arteriovenous malformation
    (E) Epidermoid

QUESTIONS 151 THROUGH 154: MARK YOUR ANSWER
SHEET TRUE (T) OR FALSE (F) FOR EACH OF THE RESPONSE
CHOICES.

151. Concerning arachnoiditis,

    (A) the lumbar area is the most common site of involvement
    (B) blunting of the nerve root sleeves is a late finding
    (C) cyst formation is the result of loculation of the subarachnoid space by adhesions
    (D) calcification or ossification detectable on CT is a frequent finding
    (E) syringohydromyelia is a complication

152. Concerning hemangioblastomas,

    (A) approximately 60% are intramedullary in location
    (B) most are associated with von Hippel-Lindau disease
    (C) they most commonly involve the conus medullaris
    (D) more than 50% of intramedullary lesions have associated syringes
    (E) most can be distinguished from spinal arteriovenous malformation by angiography

153. Concerning spinal cord arteriovenous malformations,

    (A) subarachnoid hemorrhage is the first presenting sign in approximately 80% of cases
    (B) cutaneous angiomas are present in approximately 15% of cases
    (C) they occur in the cervical area in approximately 60% of cases
    (D) most lie ventral to the spinal cord
    (E) the site of arteriovenous shunting cannot be determined myelographically

CASE 32 (Cont'd)

154. Concerning spinal cord angiography,

T (A) blood flow in the anterior spinal artery is bidirectional

(B) a substantial supply to an arteriovenous malformation from an enlarged anterior spinal artery suggests an intramedullary component

T (C) the great anterior medullary artery (the artery of Adamkiewicz) arises on the right side in two-thirds of cases

T (D) postangiographic cord damage occurs more commonly during selective bronchial arteriography than during vertebral arteriography

(E) a suspected arteriovenous malformation can be excluded by a normal aortogram

DEMOGRAPHIC DATA QUESTIONS

Please answer all of the questions below. The data you provide will be used to supply information that will allow you to compare your performance on the examination with that of others at similar levels of training and with similar backgrounds, and for purposes of planning continuing education projects. Please answer each question as accurately and as objectively as possible. Please mark the *one* BEST response for each question. Recall, of course, that we do *not* want individual names. Our analyses will reflect only categories and groups; everything will remain completely anonymous and no attempt will be made to identify any specific individual.

155. The ACR will be evaluating the questions in this examination to determine their degree of difficulty and to determine the success of the examination as an instrument of self-evaluation and continuing education. To assist the ACR, please indicate in which of the following ways you took this examination.

    (A) Used reference materials or read the syllabus portion of this book to assist in answering some portion of the examination
    (B) Did *not* use reference materials and did not read the syllabus portion of this book while taking the examination

156. How much residency and fellowship training in *Diagnostic* Radiology have you completed as of June 1990?

    (A) None
    (B) Less than 1 year
    (C) 1 year
    (D) 2 years
    (E) 3 years
    (F) 4 or more years

157. When did you *finish* your residency training in Radiology?

    (A) Prior to 1980
    (B) 1980–1984
    (C) 1985–1989
    (D) 1990
    (E) Not yet completed
    (F) Radiology is *not* my specialty

158. Have you been certified by the American Board of Radiology?

    (A) Yes
    (B) No

159. Have you completed a fellowship in Neuroradiology?

    (A) Yes
    (B) No

160. Which *one* of the practice categories listed below BEST describes your practice in the immediate past 3 years? (For residents and fellows, in which *one* did you or will you spend the major portion of your residency and fellowship?)

    (A) Community or general hospital—less than 200 beds
    (B) Community or general hospital—200 to 499 beds
    (C) Community or general hospital—500 or more beds
    (D) University-affiliated hospital
    (E) Office practice

161. In which *one* of the following general areas of Radiology do you consider yourself MOST expert?

(A) Chest
(B) Bone
(C) Gastrointestinal
(D) Genitourinary
(E) Head and neck
(F) Neuroradiology
(G) Pediatric radiology
(H) Cardiovascular Radiology
(I) Other

162. In which *one* of the following radiologic modalities do you consider yourself MOST expert?

(A) General angiography
(B) Interventional radiology
(C) Magnetic resonance imaging
(D) Nuclear medicine
(E) Ultrasonography
(F) Computed tomography
(G) Radiation therapy
(H) Other

Neuroradiology

Case 1: Dermoid Tumor

Question 1

Which *one* of the following is the MOST likely diagnosis?

(A) Arachnoid cyst
(B) Dermoid tumor
(C) Hemangioblastoma
(D) Cystic metastatic tumor
(E) Cerebellar astrocytoma

You are shown pre- and postinfusion computed tomographic (CT) scans (Figures 1-1 and 1-2) of a 44-year-old man who presented with a 1-year history of intermittent severe headaches and dizziness. The pre- and postinfusion CT scans (Figures 1-3 and 1-4) demonstrate a large, well-circumscribed, low-density lesion in the posterior fossa with no evidence of calcification or contrast enhancement. There is a heterogeneous component within the low-density lesion (arrow, Figure 1-4), and the fourth ventricle is compressed and displaced to the right side (Figure 1-4). There is minimal dilatation of the third ventricle (arrow, Figure 1-3) due to obstructive hydrocephalus. The CT findings are typical for a dermoid tumor **(Option (B) is correct).** Surgery revealed a large cerebellopontine angle cistern dermoid tumor containing a hair ball within the lesion.

The presence of an inhomogeneous mass within the low-density lesion excludes the possibility of an arachnoid cyst (Option (A)). Arachnoid cysts appear on CT as low-density, nonenhancing lesions, which may exhibit mass effect. Metrizamide CT cisternography is often helpful in differentiating dermoid and epidermoid tumors from arachnoid cysts. Dermoid and epidermoid tumors commonly have a lobulated surface outlined by the metrizamide which enters into the surface crevices or clefts of the lesion. The postinjection metrizamide CT study obtained soon after injection most commonly demonstrates an arachnoid cyst as a smoothly outlined low-density lesion that does not opacify with the contrast agent. Rarely, there is free communication between the subarachnoid space and the

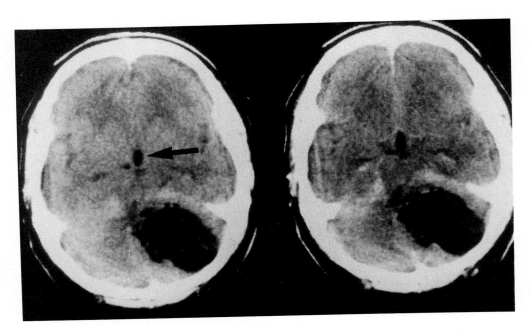

Figure 1-3

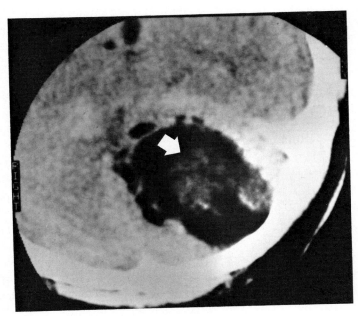

Figure 1-4
Figures 1-3 and 1-4 (Same as Figures 1-1 and 1-2, respectively).
Precontrast and postcontrast CT images demonstrate a low-density
posterior fossa lesion, which contains an irregular, heterogeneous soft
tissue density (arrow, Figure 1-4). The third ventricle is enlarged (arrow,
Figure 1-3).

arachnoid cyst, in which case the immediate postinjection metrizamide CT study demonstrates contrast opacification of the cyst. Delayed CT studies obtained 4 to 6 hours following injection of the metrizamide commonly demonstrate delayed opacification of the arachnoid cyst secondary to diffusion of the contrast material through the wall of the cyst.

The absence of an enhancing mural nodule plus the presence of a heterogeneous mass within the lesion virtually exclude the possibility of a hemangioblastoma (Option (C)). From the CT sections you are shown, it is difficult to be certain that the lesion is not intra-axial in location. Hemangioblastomas usually occur within the substance of the cerebellum. They rarely occur in the medulla, spinal cord, or supratentorial compartment. Hemangioblastomas are commonly cystic tumors with vascular mural nodules that exhibit intense enhancement following contrast administration. Hemangioblastomas do not calcify. These CT features differentiate hemangioblastomas from dermoid tumors and arachnoid cysts. Some hemangioblastomas (20 to 25%) are solid neoplasms that exhibit uniform contrast enhancement.

The most common primary tumors giving rise to metastatic brain lesions (Option (D)) include carcinomas of the lung, breast, and kidney and malignant melanoma. The typical appearance of a metastatic deposit is that of an enhancing lesion with adjacent white matter edema. However, metastasis may present a variable CT picture. The presence of multiple lesions favors the diagnosis of metastatic disease, but solitary metastasis has been reported in up to 50% of cases in CT series. The corresponding frequency in autopsy series ranges from 25 to 40%. In the present case, the appearance of a single, nonenhancing lesion, containing a nonenhancing soft tissue component and without adjacent edema, favors a diagnosis other than metastasis.

A cerebellar astrocytoma (Option (E)) may be solid or cystic. Solid astrocytomas usually involve the vermis and are more invasive than cystic astrocytomas. When solid, they tend to be slightly hypodense on the preinfusion CT study and to enhance homogeneously following infusion of contrast material (Figure 1-5). Most cerebellar astrocytomas are cystic lesions located in the cerebellar hemispheres (Figure 1-6). Following contrast agent administration, enhancement of the periphery of the lesion and of a mural nodule, if present, is usually seen on CT (Figures 1-6 and 1-7). The cystic portion of the tumor usually has attenuation values greater than that of cerebrospinal fluid (CSF) due to the elevated protein content of the fluid. About 20% of cystic astrocytomas demonstrate calcification. The lesions are often eccentric in location and

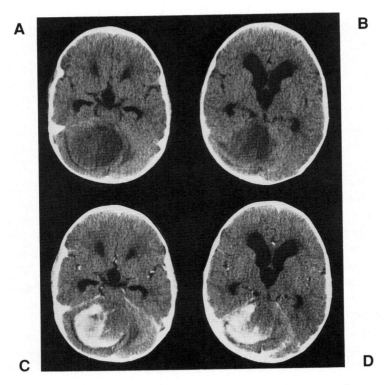

A   B

C   D

Figure 1-5. Cerebellar astrocytoma. Preinfusion CT images demonstrate a hypodense lesion with obliteration of the fourth ventricle and resulting obstructing hydrocephalus (A and B). Postinfusion CT images demonstrate fairly homogeneous contrast enhancement of the tumor (C and D).

typically cause obstructive hydrocephalus. They are usually larger than hemangioblastomas and, unlike the hemangioblastomas, they commonly exhibit contrast enhancement in the wall of the cyst. The presence of a heterogeneous mass within the lesion and the absence of contrast enhancement within the wall of the lesion make the diagnosis of cerebellar astrocytoma highly unlikely. Magnetic resonance imaging (MRI) occasionally demonstrates the mural nodule to better advantage than does CT (Figure 1-8).

Dermoid and epidermoid tumors are congenital tumors thought to arise via inclusion of epithelial elements into the neural tube prior to closure. Together, they account for 0.5 to 3.0% of all intracranial tumors.

Epidermoid tumors are composed solely of ectodermal elements and are lined with stratified squamous epithelium. They contain epithelial

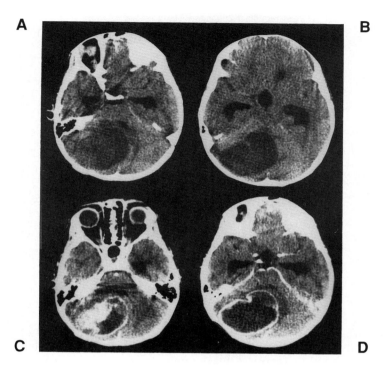

A

B

C

D

Figure 1-6. Cerebellar astrocytoma. Preinfusion CT images demonstrate a hypodense lesion with obstructive hydrocephalus (A and B). Postinfusion CT images demonstrate a ring-like pattern of contrast enhancement with a large mural nodule in the lateral aspect of the tumor (C and D).

debris and cholesterol crystals. Grossly, these tumors have a lobulated, grayish white appearance and are therefore referred to as "pearly tumors." They may be intradural or extradural in location. The extradural variety are typically situated in the diploic space. The most common intradural site is in the cerebellopontine angle cistern, as in the test case. Other sites of occurrence include the parasellar region, within the ventricles, and, rarely, within the parenchyma.

Dermoid tumors are composed of ectodermal and mesodermal elements and are lined with stratified squamous epithelium, as well as with hair follicles, sweat glands, and sebaceous glands. The presence of hair, skin, or fat elements therefore aids in differentiating dermoid tumors from epidermoid tumors. Dermoid tumors typically occur in the posterior fossa near the base of the brain. They are usually located near the midline. They may also be intraventricular in location and rarely occur in the

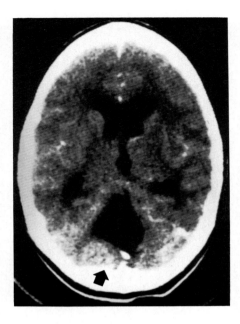

Figure 1-7. Cerebellar astrocytoma. The postinfusion CT study demonstrates a low-density lesion in the vermis and right cerebellar hemisphere with a mural nodule (arrow) that demonstrates relatively inhomogeneous contrast enhancement.

brain parenchyma. Both dermoid and epidermoid tumors are believed to grow by collecting desquamated epithelium into the interior of the tumor.

The usual CT appearance of each of these tumors is that of a low-attenuation lesion that infrequently demonstrates contrast enhancement of its capsule. The low density is accounted for by the cholesterol contained within the lesion. The CT density may be greater than 0 Hounsfield units (HU) when the relative amount of nonlipid material, such as keratin, is elevated. A distinguishing feature of dermoid tumors is the presence of an inhomogeneous density within the lesion; this density usually represents a hair ball. Partial mural calcification may occasionally be seen; it is more common with dermoid tumors. An unusual variation of both dermoid and epidermoid tumors is the CT appearance of a homogeneous high-density lesion that does not enhance. The physicochemical basis for this rare appearance is not known. One theory suggests that the homogeneous high density may be due to saponification of the keratinized debris to calcium soaps.

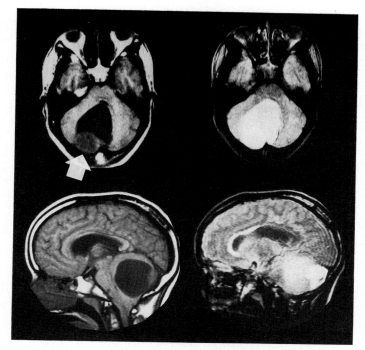

Figure 1-8. Same patient as in Figure 1-7. MRI study with T1-weighted (left) and T2-weighted images (right) reveals a cerebellar cystic tumor containing a mural nodule (arrow).

Question 2

Concerning arachnoid cysts,

(A) in a minority of cases, they are differentiated from epidermoid tumors by analysis of their CT attenuation values
(B) the most common site of occurrence in the posterior fossa is the cerebellopontine angle cistern
(C) the presence of hydrocephalus is an important factor to be considered in distinguishing them from developmentally large cisternae magnae
(D) those occurring in the cerebellopontine angle cistern do not extend above the tentorium
(E) the demonstration of contrast within the cysts on delayed positive-contrast cisternography excludes the diagnosis

Arachnoid cysts and epidermoid tumors may have a similar CT appearance; both appear as homogeneous, low-density lesions. Arachnoid cysts demonstrate attenuation values equal to those of CSF. Epidermoid

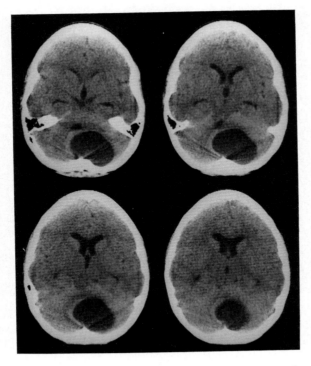

Figure 1-9. Arachnoid cyst. Preinfusion CT images demonstrate a sharply delimited low-density lesion that is retrocerebellar in location. The fourth ventricle is compressed and displaced anteriorly and to the right side. There is a minimal degree of hydrocephalus.

tumors typically have attenuation values that are equal to or slightly higher than those of CSF, with a range of −10 to +30 HU. Therefore, in most cases it is impossible to differentiate between arachnoid cysts and epidermoid tumors by analysis of CT attenuation values **(Option (A) is true).** The most common site of occurrence of arachnoid cysts in the posterior fossa is retrocerebellar in location (Figures 1-9 and 1-10) **(Option (B) is false).** Hydrocephalus occurs with arachnoid cysts of the posterior fossa, depending on the size of the lesion, but not in association with developmentally large cisternae magnae **(Option (C) is true).** It is possible for arachnoid cysts located in the cerebellopontine angle cistern to extend through the tentorial notch **(Option (D) is false).** This is also true for epidermoid tumors located in the cerebellopontine angle cistern. Metrizamide CT cisternography is useful in differentiating between arachnoid cysts and neoplasms, as discussed above. Arachnoid

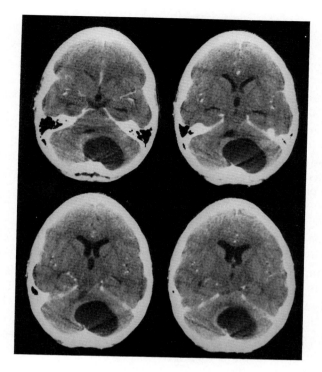

Figure 1-10. Same patient as in Figure 1-9. Postinfusion CT shows no evidence of contrast enhancement of the lesion.

cysts often contain contrast on delayed CT scans obtained after intrathecal metrizamide injection **(Option (E) is false).** However, differentiation of an arachnoid cyst from a tumor may be accomplished more easily in a noninvasive manner by MRI.

Question 3

Concerning dermoid tumors,

(A) they are usually distinguishable from arachnoid cysts on contrast-enhanced CT because their capsules are enhanced
(B) calcification of the lesions is frequently observed on CT scans
(C) they are composed of elements of one germ layer, the ectoderm
(D) they are differentiated from arachnoid cysts on magnetic resonance imaging
(E) CT demonstration of fat in the ventricular system is an indication of rupture of the lesions

If the cholesterol content of a dermoid tumor is high enough, the lesion will demonstrate increased signal on T1- and T2-weighted MR images (short T1, long T2). Arachnoid cysts, on the other hand, demonstrate reduced signal on T1-weighted images (long T1) and increased signal on T2-weighted images (long T2); this is the characteristic appearance of CSF **(Option (D) is true).** Dermoid tumors may rupture, with resulting spillage of fatty contents into the subarachnoid space and ventricles. When in the ventricle, the fatty elements will float on top of the CSF due to the higher specific gravity of CSF and will appear as a fat-CSF fluid level on CT images **(Option (E) is true).** A ruptured dermoid may present clinically as aseptic or chemical meningitis. Contrast enhancement of the capsule of a dermoid tumor is extremely rare **(Option (A) is false).** Arachnoid cysts do not demonstrate any increase in attenuation value following contrast enhancement. Dermoid and epidermoid tumors only occasionally calcify **(Option (B) is false).** Partial mural calcification, when seen, is usually found in dermoid tumors. Epidermoid tumors are composed of derivatives of one germ cell layer, the ectoderm; dermoid tumors are made up of components arising from two layers, the ectoderm and the mesoderm **(Option (C) is false)**; and teratomas are composed of tissues from all three germ cell layers.

Question 4

Concerning hemangioblastomas,

(A) calcification of the mural nodules is seen in approximately 25% of cases
(B) they are the most common primary cerebellar tumors in adults
(C) the mural nodules usually abut a pial surface
(D) they usually demonstrate ring blush on contrast-enhanced CT
(E) CT is more accurate than is angiography in demonstrating multiple small solid lesions

Metastatic lesions constitute the majority of posterior fossa neoplasms in adults. Hemangioblastomas are the most common primary intra-axial posterior fossa tumors in the adult population and account for 7 to 12% of all posterior fossa tumors **(Option (B) is true).** The mural nodules of cystic hemangioblastomas typically are located at or near a pial surface, especially the tentorial or occipital cerebellar surface (Figures 1-11 and 1-12) **(Option (C) is true).** Calcification of the mural nodule of a hemangioblastoma does not occur **(Option (A) is false).** If calcification is present in a cerebellar tumor in an adult, cystic astrocytoma is a more likely diagnostic consideration; approximately 20% of astrocytomas demonstrate calcification. Peripheral contrast enhancement is not usually seen in hemangioblastomas. Rather, the solid component of the tumor will show uniform, intense enhancement **(Option (D) is false).** Vertebral angiography with subtraction images may demonstrate small nodules of hemangioblastoma better than does CT (Figure 1-13). Angiography may also demonstrate a greater number of nodules than is seen on CT or demonstrate the presence of nodules that are missed on CT **(Option (E) is false).** With solid hemangioblastomas, angiography commonly demonstrates neovascularity, a tumor blush, and enlarged feeding arteries and draining veins (Figures 1-14 to 1-16).

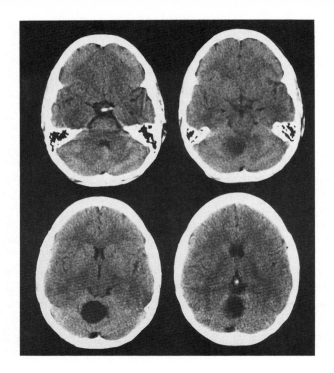

Figure 1-11. Cerebellar hemangioblastoma. Preinfusion CT images demonstrate a well-defined, low-attenuation lesion within the cerebellum.

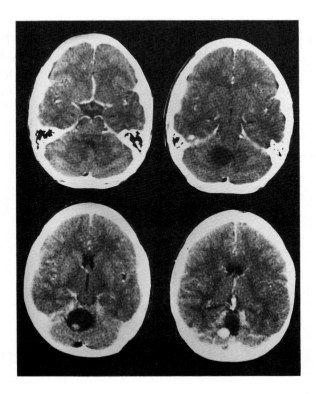

Figure 1-12. Same patient as in Figure 1-11. Postinfusion CT shows an enhancing mural nodule abutting a pial surface.

A

B

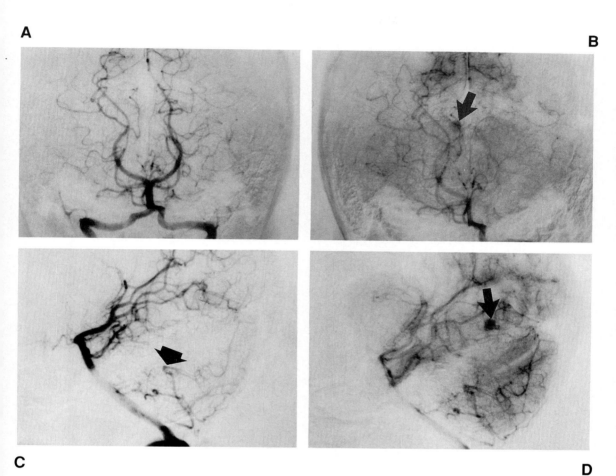

C

D

Figure 1-13. Same patient as in Figures 1-11 and 1-12. Anteroposterior (A and B) and lateral projections (C and D) of a vertebral angiogram with subtraction demonstrate the small vascular tumor nodule (arrows, panels B and D) and the anterior displacement of the choroidal point of the posterior inferior cerebellar artery (arrowhead, panel C).

A

B

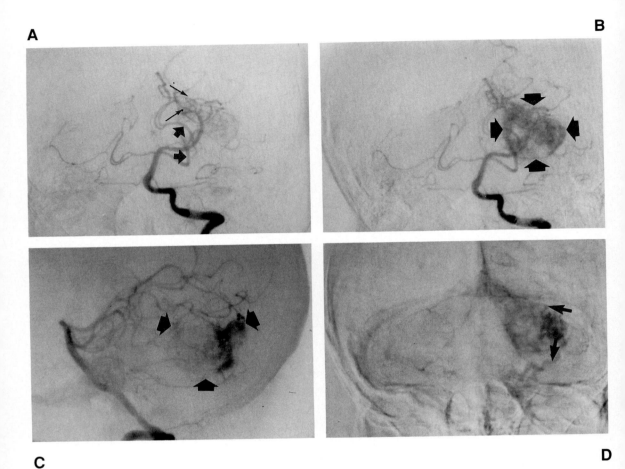

C

D

Figure 1-14. Cerebellar hemangioblastoma. A subtraction vertebral angiogram, with anteroposterior (A, B, and D) and lateral projections (C), demonstrates a large vascular tumor (arrowheads, panels B and C). The tumor is supplied by enlarged hemispheric branches (small arrows, panel A) of the superior cerebellar artery (large arrows, panel A). Enlarged veins drain the tumor (arrows, panel D).

Case 2: Subdural Hematoma

Question 6

Which *one* of the following is the MOST likely diagnosis?

(A) Infiltrating glioma
(B) Subdural hematoma
(C) Hemorrhagic infarct
(D) Cortical vein thrombosis
(E) Meningioma

Subdural hematoma (SDH) is the most likely diagnosis **(Option (B) is correct).** Pre- and postinfusion computed tomography (CT) reveals asymmetric compression of parietal cortical gyri with sulcal effacement (Figure 2-1). The mass effect has resulted in obliteration of the ipsilateral half of the interhemispheric fissure (arrows, Figure 2-2A), while the contralateral fissure is easily visible. The falx (enhanced after infusion in Figure 2-2B) prevents bilateral distribution of mass effect near the vertex. The first step in narrowing the listed differential diagnoses is deciding whether the lesion is outside the brain (extra-axial) or within it (intra-axial). In this case, the lesion is peripheral, with a broad surface adjacent to the inner table of the skull, a finding that favors an extra-axial location. Also, the density interface between gray matter and the more radiolucent white matter is preserved. Inward displacement (buckling) of this interface (arrowheads, Figure 2-2A) and the associated white matter compression are signs of an extra-axial location (Figure 2-3). The contrast-enhanced CT scan also shows punctate enhancement of surface cortical veins (arrows, Figure 2-2B), indicating inward cortical displacement and confirming the extra-axial location of the lesion. All of these findings eliminate from consideration intra-axial processes such as infiltrating glioma (Option (A)), hemorrhagic infarct (Option (C)), and cortical vein thrombosis (Option (D)). Moreover, shape and density of the mass are more consistent with a fluid collection than with a solid tumor. Solid neoplasms in an extra-axial location tend to focally invaginate brain. SDHs generally arise from torn bridging veins which bleed (under

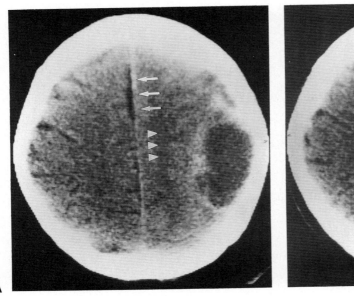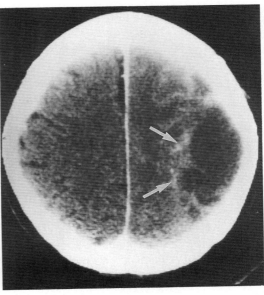

A   B

Figure 2-2 (Same as Figure 2-1). See text for description.

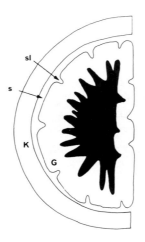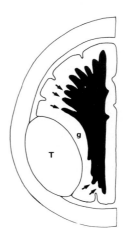

Figure 2-3. Representation of right cerebral hemisphere. (Left) Normal transverse axial CT scan at the level of the centrum semiovale above the lateral ventricles. Fronds of central white matter (black area) are insinuated into cortical gray matter (G). s = subarachnoid space; K = skull; sl = sulcus. The border between gray and white matter is the "gray-white interface." Central white matter is in the shape of a porcupine with the belly directed medially. (Right) CT gray and white matter changes associated with laterally placed extra-axial masses ("white matter buckling"). Preservation of gray matter (g) and gray matter-white matter interface. White matter fronds (arrows) are crowded. The white matter is compressed and buckled adjacent to the lesion (T). (Reprinted with permission from George et al. [3].)

22

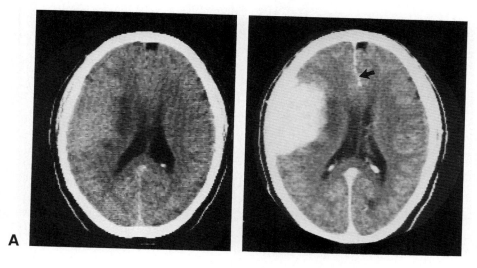

A   B

Figure 2-4. Meningioma. Noncontrast (A) and contrast-enhanced CT images (B) in a 54-year-old man with headache and right focal seizures. (A) Note the large hyperdense mass with medial focal cerebral edema and mild ventricular shift. (B) Homogeneous enhancement better demonstrates the margin of tumor and its broad base against the skull (extra-axial sign). Note the contralateral shift of the anterior cerebral artery in the interhemispheric fissure (arrow).

low pressure) within the potential space between the arachnoid and dural layers investing the brain. The hemorrhage fails to focally compress brain; instead, it coats the entire hemisphere in a crescentic fashion. Ipsilateral gyral compression and sulcal effacement result, with the asymmetric absence of surface cortical sulcal visualization being a key to diagnosis. Acute hemorrhages tend to be higher in attenuation (denser) than adjacent brain, although exceptions may occur if bleeding is accompanied by arachnoid tear and subdural hygroma. The web-like regions of higher attenuation occasionally seen within chronic SDH represent areas of recent bleeding within an older hematoma, with blood dissecting between areas of clot and along fibrous bands developing between lesional membranes. A similar inhomogeneous appearance may occur more focally in intra-axial lesions, such as hemorrhagic infarction (see Figure 2-10). Meningioma should be differentiated by its typical CT appearance: a focal extra-axial mass, uniformly hyperdense on noncontrast CT and exhibiting homogeneous enhancement after contrast infusion (Figure 2-4). Wide-window images may further aid in the diagnosis of meningioma by revealing a characteristic focal thickening

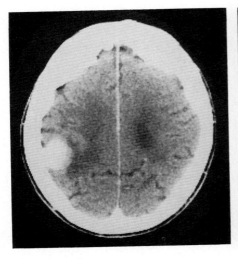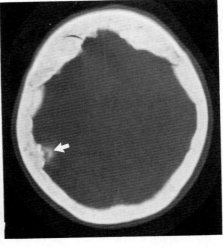

A   B

Figure 2-5. Meningioma with hyperostosis of the inner table of the skull and tumoral calcification. (A) Contrast-enhanced CT reveals enhancing tumor and adjacent lucent edema. (B) Wide-window noncontrast CT shows focal hyperostosis, indicating the extra-axial site of origin of the mass, and tumoral calcification (arrow).

(hyperostosis) of bone at the inner table of the skull adjacent to the mass in such cases (Figure 2-5). Bony hyperostosis or erosion adjacent to an intracranial mass usually indicates that the mass is extra-axial in location. The characteristics of the lesion shown in Figure 2-1 therefore exclude meningioma (Option (E)) from consideration.

Question 7

Concerning gliomatous tumors,

(A) magnetic resonance imaging (MRI) with paramagnetic contrast agents more reliably differentiates tumor growth from associated edema than does noncontrast MRI in cases of malignant glioma
(B) gliomas spread along white matter tracts
(C) hemorrhage occurs in 20% of all intracranial gliomas
(D) low-grade gliomas exhibit moderate contrast enhancement
(E) angiography demonstrates tumor vascularity in approximately 80% of malignant gliomas

Gliomatous tumors of brain vary in histologic appearance, with the most common cell of origin being the astrocyte. Astrocytomas, when malignant, are diffuse infiltrating tumors with poorly defined borders; they tend to spread along the white matter pathways connecting various cortical regions with deeper neuronal centers **(Option (B) is true).** These tumors may be heterogeneous in both gross and microscopic appearance, with observed features dependent on the degree of anaplasia, neovascularity, calcification, and degenerative changes (necrosis, hemorrhage, and cyst formation). More benign (low-grade) astrocytomas show minimal anaplasia and neither necrosis nor hypervascularity. If relatively acellular, these tumors may be hard to distinguish from gliosis (repair) or normal brain tissue. Mixed tumors with areas of higher- and lower-grade neoplasia may exist. Astrocytoma with high-grade anaplasia has also been termed glioblastoma multiforme.

Angiography is no longer used to detect and localize astrocytoma. While vascular displacement can indicate the general location of a tumor, small lesions are easily missed and telltale hypervascularity, present in less than 50% of malignant lesions, is usually absent in lower-grade tumors **(Option (E) is false).** CT and MRI indicate tumor location and extent far more accurately and are the procedures of choice at present.

CT features of supratentorial astrocytoma reflect these pathologic findings. Low-grade tumors tend to appear as homogeneous lesions of density lower than that of adjacent brain, more or less well marginated, often extending in a linear fashion along white matter tracts (Figure 2-6). These lesions only rarely show calcification, cystic change, or enhancement on contrast-enhanced CT **(Option (D) is false).** More malignant tumors tend to be more heterogeneous in density and frequently show areas of focal low density representative of necrosis, cystic change, and old hemorrhage (Figure 2-7). Hypervascularity may be observed, with the predominant blood supply arising from internal carotid or vertebral artery branches (Figure 2-8). Hemorrhage occurs in approximately 4% of cases **(Option (C) is false).** Contrast-enhanced CT will often show ring-like or nodular enhancement of solid tumor or tumoral cyst wall. Calcification, best appreciated on noncontrast CT, occurs in 10 to 15% of cases. Low-grade tumors exhibit little or no mass effect on surrounding structures, whereas high-grade tumors do so in over 90% of cases. Glioblastoma multiforme is almost uniformly accompanied by mass effect and contrast enhancement, which often takes the form of irregularly thick rings and nodules (Figure 2-7). CT features of tumors occurring within the posterior fossa are less well correlated with degree of malignancy than those occurring within the supratentorial region.

MRI is a technique exquisitely attuned to subtle changes in cellular environment and is more sensitive to the presence of many lesions than

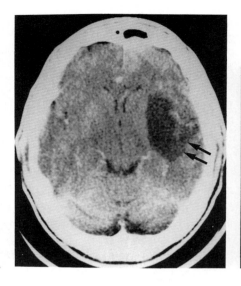

A

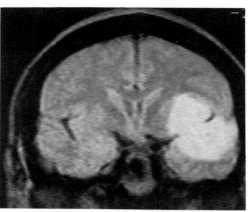

B

Figure 2-6. Infiltrating astrocytoma (grade II). (A) Axial contrast-enhanced CT scan reveals a focal low-density mass in the left frontal lobe and insula, extending via the uncinate fasciculus (white matter) into the temporal lobe (arrows). (B) T2-weighted spin-echo MR image in the coronal plane shows a high-signal mass extending within the temporal lobe, insular cortex, and frontal operculum. Biopsy revealed infiltrating astrocytoma.

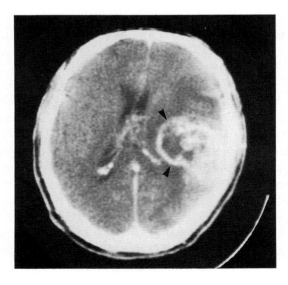

Figure 2-7. Glioblastoma multiforme. Contrast-enhanced CT reveals ring-like enhancement at the medial portion of the tumor (arrowheads), with nodular enhancement laterally and central lucency indicating tumoral necrosis. Edema surrounds the tumor margin.

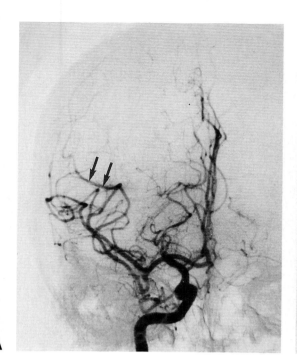

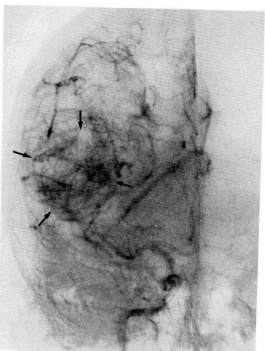

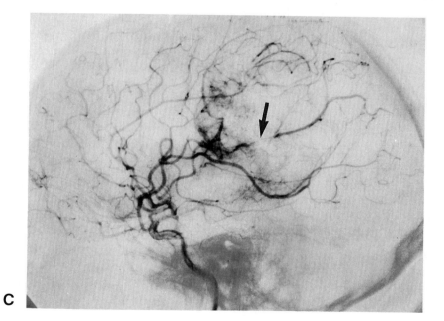

Figure 2-8. Glioblastoma multiforme with cortical extension. Internal carotid angiography in frontal (A and B) and lateral (C) projections. Arterial-phase films show displacement of the middle cerebral artery and its branches (arrows, panel A) and constriction of a cortical branch (arrow, panel C), indicating mass effect and cortical invasion, respectively. (B) Capillary-phase film shows a patchy hypervascular blush (arrows) found with some aggressive malignant gliomas.

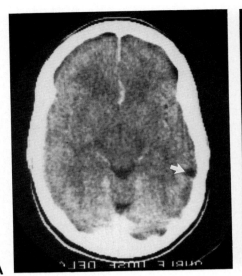 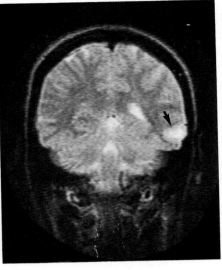

A   B

Figure 2-9. A 15-year-old girl with focal seizure disorder revealing low-grade astrocytoma. (A) Contrast-enhanced CT study initially interpreted as normal. Focal cortically oriented lucency (arrow) represents cystic glioma (grade I) found at surgery. (B) T2-weighted MR image (SE, 2,000/90) clearly indicates the site of the temporal lobe lesion (arrow), although both tumor and focal cystic lesions are diagnostic considerations.

is CT. While detection can be accomplished easily by many pulse sequence techniques weighted for sensitivity to changes in T2 relaxation (Figures 2-9 and 2-10), only certain T2-weighted techniques are effective for differentiating tumor from surrounding brain edema (Figure 2-11), and even these methods may be unsuccessful. MRI performed after the administration of paramagnetic blood-brain barrier contrast agents, such as gadopentetate dimeglumine, combines the sensitivity of T2-weighted studies with improved detection of active tumor margin and differentiation of tumor from edema **(Option (A) is true).** The specificity of MR (and CT) is lower than the corresponding sensitivity. Many lesions may mimic the CT or MRI appearance of tumor. For example, cortically oriented infarcts (Figure 2-12) of venous etiology can closely resemble tumor (Figure 2-10), although attention to the clinical history may allow easy differentiation of these processes.

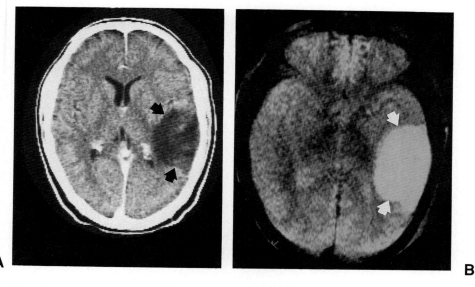

A

B

Figure 2-10. Grade II astrocytoma. (A) Contrast-enhanced CT study reveals a focal cortically oriented mass (arrows). Note the compression of adjacent ventricular choroid plexus. (B) T2-weighted (SE, 3,000/120) MR image reveals high signal of tumor relative to adjacent cerebral parenchyma (arrows). Tumor tissue has a relatively long T2 relaxation time.

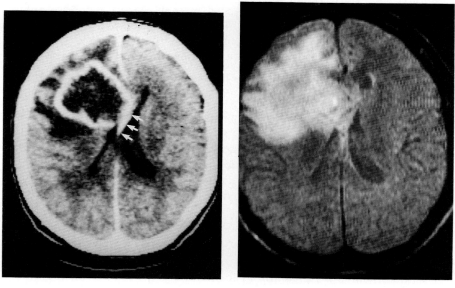

A

B

Figure 2-11. Cystic malignant glioma. (A) Contrast-enhanced CT reveals a ring-enhancing mass with central necrosis and peritumoral edema. A spike of enhancing tumor can be readily seen in the septum pellucidum, suggesting early contralateral spread of tumor (arrows). (B) Axial T2-weighted MR image reveals high signal, highest from the edematous white matter, fairly high from the necrotic center, and lower in the region of the ring-like tumor margin seen in panel A. The high signal from the septum pellucidum could represent tumor or edema, and MRI cannot reliably distinguish between these possibilities. CT is more accurate than MRI in this case for delineating contralateral (septal) tumor extension, a key finding for determining operability.

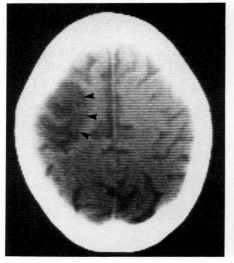
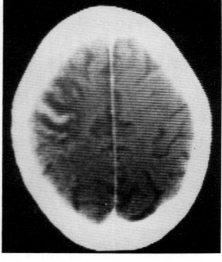

Figure 2-12. Focal infarction due to venous occlusion. (A) A focal area of low attenuation is visible on noncontrast CT (arrowheads). There is regional cortical sulcal effacement (mass effect) and a lack of specific vascular territorial distribution. The image closely resembles that of the low-grade glioma shown in Figure 2-10. (B) Contrast-enhanced CT at the same level as that of panel A reveals linear (gyral) enhancement, which is characteristic of infarction. Regions of cortical infarction due to venous thrombosis may closely mimic the CT features of tumor.

Question 8

Concerning CT findings of subdural hematoma (SDH),

(A) the density of the hematoma is an accurate indicator of its age
(B) unilateral obliteration of cortical sulci is a reliable finding for differentiation between isodense SDH and acute infarction
(C) buckling of the gray matter-white matter interface is seen with both SDH and meningioma
(D) MRI is more sensitive than CT for the detection of subacute SDH
(E) rebleeding into a chronic SDH simulates a hemorrhagic infarct

CT and MRI are complementary for the evaluation of SDH. Most acute lesions (0 to 2 days old) appear hyperdense on CT and isointense or slightly hyperintense with brain on T1-weighted MR scans. Heavily T2-weighted MR scans may show low intensity (T2 shortening) in cases of acute SDH. Hematomas 2 to 3 weeks old, which are easily detected as

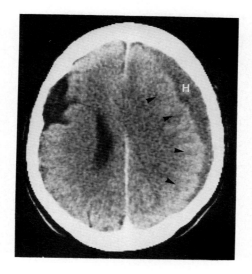

Figure 2-13. Chronic SDH with white matter buckling in a 58-year-old woman. Contrast-enhanced CT at the level of the lateral ventricles reveals a crescentic fluid collection (H) with less attenuation than that of adjacent cerebral cortex. The interface between more lucent white matter and the denser cortical gray matter is preserved (arrowheads) and is anteriorly flattened or buckled inward. Note also the sulcal effacement and ventricular compression (ventricle not seen) and contralateral ventricular dilatation due to subfalcine brain herniation and ventricular obstruction at the level of the foramen of Munro. Fluid with "crankcase oil" consistency was removed after placement of a left frontal burrhole.

bright signal in T1- and T2-weighted MR studies, may be isodense with brain and therefore difficult to detect in CT studies **(Option (D) is true).** CT density alone is not always a reliable indicator of the age of a hemorrhage. A hyperacute SDH may appear low in density if cerebrospinal fluid becomes mixed with the blood or if the patient's hematocrit level is extraordinarily low **(Option (A) is false).** Buckling of white matter (Figure 2-13; see also Figures 2-2B and 2-3) may occur with any laterally placed extra-axial mass, including convexity meningioma, and therefore is not a specific sign of SDH **(Option (C) is true).** The presence of sulcal obliteration alone (mass effect) is also not specific for SDH, since any cortically oriented lesion, including acute cortical infarction, may create similar effacement **(Option (B) is false).** Subdural hemorrhages will decrease in density over time on serial CT studies, as X-ray attenuation decreases with the structural breakdown of hemoglobin. When the density of the clot has decreased so that it equals that of adjacent cerebral

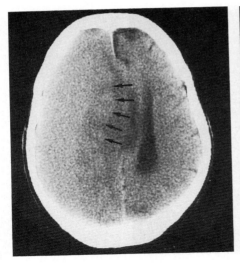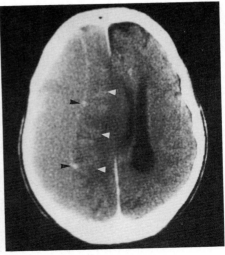

A

B

Figure 2-14. Large acute SDH, indicating the value of contrast enhancement. (A) Noncontrast CT shows midline and ventricular shift from right to left. Note that a homogeneously hyperdense crescentic fluid collection is present on the right. The margin of the SDH is poorly defined since the collection is only slightly denser than cerebral gray matter. Note the inward buckling of the gray matter-white matter interface (arrows), suggesting the extra-axial location of the lesion. (B) Contrast-enhanced CT at the same level as that of panel A. Cortical venous enhancement (black arrowheads) more clearly demarcates the surface of the brain and its interface with the SDH than does noncontrast CT, although the diagnosis is possible without infusion in this case. Again, note the inwardly buckled gray matter-white matter interface (white arrowheads; see also Figure 2-3).

cortex (i.e., it is isodense), the lesion may be difficult to detect on CT. Careful attention to evidence of white matter buckling, mass effect, and subtle differences in attenuation will allow most diagnoses to be made on noncontrast CT; however, contrast-enhanced CT may further aid in detecting such lesions by differentially enhancing convexity cortical veins and the cortical surface of the brain (Figures 2-2, 2-13, and 2-14). Bilaterally isodense SDH may be particularly difficult to diagnose because mass effect may be symmetrically distributed. Attention to ventricular size relative to the patient's age, as well as a differential gradient in lesional density due to positional layering of erythrocytes and blood serum, may aid in the detection by CT in such cases (Figure 2-15). Patients with unclotted collections who lie supine for relatively long

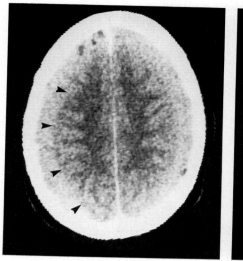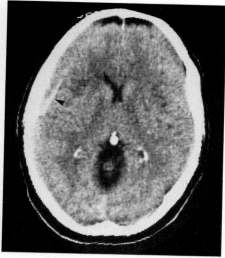

A

B

Figure 2-15. Bilateral isodense SDH in a 68-year-old man with headaches 2 weeks after minor head trauma (surgically proven). (A) Noncontrast CT at the level of the corona radiata-centrum semiovale. The inward buckling of white matter is the best clue to the presence of bilateral subdural fluid collections. The interface between the hematoma on the right and the brain surface is extremely difficult to appreciate (arrowheads). (B) More inferiorly, a noncontrast CT cut shows a thin linear area of high attenuation (arrowhead) representing fresh bleeding within the subacute hematoma. The small size of the frontal horns and their midline crowding suggest bilateral compression in this elderly patient.

periods of time may exhibit extreme erythrocyte layering phenomena (Figure 2-16).

High-density acute subdural clots may also be difficult to detect unless careful attention is paid to image exposure factors. Clots may appear to be as dense as bone on images obtained with narrow CT window settings, so detection may depend on the appreciation of apparent asymmetric "thickening" of the calvarium (Figure 2-17). Hematoma extending to the superior surface of the tentorium cerebelli may mimic intraparenchymal (intracerebral) hemorrhage, unless the marginal configuration of the limiting free tentorial edge (at the incisura) is appreciated (Figure 2-17C). While the differential diagnosis of SDH is usually not a problem, cortically based tumors or hemorrhagic infarcts may simulate some features of SDH, and vice versa, particularly if rebleeding occurs within the hematoma (Figure 2-18 [compare with Figure 2-2]) **(Option (E) is**

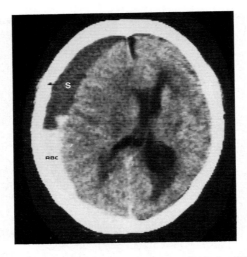

Figure 2-16. "Hematocrit level" within a subacute SDH. Noncontrast CT scan in a comatose patient 10 days after a motor vehicle accident. Note the crescentic SDH on the right. The more posterior portion of the collection is hyperdense (white) due to settling of the cellular elements of blood (RBC) with the patient lying supine. The more lucent region anteriorly (S) represents supernatant serum.

true). Although logistically limited in its application for the diagnosis of acute trauma, MRI is more accurate than CT for detecting very small extra-axial fluid collections in the subacute and chronic phases, particularly those collections at the base of the brain. Also, variation of pulse sequences may allow MRI to show more clearly collections that are "isodense" on CT and to separate pure cerebrospinal fluid collections (hygromas) from those with higher protein content (Figure 2-19).

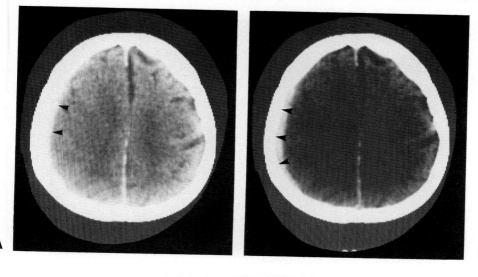

A

B

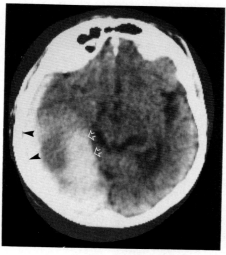

C

Figure 2-17. The asymmetric "skull thickness" sign of acute SDH. (A) Noncontrast CT image above ventricular level appears to show asymmetric skull thickness on the right (arrowheads). In reality, this represents a combination image of skull and underlying acute (white) subdural hemorrhage. (B) The differentiation of bone from less-dense acute blood is more easily appreciated at a wide-window CT setting. Note the true margin of the inner calvarial table (arrowheads). (C) Extension of subdural hemorrhage over the superior surface of the tentorium cerebelli. The characteristic sloping margin of the free edge of the tentorium (open arrows) (half of a "wine goblet" shape) defines the medial-most extension of the tentorial component of the convexity SDH. Failure to appreciate this border might result in the mistaken diagnosis of an intraparenchymal cerebral hematoma. Also shown is the high-density SDH over the lateral convexity surface adjacent to the inner calvarial table (black arrowheads).

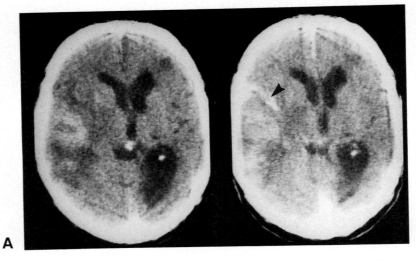

Figure 2-18. Hemorrhagic infarction in the distribution of the right middle cerebral artery. (A) Noncontrast CT reveals a mixed-density lesion in the right hemisphere, associated with mass effect (contralateral midline shift). Focal high density within the larger lucent lesion represents focal hemorrhage within a larger area of cerebral infarction. The appearance superficially resembles that of SDH with rebleeding (see Figure 2-1), although the absence of preservation of the gray matter-white matter junction should be noted in this case (intra-axial lesion). (B) Contrast-enhanced CT at the same level as that of panel A shows patchy and linear enhancement (arrowhead), indicating areas of blood-brain barrier breakdown and a loss of vascular autoregulation.

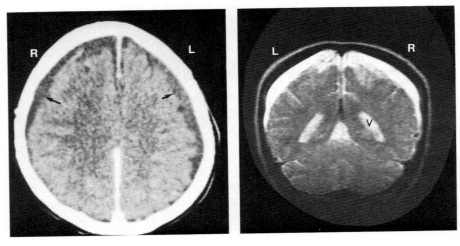

Figure 2-19. Demonstration of bilateral subdural fluid collections of varied etiology by CT and MRI. (A) Axial contrast-enhanced CT scan reveals extra-axial lucent fluid collections bilaterally (arrows). The collections are grossly similar in density. (B) Coronal-plane, T2-weighted MR image (SE, 3,120/120) shows a clear difference in the intensity of the fluid collections and shows each to be an area of higher signal than the adjacent brain. The right-sided collection is of the same intensity as ventricular cerebrospinal fluid (V) and was found to be a subdural hygroma. The left-sided collection is higher in signal (longer T2) and was found to be a chronic SDH at surgery.

Question 9

Concerning cerebral infarcts,

(A) mass effect on CT is seen in approximately 60% of all infarcts during the first week
(B) the combination of mass effect and associated contrast enhancement on CT virtually excludes the diagnosis
(C) approximately 20% are demonstrated only on the contrast-enhanced scan
(D) ring enhancement on CT is uncommon unless there is associated hemorrhage
(E) those secondary to occlusion of a superficial cortical vein involve the white matter

CT is a highly accurate and rapid method for the investigation of patients with acute stroke syndrome. The clinical management of such patients is simplified by the ease of CT differentiation of bland ischemic infarction from intracerebral hemorrhage and grossly hemorrhagic stroke. The high density of fresh blood easily distinguishes it on CT from the poorly marginated region of low density most commonly seen with acute infarct. Although routine MR pulse sequences are insensitive to infarctive hemorrhage, recent evidence suggests that low flip angle gradient echo sequences may dramatically improve the MR detection of bleeding within recent infarcts. Within the first 8 to 24 hours after clinical stroke, CT results are commonly negative. After this time, noncontrast CT reveals focal low density involving gray and subcortical white matter in a vascular distribution, often triangular in shape, corresponding to the affected territory supplied by a branch or branches of the carotid or vertebrobasilar arterial system (Figure 2-20). Mass effect due to associated edema is usually mild but occurs in 25% of acute strokes **(Option (A) is false).** Edema may arise during the first 24 hours, is usually maximal at 5 days, and may persist for up to 3 to 4 weeks. The minor degree of mass effect and typical vascular distribution tend to distinguish infarctions from tumors, which do not follow such a pattern. Weeks after the ictus, edematous but viable tissue recovers and the infarct may become more sharply defined. Subsequent resorption of necrotic tissue 1 to 2 months later leads to local ventricular dilatation and focal brain atrophy (encephalomalacia). Contrast-enhanced CT is generally not required for the diagnosis of cerebral infarction unless the clinical pattern is atypical or exact definition of the extent of involvement is considered essential. There is some evidence that the prognosis of infarction is poorer in patients receiving intravenous contrast infusion; thus, this procedure should not be used unless it will provide truly

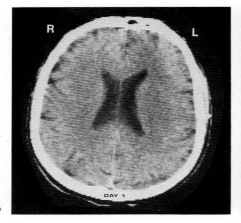
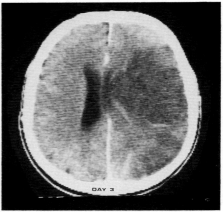

A   **B**

Figure 2-20. CT studies in a patient with clinical signs of acute left hemispheric stroke. (A) On the day of the stroke, noncontrast CT reveals only a very slight left hemispheric lucency, which might be interpreted as normal. (B) Two days later, contrast-enhanced CT shows a clearly lucent infarct involving much of the left hemisphere (middle cerebral artery distribution). Increasing cerebral edema has resulted in ventricular compression and midline shift.

essential information. Although noncontrast CT findings may occasionally be subtle and although about 20% of infarcts may be detected only by contrast-enhanced CT **(Option (C) is true)**, the finding of a "normal" CT result in a patient with an obvious clinical infarction may be all that is needed for therapeutic decision-making. On contrast-enhanced CT, the typical cortical infarction exhibits linear surface enhancement following a gyral pattern corresponding to the territory of the involved vessel (Figures 2-12, 2-18, and 2-21). Gyral enhancement may be the only clue to the position of the infarct on CT scans (Figure 2-21). Angiography may reveal a similar "gyral blush" when performed in such cases (Figure 2-22). Occlusion of deep penetrating arteries (such as lenticulostriate branches) may lead to lacunar infarcts and to a CT pattern of ring enhancement or nodular blush (Figure 2-23) **(Option (D) is false).** The presence and degree of enhancement depend upon the method of contrast administration and the time at which it is administered postictus. It is likely that all infarcts will enhance at some point during the first 6 weeks after onset of symptoms. Hence, the combination of mass effect and contrast enhancement is not unusual and does not exclude a diagnosis of infarction **(Option (B) is false).** About 10% of infarcts enhance during the first week, 25% enhance during the second week, 60% enhance during

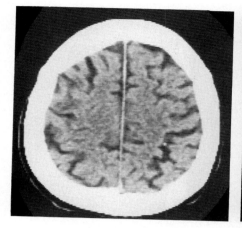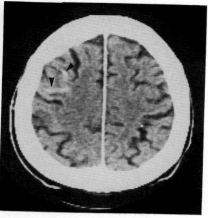

A

B

Figure 2-21. Infarct with gyral enhancement in a patient with mild weakness of the left upper extremity and left face. (A) Noncontrast CT was interpreted as normal. A normal CT scan in a patient with an acute stroke may be sufficient for the determination of prognosis and immediate therapy. (B) Contrast-enhanced CT in the same patient, performed at the same level as that of the noncontrast CT in panel A, immediately following the preinfusion study. Note linear or gyral enhancement of the infarct (arrowheads).

the third week, and 65 to 70% enhance during the fourth week. Enhancement may occasionally inhibit the detection of an area of infarction by raising the attenuation value of a hypodense lesion to that of adjacent brain, thus rendering it isodense (Figure 2-24). Hemorrhage within an otherwise bland infarct may appear as a focus of hyperdensity within a larger lucency (Figures 2-18 and 2-25). Old areas of infarction may calcify. Infarcts due to cortical venous thrombosis (Figure 2-12) tend to follow no specific vascular territory, are more frequently hemorrhagic, and may involve predominantly white matter **(Option (E) is true).**

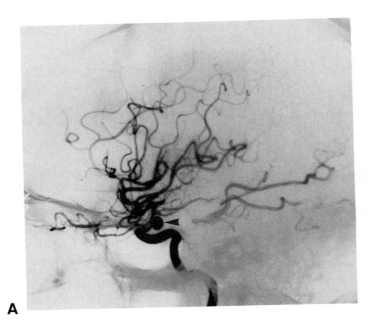

A

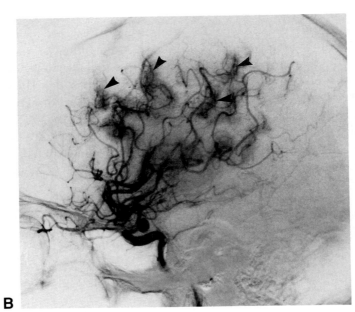

B

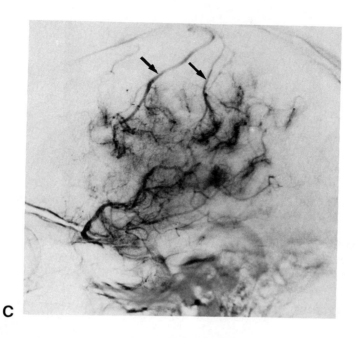

C

Figure 2-22. Gyral pattern blush at angiography in a patient with infarcts due to arterial spasm induced by subarachnoid hemorrhage from a posterior communicating artery aneurysm. Early arterial (A), late arterial (B), and capillary venous phase (C) lateral subtraction views of an internal carotid artery injection are shown. Note the aneurysm (arrowhead, panel A) and the vascular blush along the course of many infarcted posterior frontal and parietal lobe gyri (arrowheads, panel B). Early venous drainage can also be seen from this region (arrows, panel C). These findings indicate a loss of vascular autoregulation in the infarcted region of the brain.

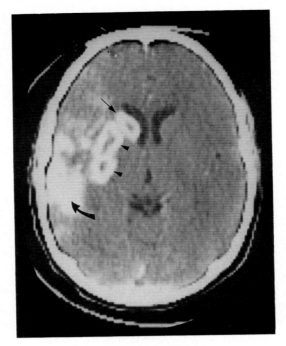

Figure 2-23. Contrast-enhanced CT. Ring-enhancing infarcts in the distribution of the lenticulostriate branches of the middle cerebral artery. Note the involvement of the head of the caudate nucleus (straight arrow) and the lateral ganglionic (putamenal) region (arrowheads). Note also the involvement of the more distal territory (patchy enhancement, curved arrow). The clinical stroke occurred 4 weeks prior to this study.

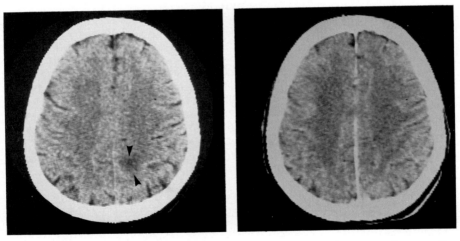

A

B

Figure 2-24. Acute infarct seen on noncontrast CT, hidden by patchy enhancement after contrast infusion. Note the focally lucent infarct (arrowheads on noncontrast CT, panel A) not seen on contrast-enhanced CT (B). The infarcted area enhances so that its attenuation is equal to that of normal adjacent brain tissue on contrast-enhanced CT.

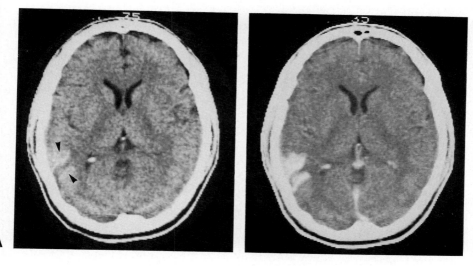

Figure 2-25. Hemorrhagic infarction with gyral enhancement: noncontrast CT (A) and contrast-enhanced CT (B). Note the focal hyperdensity indicative of hemorrhage (arrowheads, panel A) in the same area as the more well-defined enhancement seen on contrast-enhanced CT (B).

Question 10

Concerning meningiomas,

   (A) a low-density area adjacent to the tumor is most frequently caused by atrophy
   (B) nonenhancing low-density areas can be seen in 15% of benign meningiomas
   (C) tumor vessels usually arise only from internal carotid artery branches
   (D) extensive white matter edema occurs
   (E) intratumoral hemorrhage is highly specific for malignant meningioma

Meningiomas arise from arachnoidal cells adjacent to the dura mater and occur most frequently in the parasagittal region near the pacchionian granulations. The tumors grow from sites of dural attachment and are extra-axial, indenting the surface of the brain and only rarely invading it. Morphologically, tumors grow in either a globular or flat (en plaque) configuration. Blood supply primarily arises from dural arteries, generally arising from branches of the external carotid artery **(Option (C) is false).** Angiography characteristically demonstrates radiating tumor vessels and a dense, sharply marginated tumor blush, which lasts well into the venous phase of the study (Figure 2-26). Selective injection

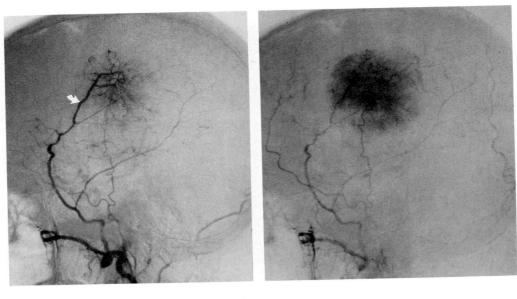

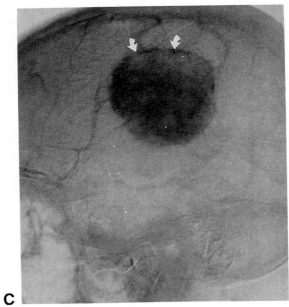

Figure 2-26. Angiographic demonstration of convexity meningioma. Lateral subtraction images of a selective external carotid artery injection obtained during early arterial (A), late arterial (B), and venous (C) phases. (A) The middle meningeal artery enlarges distally (arrow) and gives rise to a number of radiating distal branches feeding the meningioma. (B and C) The tumor blush is well marginated and homogeneous. Capsular veins are seen as marginal, densely blushing linear structures in the venous phase (arrows, panel C).

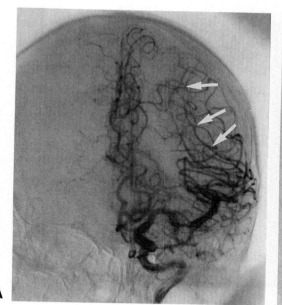
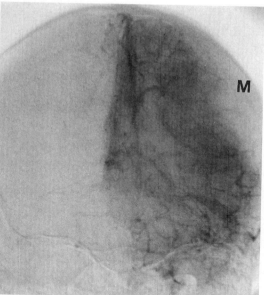

A

B

Figure 2-27. Same patient as in Figure 2-26. Frontal subtraction images during arterial (A) and venous (B) phases of an internal carotid artery injection. The lack of a vascular blush from normal brain displaced medially (arrows) by the tumor results in a clear space (M, panel B), indicating the site of the mass. The tumor is vascular, however, as demonstrated by the external carotid study (Figure 2-26).

into the internal carotid artery may give the false impression of an avascular mass displacing brain inward (Figure 2-27), although dural branches arising from the internal carotid or ophthalmic arteries may also directly supply the tumor and result in the characteristic "blush" (Figure 2-28). Tumor-related brain edema is not directly proportional to tumor size, since very small tumors may incite extensive white matter edema **(Option (D) is true).**

CT is an excellent method for detecting meningioma; contrast-enhanced CT was accurate in 96.2% of cases in a study done by the National Cancer Institute. MR studies may miss small isointense tumors unless supplemented by T1-weighted imaging performed after gadolinium contrast infusion. Meningioma (on CT) generally appears as a focal mass with a density higher than that of adjacent brain due to vascularity and scattered psammomatous calcifications (Figure 2-4). Associated bony hyperostosis and confluent tumoral calcification (Figure 2-5) may be

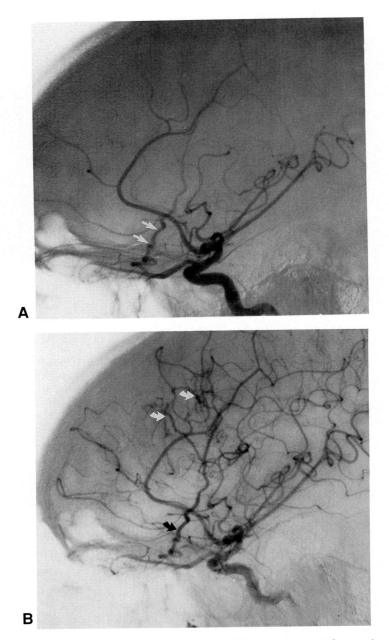

Figure 2-28. Lateral subtraction views of internal carotid arteriography. Convexity meningioma supplied by the recurrent meningeal branch of the ophthalmic artery (arrows, panel A; black curved arrow, panel B). Note the small branches supplying the tumor (white curved arrows, panel B).

detected by radiography or CT. Adjacent bone thickening confirms the extra-axial location of the tumor, since lesions arising from within the brain do not produce such sclerosis. Homogeneous enhancement on CT generally follows intravenous contrast infusion. Adjacent areas of low density may surround a part of the tumor margin and are usually due to edema or, less frequently, adjacent subarachnoid cyst formation. It is rare for perifocal brain atrophy to have such an appearance **(Option (A) is false).** In about 15% of cases, meningioma will show regions of inhomogeneous enhancement on contrast-enhanced CT **(Option (B) is true).** Causes of such focal nonenhancing areas include necrosis, central cyst formation due to old hemorrhage, and focal intratumoral scarring. Diffuse fatty infiltration within an otherwise typical meningioma may explain a primarily lucent appearance on noncontrast CT with a more classic homogeneous appearance on contrast-enhanced CT (Figure 2-29). Intratumoral hemorrhage may occur in either benign or malignant meningiomas **(Option (E) is false).** Necrosis is more frequent but is not found exclusively in malignant tumors.

Contrast infusion is an essential part of the CT study for detecting meningioma, since some tumors appear isodense with brain on noncontrast CT and are not detected. Similar problems may arise with MRI. Most meningiomas are isointense with brain on standard T1- and T2-weighted pulse sequences. Inversion recovery is the best sequence for meningioma detection because the extra-axial nature of the mass is best appreciated by secondary signs of cortical displacement and white matter buckling. The use of a paramagnetic contrast material for MRI aids in detecting some small tumors that might otherwise be missed by noncontrast MRI studies.

Eric J. Russell, M.D.

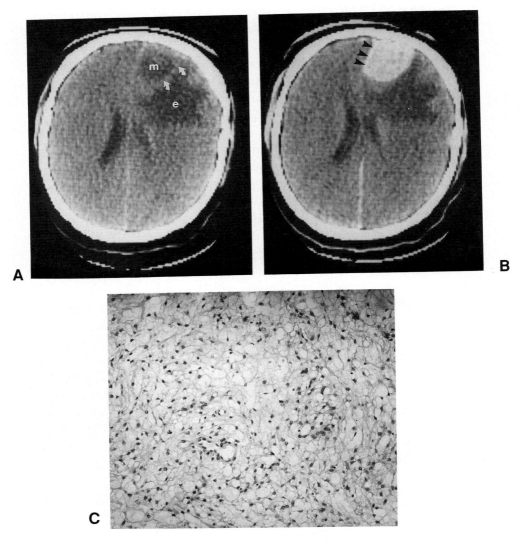

Figure 2-29. Lipomatous meningioma. (A) Noncontrast CT reveals central lucency within the tumor (m). The tumor margin is relatively dense (arrows), separating fatty tumor from white matter edema (e). (B) Axial contrast-enhanced CT scan shows the characteristic features of a meningioma arising from the anterior falx cerebri (arrowheads) and frontal convexity bone. The homogeneous blush is broadly based on dura and the adjacent inner table. Peritumoral edema is shown as focal low attenuation within adjacent white matter. (C) Fat was evenly distributed within an otherwise typical non-necrotic meningothelial meningioma (histologic section). (Reprinted with permission from Russell et al. [29].)

SUGGESTED READINGS

SUBDURAL HEMATOMA

1. Cornell SH, Chiu LC, Christie JH. Diagnosis of extracerebral fluid collections by computed tomography. AJR 1978; 131:107–110
2. Forbes GS, Sheedy PF II, Piepgras DG, Houser OW. Computed tomography in the evaluation of subdural hematomas. Radiology 1978; 126:143–148
3. George AE, Russell EJ, Kricheff II. White matter buckling: CT sign of extraaxial intracranial mass. AJR 1980; 135:1031–1036
4. Kim KS, Hemmati M, Weinberg PE. Computed tomography in isodense subdural hematoma. Radiology 1978; 128:71–74
5. Lau LS, Pike JW. The computed tomographic findings of peritentorial subdural hemorrhage. Radiology 1983; 146:699–701
6. Reed D, Robertson WD, Graeb DA, Lapointe JS, Nugent RA, Woodhurst WB. Acute subdural hematomas: atypical CT findings. AJNR 1986; 7:417–421
7. Zimmerman RA, Bilaniuk LT, Gennarelli T, Bruce D, Dolinskas C, Uzzell B. Cranial computed tomography in diagnosis and management of acute head trauma. AJR 1978; 131:27–34
8. Zimmerman RD, Heier LA, Snow RB, Liu DPC, Kelly AB, Deck MDF. Acute intracranial hemorrhage: intensity changes on sequential MR scans at 0.5 T. AJNR 1988; 9:47–57
9. Zimmerman RD, Russell EJ, Yurberg E, Leeds NE. Falx and interhemispheric fissure on axial CT. II: recognition and differentiation of interhemispheric subarachnoid and subdural hemorrhage. AJNR 1982; 3:635–642

GLIOMATOUS TUMORS

10. Butler AR, Horii SC, Kricheff II, Shannon MB, Budzilovich GN. Computed tomography in astrocytomas. A statistical analysis of the parameters of malignancy and the positive contrast-enhanced CT scan. Radiology 1978; 129:433–439
11. Earnest F IV, Kelly PJ, Scheithauer BW, et al. Cerebral astrocytomas: histopathologic correlation of MR and CT contrast enhancement with stereotactic biopsy. Radiology 1988; 166:823
12. Russell EJ, Naidich TP. The enhancing septal/alveal wedge: a septal sign of intraaxial mass. Neuroradiology 1982; 23:33–40
13. Steinhoff H, Lanksch W, Kazner E, et al. Computed tomography in the diagnosis and differential diagnosis of glioblastomas. A qualitative study of 295 cases. Neuroradiology 1977; 14:193–200
14. Tchang S, Scotti G, Terbrugge K, et al. Computerized tomography as a possible aid to histological grading of supratentorial gliomas. J Neurosurg 1977; 46:735–739
15. Thomson JLG. Computerized axial tomography and the diagnosis of glioma: a study of 100 consecutive histologically proven cases. Clin Radiol 1976; 27:431–441

16. Weisberg LA. Cerebral computed tomography in the diagnosis of supratentorial astrocytoma. Comput Tomogr 1980; 4:87–105

CEREBRAL INFARCTION

17. Brant-Zawadzki M, Weinstein P, Bartkowski H, Moseley M. MR imaging and spectroscopy in clinical and experimental cerebral ischemia: a review. AJNR 1987; 8:39–48
18. Caillé JM, Guibert F, Bidabé AM, Billerey J, Piton J. Enhancement of cerebral infarcts with CT. Comput Tomogr 1980; 4:73–77
19. Campbell JK, Houser OW, Stevens JC, Wahner HW, Baker HL, Folger WN. Computed tomography and radionuclide imaging in the evaluation of ischemic stroke. Radiology 1978; 126:695–702
20. Davis KR, Taveras JM, New PF, Schnur JA, Roberson GH. Cerebral infarction diagnosis by computerized tomography. Analysis and evaluation of findings. AJR 1975; 124:643–660
21. Hecht-Leavilt C, Gomori JM, Grossman RI, Goldberg HI, Hackney DB, Zimmerman RA, Bilaniuk LT. High-field MRI of hemorrhagic cortical infarction. AJNR 1986; 7:581–585
22. Kendall BE, Pullicino P. Intravascular contrast injection in ischaemic lesions. II: effect on prognosis. Neuroradiology 1980; 19:241–243
23. Pullicino P, Kendall BE. Contrast enhancement in ischaemic lesions. I: relationship to prognosis. Neuroradiology 1980; 19:235–239
24. Skriver EB, Olsen TS. Contrast enhancement of cerebral infarcts. Incidence and clinical value in different states of cerebral infarction. Neuroradiology 1982; 23:259–265
25. Takahashi S, Goto K, Fukasawa H, Kawata Y, Uemura K, Yaguchi K. Computed tomography of cerebral infarction along the distribution of the basal perforating arteries. Part II: thalamic arterial group. Radiology 1985; 155:119–130

MENINGIOMA

26. Bydder GM, Kingsley DP, Brown J, Niendorf HP, Young IR. MR imaging of meningiomas including studies with and without gadolinium-DTPA. J Comput Assist Tomogr 1985; 9:690–697
27. Helle TL, Conley FK. Haemorrhage associated with meningioma: a case report and review of the literature. J Neurol Neurosurg Psychiatry 1980; 43:725–729
28. New PF, Aronow S, Hesselink JR. National Cancer Institute study: evaluation of computed tomography in the diagnosis of intracranial neoplasms. IV: meningiomas. Radiology 1980; 136:665–675
29. Russell EJ, Cybulski G, Memoli V. Adjacent cerebral and paranasal sinus masses. Invest Radiol 1983; 18:317–321
30. Russell EJ, George AE, Kricheff II, Budzilovich G. Atypical computed tomography features of intracranial meningioma. Radiological-pathological correlation in a series of 131 consecutive cases. Radiology 1980; 135:673–682

31. Smith HP, Challa VR, Moody DM, Kelly DL Jr. Biological features of meningiomas that determine the production of cerebral edema. Neurosurgery 1981; 8:428–433
32. Spagnoli MV, Goldberg HI, Grossman RI, et al. Intracranial meningiomas: high-field MR imaging. Radiology 1986; 161:369–375
33. Zimmerman RD, Fleming CA, Saint-Louis LA, Lee BC, Manning JJ, Deck MD. Magnetic resonance imaging of meningiomas. AJNR 1985; 6:149–157

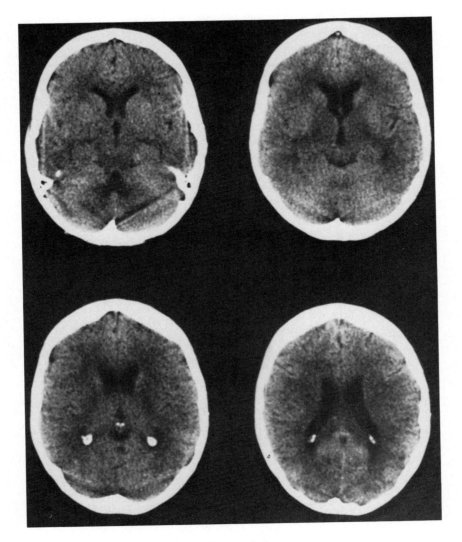

Figure 3-1

Figures 3-1 and 3-2. This 66-year-old man presented with severe headaches. You are shown pre- and postcontrast computed tomographic (CT) scans.

Case 3: Diffuse Leptomeningeal Metastatic Neoplasm

Question 11

Which *one* of the following is the MOST likely diagnosis?

(A) Subarachnoid hemorrhage
(B) Cerebellar infarction
(C) Diffuse leptomeningeal metastatic neoplasm
(D) Arteriovenous malformation
(E) Metastatic parenchymal tumors

Selected computed tomographic (CT) images of the brain in the axial plane without contrast infusion (Figure 3-1) demonstrate the cortical sulci bilaterally to be much less prominent than expected for a 66-year-old patient. The left Sylvian fissure is also less prominent than usual for this age group, and the right Sylvian fissure is virtually completely obliterated. No area of abnormal parenchymal density can be seen. The quadrigeminal and pineal cisterns appear to be normal. The ventricular system is within normal limits for the patient's age. Postcontrast CT images (Figure 3-2) demonstrate multiple areas of abnormal enhancement. There is diffuse enhancement of the cortical sulci and Sylvian fissures bilaterally. The tentorium cerebelli appears thickened, and there is diffuse enhancement of the subarachnoid space within the posterior fossa. In addition, there is enhancement in the ependymal lining of the frontal horns and bodies of the lateral ventricles bilaterally. No area of abnormal parenchymal enhancement can be seen. These CT findings are most consistent with diffuse leptomeningeal metastatic disease **(Option (C) is the correct answer)**. Additionally, the patient's history of headache is entirely consistent, since headache is one of the most common presenting symptoms of diffuse leptomeningeal metastases.

Although headache is the most common presenting symptom of acute subarachnoid hemorrhage (Option (A)), the CT findings in Figures 3-1 and 3-2 are not consistent with this diagnosis. Noncontrast CT images

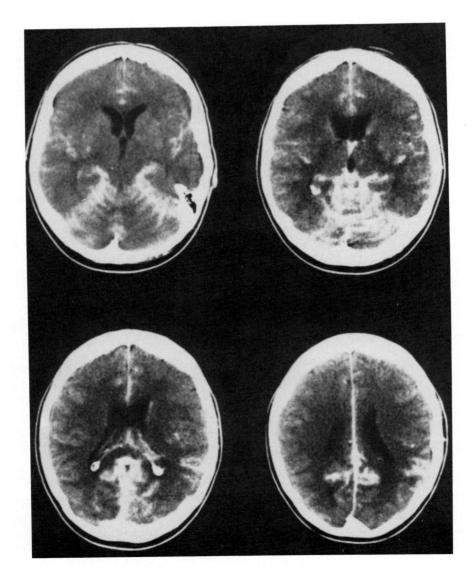

Figure 3-2

would demonstrate increased density in the subarachnoid pathways
immediately following a subarachnoid hemorrhage (Figures 3-3 and 3-4).
This increased density usually persists for a period ranging from 1 day
to 1 week. At the end of this period, the hemorrhage becomes isodense
on noncontrast CT images, resulting in the apparent obliteration of the

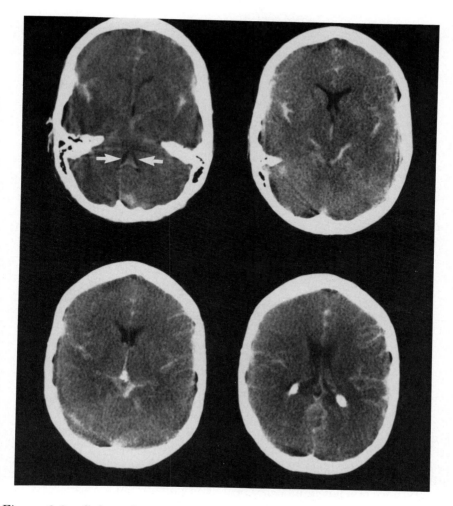

Figure 3-3. Subarachnoid hemorrhage. Noncontrast CT scans demonstrate diffuse subarachnoid hemorrhage in this patient with a history of trauma. Blood is also present within the fourth ventricle (arrows).

basal cisterns and cortical sulci. Postcontrast CT images obtained during this isodense stage may reveal leptomeningeal enhancement in the areas of hemorrhage. Acute subarachnoid hemorrhage may also appear isodense initially if the amount of hemorrhage is small or if the blood hemoglobin level is low. Approximately 1 to 2 weeks after the acute event, subarachnoid hemorrhages are of low density and therefore not directly detectable by CT. Ruptured saccular aneurysms are responsible for approximately 75% of subarachnoid hemorrhages in the absence of

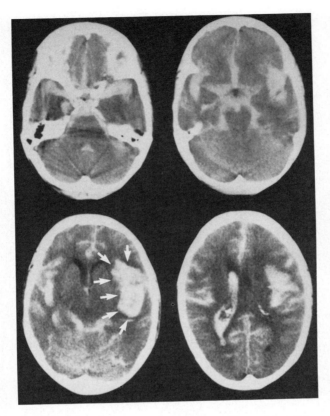

Figure 3-4. Subarachnoid hemorrhage. Noncontrast CT scans demonstrate considerable subarachnoid and intraventricular hemorrhage. A focal collection of blood in the left Sylvian fissure region represents an intracerebral hematoma (arrows). Cerebral angiography demonstrated the presence of a left middle cerebral artery aneurysm.

trauma. Less common causes of subarachnoid hemorrhage include ruptured arteriovenous malformation (AVM), hypertensive hemorrhage, hypocoagulable states, arteritis, hemorrhagic infarction, and venous thrombosis.

Patients with acute cerebellar infarction (Option (B)) may present with the onset of headaches. However, this complaint is relatively nonspecific and is usually accompanied by symptoms more directly referable to the posterior fossa. Although noncontrast CT images obtained immediately postinfarction are frequently normal, follow-up studies are likely to demonstrate an area of low density in the area of infarction. Postcontrast CT images may demonstrate abnormal contrast enhancement within the low-density area. A characteristic CT finding in cerebellar infarction is a discrete linear pattern of enhancement strictly corresponding to the cerebellar folia. This is distinct from the coarser pattern of enhancement of the posterior fossa subarachnoid space seen in leptomeningeal metastases (Figure 3-2). In addition, the supratentorial abnormalities identified in Figures 3-1 and 3-2 cannot be explained on the basis of cerebellar infarction, and thus cerebellar infarction is not likely.

Most patients with AVMs (Option (D)) present clinically with acute parenchymal hemorrhage and commonly have focal neurological findings. Less frequently, these patients present with headache alone. Figure 3-1 demonstrates no evidence of acute parenchymal hemorrhage. In the presence of an AVM without associated hemorrhage, noncontrast CT is likely to demonstrate a mixed pattern of high and low density, possibly involving an entire cerebral or cerebellar hemisphere. The postcontrast CT study typically reveals a heterogeneous pattern of contrast enhancement, usually in a serpiginous configuration, with visualization of enlarged feeding and draining vessels. The pattern of contrast enhancement in the posterior fossa in Figure 3-2 may superficially resemble that of an AVM. However, no feeding or draining vessels can be identified. In addition, the vascular nidus of an AVM is limited to a single hemisphere, although feeding vessels may be derived from the contralateral side. Finally, the multiple supratentorial abnormalities seen in Figure 3-2 cannot be accounted for by a posterior fossa AVM; thus, AVM is also unlikely.

The absence of areas of abnormal parenchymal density or contrast enhancement on CT precludes the diagnosis of metastatic parenchymal tumors (Option (E)) in this patient. Parenchymal metastases account for approximately 10 to 20% of all intracranial neoplasms. They occur at some time during the course of the disease in 10 to 40% of patients with cancer and are usually preceded by pulmonary metastases. The mode of tumor spread is believed to be hematogenous in the majority of cases. Patients with parenchymal metastases most commonly present with headache in addition to focal neurologic deficit(s). In adults, the most common primary tumor sites are the lung, breast, skin (melanoma), kidney, colon, and rectum. When the patient's initial presentation is the result of intracranial parenchymal metastases, the occult primary tumor site is most commonly a carcinoma of the lung. Neuroblastoma, rhabdomyosarcoma, and Wilms' tumor are the primary neoplasms responsible for most childhood intracranial parenchymal metastases. On noncontrast CT, parenchymal metastases frequently present as multiple round lesions of variable density at the cortical-medullary

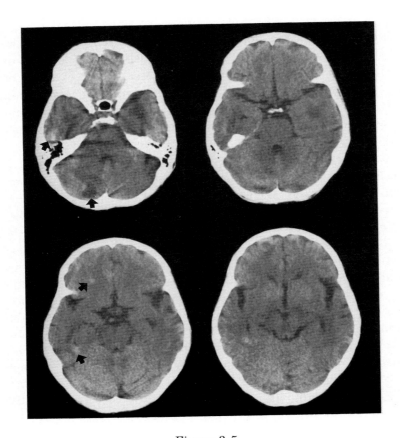

Figure 3-5

Figures 3-5 and 3-6. Parenchymal metastases. Noncontrast CT scans (Figure 3-5) demonstrate multiple lesions both supra- and infratentorially. They range in appearance from hypo- to hyperdense (arrows). There is relatively little associated edema. Postcontrast CT scans (Figure 3-6) demonstrate innumerable areas of enhancement. Both nodular and ring lesions are present.

junction with moderate to marked white matter (vasogenic) edema (Figure 3-5). Hemorrhagic metastases are most frequently the result of choriocarcinoma, melanoma, bronchogenic carcinoma, and renal cell carcinoma. Calcified metastases, although uncommon, may be seen with carcinomas of the lung, breast, and colon, among others. High-dose contrast enhancement with up to 80 g of iodine increases the diagnostic accuracy of CT for detecting intracranial parenchymal metastases. The most common appearance on postcontrast CT is that of multiple lesions with nodular or ring-like enhancement (Figures 3-6 to 3-8). However,

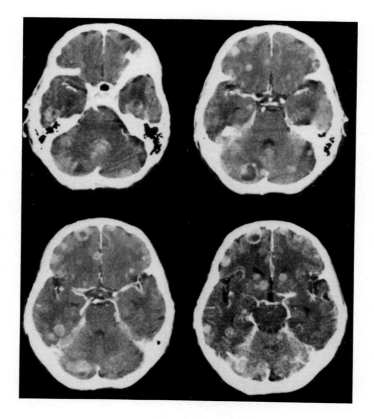

Figure 3-6

approximately 15 to 35% of metastases are solitary. Primary tumors of the breast and kidney account for most solitary lesions. The differential diagnosis of multiple intracranial metastases includes such entities as multiple abscesses, multiple areas of infarction, and multiple areas of demyelination (multiple sclerosis). The main differential diagnosis of a solitary metastatic lesion is that of a primary intracranial tumor.

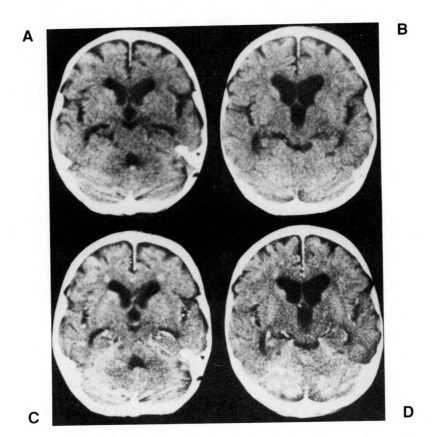

Figure 3-7. Parenchymal metastases. Comparison of precontrast (A and B) and postcontrast (C and D) CT scans allows demonstration of multiple contrast-enhancing nodules within the cerebellar hemispheres bilaterally. Additional lesions are identified adjacent to the frontal horns of the lateral ventricles.

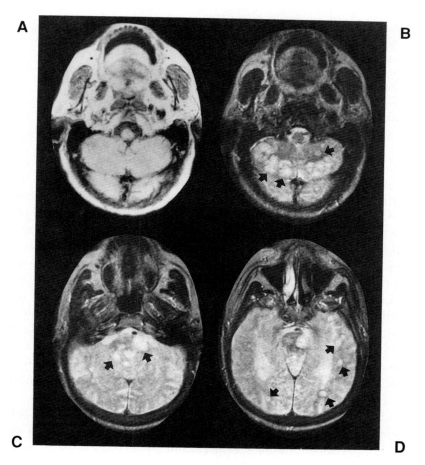

Figure 3-8. Same patient as in Figure 3-7. Parenchymal metastases. T1-weighted (A) and T2-weighted (B, C, and D) MR images of the brain. The T1-weighted image reveals no definite abnormality. The T2-weighted images show innumerable lesions with increased signal intensity involving the cerebral hemispheres, cerebellum, and brain stem (arrows).

Question 12

Concerning cerebellar infarction,

(A) cerebellar arteries do not freely communicate over the surface of the cerebellum
(B) a common presenting symptom is vertigo
(C) the superior cerebellar artery is the most common vessel involved
(D) absent filling of the posterior inferior cerebellar artery on angiography confirms the diagnosis
(E) nodular and ring-like enhancement on CT makes differentiation from neoplasm difficult
(F) obliteration of posterior fossa cisterns on CT suggests poor prognosis

The true overall incidence of cerebellar infarction has not been determined with certainty. However, relatively large cerebellar infarctions involving at least one-third of a cerebellar hemisphere, referred to as acute massive cerebellar infarction, appear to account for slightly less than 1% of all cerebrovascular accidents. Smaller cerebellar infarctions probably account for a similar percentage of the total number of accidents. The fact that cerebellar infarctions are significantly less common than either cerebral or brain stem infarctions may be due, in part, to the free communication of the cerebellar arteries over the surface of the cerebellum **(Option (A) is false).** Frequent anastomoses include those between the two posterior inferior cerebellar arteries (PICAs), between each PICA and the ipsilateral anterior inferior cerebellar artery (AICA), between the vermian branches of each PICA and the ipsilateral superior cerebellar artery (SCA), and between branches of an AICA and the ipsilateral SCA within the horizontal fissure of the cerebellum.

Cerebellar infarction is usually the result of atherosclerotic arterial occlusion. Approximately 25% of the occlusions were embolic in nature in one autopsy series. Cerebellar infarction occurs more often in men, and most patients are in late middle age or older. Predisposing factors include cardiovascular disease, hypertension, diabetes mellitus, previous cerebrovascular disease, blood dyscrasias, contraceptive pill use, and trauma.

Vertigo is a common presenting symptom in patients with cerebellar infarction **(Option (B) is true).** Occlusion of the PICA, AICA, or SCA may result in vertigo, and it may be the only presenting symptom in patients with small cerebellar infarctions. However, such signs and symptoms as ataxia, headache, nausea, and vomiting frequently accompany vertigo in patients with small cerebellar infarctions and in patients in the initial stage of acute massive cerebellar infarction. After a so-called "latent period" of roughly 12 to 96 hours characterized by clinical stability, patients with acute massive cerebellar infarction will probably develop progressive neurological deterioration. As opposed to the earlier signs and symptoms related directly to cerebellar destruction, this further deterioration arises mainly as a result of brain stem compression. Clinical findings may include nystagmus, decreased consciousness, ocular muscle paresis (cranial nerves III, IV, and VI), facial weakness (cranial nerve VII), hearing loss and tinnitus (cranial nerve VIII), pupillary dilatation (cranial nerve III), dysarthria and dysphasia (cranial nerve X), and motor dysfunction. This may ultimately lead to quadriplegia, coma, and death within hours or days. Although a primary vestibular process, such as a labyrinthine disorder, is another diagnostic consideration in a patient with the acute onset of vertigo, the presence of associated cerebellar and brain stem findings excludes this possibility.

Various studies demonstrate that approximately 70 to 90% of cerebellar infarctions occur in the distribution of the PICA **(Option (C) is false).** CT images show the area of abnormality to be in the posteroinferior aspect of the cerebellar hemisphere. However, angiography usually reveals the actual site of arterial occlusion or stenosis to be within the vertebral artery rather than within the PICA itself. It should also be noted that failure to demonstrate a PICA angiographically may not be the result of an arterial occlusion. In an estimated 20% of vertebral angiograms, there is nonvisualization of the PICA on the basis of congenital absence **(Option (D) is false).** The vascular territory of the PICA is supplied by the ipsilateral AICA in such cases. Most of the remaining 10 to 30% of cerebellar infarctions occur in the distribution of an SCA, with CT showing the area of abnormality to be in the superior aspect of the hemisphere and/or vermis. Again, angiography is more likely to reveal disease in the vertebrobasilar system than in the SCA itself. Cerebellar infarctions less frequently occur in the distribution of the AICA. CT may show an abnormality in the anteroinferior aspect of the cerebellar hemisphere. Failure to demonstrate an area of significant arterial stenosis or a complete arterial occlusion by angiography in a patient with cerebellar infarction raises the possibility of arterial recanalization or embolic fragmentation.

The CT appearance of cerebellar infarction without contrast infusion is usually that of an area of low attenuation within a cerebellar hemisphere corresponding in location to a specific vascular territory (Figure 3-9). The involvement of multiple vascular territories, possibly bilaterally, is less common. The low-attenuation area frequently

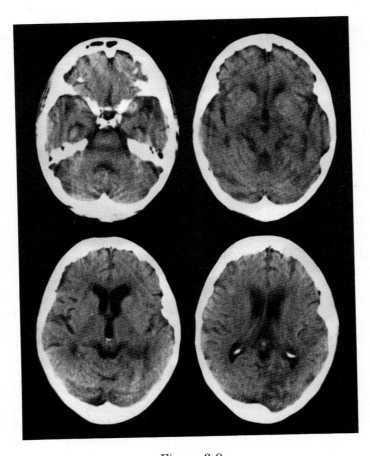

Figure 3-9

Figures 3-9 and 3-10. Cerebellar infarction. Noncontrast CT scans (Figure 3-9) demonstrate a poorly defined area of decreased density involving the lateral and superior aspects of the left cerebellar hemisphere. There is no significant associated mass effect. Postcontrast CT scans (Figure 3-10) demonstrate a characteristic enhancement pattern in the left cerebellar hemisphere conforming to the cerebellar folia.

demonstrates a wedge-shaped configuration with the apex directed centrally. In less than 25% of cases, the area of infarction is isodense or hyperdense with respect to the normal cerebellum. This reflects the presence of hemorrhagic infarction and/or an infarction associated with frank hematoma formation. Findings consistent with cerebellar infarction are usually identified on noncontrast CT studies within 12 to 48 hours after the initial onset of symptoms. False-negative findings may

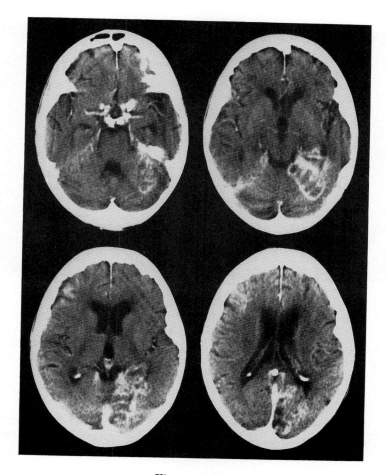

Figure 3-10

be the result of beam-hardening artifacts arising from the skull base which obscure the posterior fossa.

Approximately 15 to 25% of cerebellar infarctions demonstrate enhancement on CT following contrast material infusion. As is true of supratentorial infarctions, the enhancement is most likely to be evident during the period from 1 to 4 weeks following the onset of symptoms. The pattern of contrast enhancement most characteristic of cerebellar infarction is one in which the enhancement corresponds to the cerebellar folia (Figure 3-10). This type of enhancement is analogous to the gyral pattern often observed in supratentorial infarctions. However, other types of contrast enhancement, including nodular and ring-like patterns, may also be seen with cerebellar infarctions. These latter patterns of

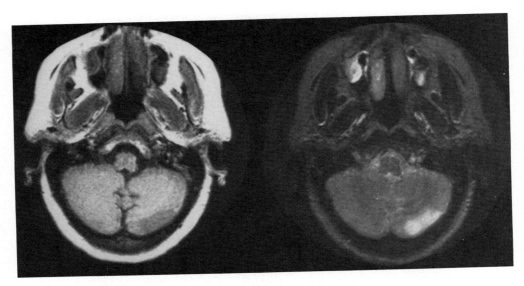

Figure 3-11. Cerebellar infarction. T1-weighted (left) and T2-weighted (right) MR images of the posterior fossa. The T1-weighted image demonstrates a focally decreased signal intensity in the posterolateral aspect of the left cerebellar hemisphere without associated mass effect. The T2-weighted image demonstrates a corresponding area of increased signal intensity.

contrast enhancement make the differentiation between cerebellar infarction and neoplasm difficult **(Option (E) is true).** Several factors may play a role in the differentiation between cerebellar infarctions with unusual patterns of enhancement and neoplasms. These factors include clinical symptoms, CT findings other than the pattern of contrast enhancement, and follow-up studies. Symptoms related to infarction are generally more sudden in their onset than those related to neoplasm. On CT, gray matter enhancement is more characteristic of an infarction, whereas white matter enhancement, particularly in a nodular or ring-like pattern, is more commonly observed with neoplasm. White matter edema, also referred to as vasogenic edema, is another CT finding in favor of neoplasm. However, follow-up studies often play the most definitive role in the differentiation between cerebellar infarction and neoplasm. The subsequent development on CT of a well-circumscribed area of decreased attenuation with no mass effect and no contrast enhancement strongly favors the diagnosis of infarction rather than neoplasm.

Magnetic resonance imaging (MRI) can reveal infarctions more clearly (Figure 3-11) than CT. MRI provides more-precise information regarding the anatomy of infarcts, since this modality can display the brain in multiple planes. High-resolution MRI also provides a noninvasive way of evaluating both the extracranial vessels and the major intracranial arteries, including the internal carotid, basilar, and proximal middle cerebral artery branches.

Cerebellar infarction involving a small portion of the hemisphere, usually in a PICA distribution, is associated with a good prognosis. The affected patient is likely to demonstrate only the relatively minor cerebellar signs and symptoms described above. As a general rule, clinical recovery is fairly rapid and usually complete, with little or no medical intervention required. However, acute massive cerebellar infarction involving at least one-third of a hemisphere is associated with a significantly different clinical course. In this type of infarction, considerable fluid accumulation occurs in the area of ischemic necrosis. This developing cerebellar edema, possibly in conjunction with hemorrhage, acts as a rapidly expanding posterior fossa mass lesion. CT findings consistent with significant mass effect may include fourth ventricular or aqueductal compression with associated hydrocephalus (Figure 3-12), supratentorial or tonsillar herniation, and obliteration of posterior fossa cisterns. These CT findings suggest a poor prognosis **(Option (F) is true)** since they indicate the presence of a mass effect capable of producing neurologic deterioration secondary to brain stem compression. Mortality estimates range as high as 80% for cerebellar infarctions associated with the signs and symptoms of brain stem compression. However, greater clinical awareness, prompt CT diagnosis, and various treatment modalities (medical decompression, surgical decompression, and/or ventricular drainage) can significantly improve the prognosis.

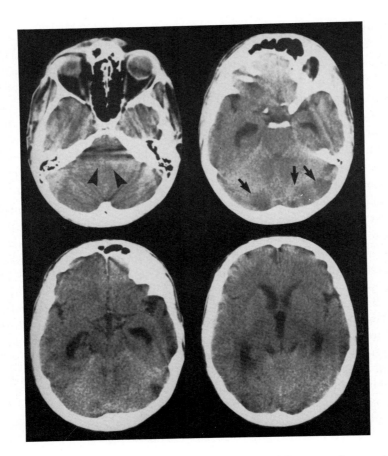

Figure 3-12. Cerebellar infarction. Noncontrast CT scans demonstrate areas of decreased density involving the posterior aspects of the cerebellar hemispheres bilaterally (arrows). Mass effect producing compression of the fourth ventricle (arrowheads) with resultant mild hydrocephalus indicates the acute nature of the process.

Question 13

Concerning leptomeningeal spread of neoplasm,

(A) leptomeningeal metastases are usually not diagnosed on CT unless they produce hydrocephalus and obliteration of the cisterns
(B) squamous cell carcinoma commonly invades the leptomeninges
(C) most lymphomas demonstrate involvement of both the leptomeninges and deep-brain structures on contrast-enhanced CT
(D) in the majority of cases, leptomeningeal carcinomatosis cannot be differentiated from bacterial meningitis by CT

Leptomeningeal spread of neoplasm, variously referred to as leptomeningeal metastases, leptomeningeal carcinomatosis, or carcinomatous meningitis, involves the diffuse infiltration of the leptomeninges and subarachnoid space by metastatic tumor. The most likely pathologic basis for the leptomeningeal spread of neoplasm appears to be the hematogenous spread of tumor directly to the arachnoid itself, although several other theories exist. The clinical diagnosis of leptomeningeal metastases may be suspected when varied neurologic signs and symptoms are encountered in conjunction with an abnormal cerebrospinal fluid (CSF) examination in a patient with a known malignancy. Approximately 50% of patients with leptomeningeal metastases present with signs and symptoms related to the cerebral hemispheres. These symptoms include headache, change in mental status, difficulty in walking, nausea and vomiting, and seizures. Cranial nerve signs and symptoms are noted in approximately 40% of patients and include diplopia secondary to ocular muscle paresis (cranial nerves III, IV, and VI), facial weakness (cranial nerve VII), and diminished hearing (cranial nerve VIII). However, a CSF analysis demonstrating the presence of malignant cells, usually in association with decreased glucose concentration and an increased protein content, is required for the definitive diagnosis of leptomeningeal metastases. More than one CSF analysis may be required in some patients to avoid false-negative results. It should be noted that the CSF rarely demonstrates positive cytology with only focal leptomeningeal involvement by tumor and is virtually never positive with parenchymal metastases alone.

CT is a valuable modality in the radiographic evaluation of patients with suspected leptomeningeal spread of neoplasm. In one recent study of leptomeningeal metastatic disease due to hematologic or nonhematologic primary tumors, more than 30% of patients with positive CSF cytology demonstrated definite abnormalities on CT that were directly related to the presence of leptomeningeal metastases. The two most common CT abnormalities seen with leptomeningeal metastases are obliteration of the cisterns and hydrocephalus **(Option (A) is true).** Obliteration of the cisterns is associated with obliteration of the cortical subarachnoid space as well. Following infusion of contrast material, there is often enhancement of the obliterated cisterns and cortical subarachnoid space. This finding is usually most prominent in the basal cisterns, Sylvian fissures, and inferior convexity cortical sulci. Tumor neovascularization alone may account for the contrast enhancement. However, the enhancement may also be due in part to a nonspecific leptomeningeal reaction to the presence of tumor. This nonspecific reaction may account for the persistence of abnormal contrast enhancement in some patients with negative CSF cytology following treatment. The hydrocephalus associated with leptomeningeal metastases is usually of the communicating type and is mild to moderate in severity. The presence of communicating hydrocephalus in a patient with a known neoplasm should strongly suggest the possibility of leptomeningeal spread of tumor.

Other CT findings, less sensitive than those of obliteration of the cisterns and hydrocephalus, may also be seen with leptomeningeal spread of neoplasm. Although tentorial enhancement is normally identified on CT following contrast infusion, it should suggest leptomeningeal metastases when the area of enhancement is widened and irregular, a finding indicative of a thickened tentorium cerebelli. As with enhancement of the cisterns, this abnormal tentorial enhancement may represent tumor neovascularity and/or a nonspecific leptomeningeal reaction. CT also demonstrates enhancement in the ependymal-subependymal region, representing periventricular leptomeningeal metastases. This finding may be either localized or diffuse and is generally not associated with surrounding edema. Certain primary brain tumors, including medulloblastoma, ependymoma, and pinealoblastoma, may also demonstrate periventricular spread, which results in ependymal-subependymal enhancement. The nonhematologic malignancies most likely to produce leptomeningeal metastases are breast carcinoma, bronchogenic carcinoma, and melanoma. In general, adenocarcinomas are far more likely to result in leptomeningeal metastases than are squamous cell carcinomas or sarcomas **(Option (B) is false).** Thus, while the most common histologic type of lung neoplasm is the squamous cell carcinoma, the less common adenocarcinoma is responsible for most leptomeningeal metastases that occur in patients with primary lung tumors. Regardless of the specific type of primary malignancy, patients with leptomeningeal

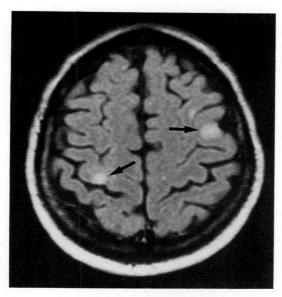

Figure 3-13. Parenchymal metastases. A T1-weighted MR scan obtained following injection of gadolinium DTPA demonstrates lesions involving both cerebral hemispheres (arrows).

metastases are likely to have widespread tumor dissemination throughout the body.

CT can detect the leptomeningeal spread of neoplasm in slightly less than one-half of patients with nonhematologic malignancies and positive CSF cytology. The sensitivity of CT appears to be significantly decreased in those instances in which leptomeningeal metastases are not accompanied by parenchymal metastases. However, this has limited clinical significance since leptomeningeal metastases are usually associated with the presence of parenchymal brain metastases in patients with nonhematologic malignancies.

Magnetic resonance imaging can be expected to play an increasing role in the detection of leptomeningeal spread of tumor. Early studies employing routine T1- and T2-weighted spin echo sequences demonstrated that the sensitivity of unenhanced MRI actually was less than that of postcontrast CT. However, MR studies obtained following the intravenous administration of gadolinium DTPA are likely to demonstrate significantly greater sensitivity than postcontrast CT when evaluating for leptomeningeal carcinomatosis (Figures 3-13 and 3-14).

The hematologic malignancy most likely to produce leptomeningeal involvement is lymphoma. Intracranial involvement in general is estimated to occur in slightly less than 10% of patients with diffuse

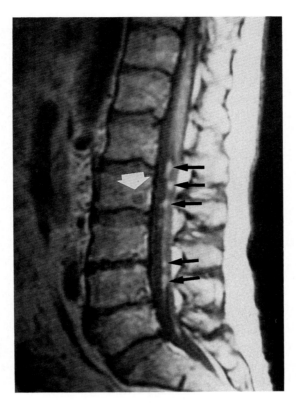

Figure 3-14. Same patient as in Figure 3-13. Spinal leptomeningeal carcinomatosis. A T1-weighted postcontrast MR scan demonstrates many small tumor nodules (black arrows) studding the cauda equina. Lesions are also present in the lower thoracic region. Incidentally noted is a metastatic focus involving the L2 vertebral body (white arrow).

histiocytic lymphoma, a type of non-Hodgkin's lymphoma. The frequency of intracranial involvement is considerably less with the other types of non-Hodgkin's lymphoma and with Hodgkin's disease (Hodgkin's lymphoma). As documented by CSF analyses and by autopsy series, the most common intracranial manifestation of lymphoma (excluding primary lymphoma of the brain) is leptomeningeal metastasis. However, multiple studies demonstrate that visualization by CT of the leptomeningeal infiltration is generally unreliable, with the various reported detection rates ranging from 0% to approximately 15%. CT protocols involving the use of high-dose contrast infusion and delayed scanning fail to significantly increase the sensitivity of detection. Lymphomatous masses within the brain, although pathologically less common than leptomeningeal metastases, are more likely to be detected by CT in the patient with lymphoma. In a recent series, approximately one-third of patients with lymphoma and positive CSF cytology demonstrated lymphomatous brain masses. These masses are isodense to slightly hyperdense on precontrast infusion images and enhance homogeneously following contrast infusion. The amount of associated edema and mass effect is proportional to the size of the lesions. It is significant that these lymphomatous masses tend to be contiguous with cortical or ependymal surfaces, suggesting that they arise as a result of direct spread from the meninges or the CSF, respectively. The presence of these masses in the periventricular regions adjacent to ependymal surfaces accounts for the involvement of the deep-brain parenchyma that may be observed on CT. However, neither involvement of the leptomeninges nor involvement of the deep-brain parenchyma is demonstrated on CT in most patients with lymphoma that has spread intracranially **(Option (C) is false).**

Leptomeningeal carcinomatosis and bacterial meningitis share many of the same CT features and therefore cannot be reliably differentiated by CT alone in the majority of cases **(Option (D) is true).** Patients, particularly children, with bacterial meningitis may develop hydrocephalus either early or late in the course of the disease. Hydrocephalus is usually of the communicating type, although noncommunicating hydrocephalus occurs as well. Diffuse leptomeningeal enhancement following contrast infusion is another CT feature of bacterial meningitis. This finding may be noted several days after the onset of the illness. Finally, ventriculitis may be observed as a late complication of bacterial meningitis, resulting in ependymal-subependymal enhancement on postinfusion CT images. Thus, it is apparent that both leptomeningeal carcinomatosis and bacterial meningitis may demonstrate hydrocephalus, leptomeningeal enhancement, and ependymal-subependymal enhancement on CT. Reliable differentiation between these two entities must therefore be based on clinical and laboratory criteria. Headache, mental disturbance, nausea and vomiting, and cranial nerve dysfunction are clinical symptoms common to both leptomeningeal carcinomatosis and bacterial meningitis. However, fever and intact deep tendon reflexes are usually present in the infectious process but absent in the neoplastic one. The most definitive diagnostic study is laboratory analysis of the CSF. The CSF in leptomeningeal carcinomatosis is usually characterized by 100 or fewer leukocytes (predominantly lymphocytes) per mm^3, an increased protein level, decreased glucose concentration, and cytology positive for neoplastic cells. In contrast, the CSF in bacterial meningitis is usually characterized by 1,000 to 10,000 leukocytes (predominantly polymorphonuclear) per mm^3, increased protein content, decreased glucose level, and microscopic as well as culture evidence of a bacterial agent. In addition to infectious meningitis, other entities to be considered in the differential diagnosis of leptomeningeal carcinomatosis on CT studies include subarachnoid hemorrhage, subacute infarction with associated gyral enhancement, AVM, and gyral enhancement following a seizure.

The leptomeningeal spread of neoplasm is currently estimated to account for 8 to 10% of all intracranial metastases. Because of improved diagnostic and treatment modalities that have prolonged survival for cancer patients, the incidence of leptomeningeal tumor spread appears to be increasing. This seems to be particularly true for carcinoma of the breast, lung, and ovary, as well as lymphoma and sarcomas. Until fairly recently, the prognosis for patients with leptomeningeal metastases was uniformly poor. Progressive deterioration could be expected to lead to death, with a mean survival time of only about 4 to 6 weeks. However, with more-aggressive treatment, including such measures as intrathecal chemotherapy and radiation therapy, symptomatic improvement and survival in the range of months to years following initial diagnosis can be expected.

Question 14

Concerning arteriovenous malformations,

(A) in the absence of hemorrhage, mass effect is not seen on CT
(B) noncontrast CT demonstrates mixed increased and decreased densities only when hemorrhage is present
(C) on CT, low-density areas in the parenchyma adjacent to an arteriovenous malformation most commonly represent edema
(D) CT evidence of calcification is seen in less than one-third of cases
(E) the predominant site of hemorrhage is the subarachnoid space

Vascular malformations of the brain include AVMs, capillary telangiectasias, cavernous angiomas, and venous angiomas. However, only AVMs involve the rapid arteriovenous shunting of blood. The median time of onset of symptoms in patients with AVMs is the fourth decade. Most patients initially present as a result of acute hemorrhage. In the absence of hemorrhage, other symptoms, in order of decreasing frequency, are seizure, headache, progressive neurologic deficit, dementia, and audible intracranial bruit.

AVMs are congenital in nature. Their embryogenesis is believed to occur at about 3 weeks' gestation. At that time, there is formation of the primitive intracranial arteries, capillaries, and veins. A localized developmental arrest results in a direct arteriovenous communication. Thus, the fundamental abnormality responsible for the presence of an AVM is the absence of an intervening capillary bed between essentially normal feeding arteries and draining veins. The subsequent dilatation of the feeding and draining vessels is the result of increased flow through a low-pressure system rather than any intrinsic abnormality.

AVMs most commonly occur in the supratentorial region and usually involve the cerebral hemispheres, particularly the parietal lobe, and are usually 2 cm or larger in diameter. Other relatively common sites for supratentorial AVMs include the basal ganglia, internal capsule, and thalamus. Approximately 20% of AVMs are infratentorial in location, usually within the cerebellum or pons. Anatomic specimens typically demonstrate the presence of a nidus of vascular channels supplied by a variable number of dilated arteries and drained by multiple dilated veins. The interstitial neural tissue within the AVM usually demonstrates gliosis and is largely nonfunctional. In the absence of recent hemorrhage, the most common pattern observed on noncontrast CT in the case of an AVM is a poorly defined area of mixed increased and decreased densities (Figure 3-15) **(Option (B) is false)**. AVMs are less commonly observed to be isodense or of relatively homogeneous increased density. The low-density areas within the parenchyma observed in the mixed pattern most commonly represent atrophy **(Option (C) is false)**. The atrophy is most likely to occur at the actual site of the AVM or within the immediately surrounding parenchyma, but it may also occur in relatively remote areas. The atrophy is usually due to ischemia resulting from a vascular "steal" by the AVM. The pulsatile nature of the AVM may also play a mechanical role in the development of this atrophy. Less commonly, the low-density areas may be due to infarction, resolving hematoma, or edema. The areas of increased density in and around the site of an AVM that has not recently hemorrhaged may be due to vascular and/or parenchymal calcifications. CT evidence of calcification is seen in less than one-third of cases **(Option (D) is true)**. Areas of increased density may also be the result of previous microscopic hemorrhages, mural thrombi, or blood within dilated vessels. Mass effect may be present in the absence of recent hemorrhage **(Option (A) is false)**. The mass effect, usually mild, may be attributed to the vascular nidus and/or to the enlarged feeding or draining vessels. CT findings of mass effect may include focal obliteration of the sulci or ventricular compression (Figures 3-15 and 3-16). In the case of AVMs draining into the galenic system (vein of Galen aneurysm), noncommunicating hydrocephalus may result from compression of the aqueduct of Sylvius.

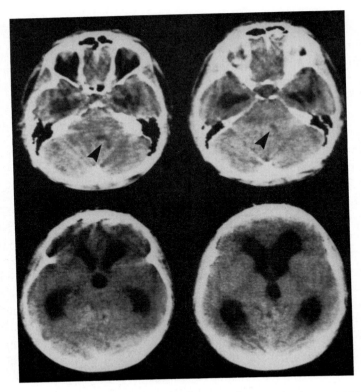

Figure 3-15. AVM. Noncontrast CT scans domonstrate compression of the posterolateral aspect of the fourth ventricle on the right side (arrowheads). Hydrocephalus may be the result of previous intraventricular hemorrhage and/or fourth ventricular compression.

Since approximately 20 to 25% of noncontrast CT studies fail to provide either direct or indirect evidence of an AVM, high-dose contrast infusion is recommended for complete evaluation. Almost all AVMs can be expected to demonstrate enhancement on postcontrast CT. The enhancement pattern is usually heterogeneous with a serpiginous, tubular, or linear configuration. Less common is a homogeneous pattern with diffuse or nodular enhancement. The visualized structures are more likely to represent the central vascular nidus and adjacent draining veins than the feeding arteries (Figure 3-16). Failure to demonstrate enhancement on postcontrast CT may be the result of thrombosis or the small size of an AVM, or a dural location, in which case the enhancement of the dura itself obscures the lesion.

Diagnostic modalities other than CT may play a role in the detection and evaluation of AVMs. Conventional radiographs of the skull may demonstrate enlarged vascular channels, abnormal intracranial calcifica-

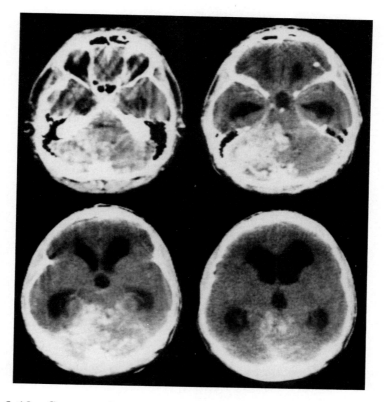

Figure 3-16. Same patient as in Figure 3-15. Postcontrast CT scans demonstrate abnormal enhancement throughout the right cerebellar hemisphere and in the region of the vermis. Differing patterns of enhancement are present in the various portions of the AVM.

tion, erosion of the inner table, asymmetry of the cranial fossae, and shift of a calcified pineal gland. However, it is angiography that usually makes the definitive diagnosis following an initial CT evaluation that suggests the presence of an AVM. In addition, angiography can be used to evaluate nonspecific CT findings more fully and also to provide the surgeon with a vascular "road map" of the AVM site. The typical angiographic appearance of an AVM is that of a racemose tangle of vessels supplied by large arterial feeders and drained by relatively larger veins (Figures 3-17 to 3-22). The rapid arteriovenous shunting of blood requires the use of a rapid filming sequence to visualize all of the feeding and draining vessels. The AVM often has a wedge-shaped configuration, with the base oriented along the cortical or subcortical margin and the apex directed centrally. Approximately 75% of AVMs are supplied exclusively by cerebral or cerebellar arteries (pial AVMs), 10% are supplied exclusively

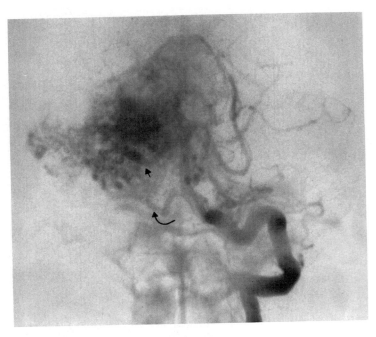

Figure 3-17

Figures 3-17 through 3-20. Same patient as in Figures 3-15 and 3-16. Subtraction views from a vertebral angiogram are shown. An anteroposterior view in the arterial phase (Figure 3-17) shows that there are multiple enlarged arterial branches that supply the AVM. Some of these feeders arise from an enlarged right anterior inferior cerebellar artery (curved arrow), and others arise from an enlarged right superior cerebellar artery (straight arrow). A lateral view in the arterial phase (Figure 3-18) shows enlarged arterial branches arising from the right anterior inferior cerebellar artery (curved arrow) and right superior cerebellar artery (straight arrow). The anteroposterior view in the venous phase (Figure 3-19) demonstrates multiple enlarged venous tributaries which drain the AVM. A lateral projection in the venous phase (Figure 3-20) shows multiple enlarged venous tributaries and an enlarged straight sinus and vein of Galen.

by dural meningeal arteries (dural AVMs), and 15% are supplied by a combination of both types of arterial feeders (mixed pial-dural AVMs). A disproportionately large number of dural and mixed pial-dural AVMs are located in the posterior fossa. Interestingly, one or more aneurysms may be identified arising from the feeding arteries in up to 10% of AVMs. These most likely result from a combination of atherosclerotic changes and high flow within these arteries. The angiographic differentiation between an AVM and tumor is usually straightforward. The presence of

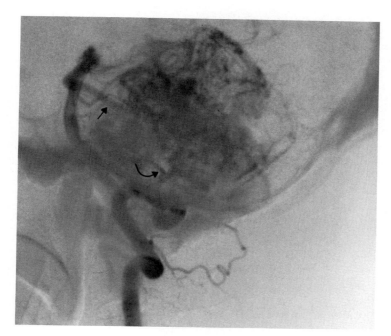

Figure 3-18

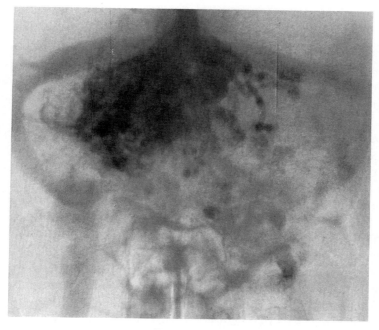

Figure 3-19

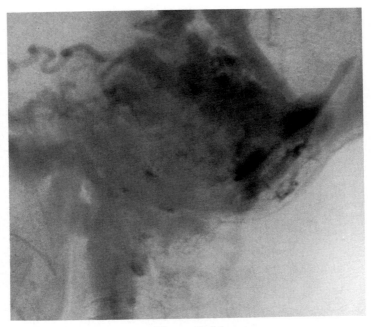

Figure 3-20

dilated, undulating feeding vessels, tightly packed vascular channels having a uniform caliber, enlarged draining veins, and minimal mass effect are findings that favor the diagnosis of an AVM. In contrast, minimally dilated and stretched feeding vessels, irregular tumor vessels with intervening avascular spaces, normal-caliber early draining veins, and more-pronounced mass effect favor the diagnosis of a malignant tumor.

As previously mentioned, most patients with AVMs present as a result of an acute hemorrhage and its sequelae. At least one episode of hemorrhage is likely to occur in an estimated 50 to 85% of patients with AVMs. The risk of subsequent hemorrhages substantially increases following the first episode. The usual site of hemorrhage is intraparenchymal, resulting in the formation of an intracerebral hematoma. Intraventricular hemorrhage occurs less commonly and may be secondary to either a deep parenchymal or ependymal AVM. Subarachnoid hemorrhage is an uncommon presentation for an AVM **(Option (E) is false).** Saccular aneurysms, which are much more common than AVMs, are more often the cause of subarachnoid hemorrhage. However, since most aneurysmal subarachnoid hemorrhages occur during the fifth and sixth decades of life, an AVM is the most common cause of subarachnoid hemorrhage in patients under the age of 20 years. Regardless of the exact

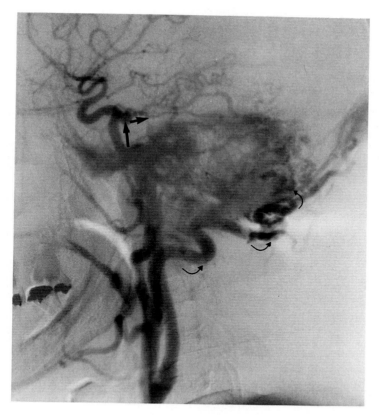

Figure 3-21

Figures 3-21 and 3-22. Same patient as in Figures 3-15 through 3-20. A subtraction lateral view of the right common carotid angiogram in the early arterial phase (Figure 3-21) shows enlargement of the occipital branch of the external carotid artery (curved arrows), which in turn leads to multiple feeders supplying the AVM. There is also an aneurysm (large arrow) arising from the site of origin of an enlarged meningohypophyseal trunk branch (small arrow) which also contributes to the supply of the AVM. In the midarterial phase (Figure 3-22), there are enlarged vessels which represent veins draining the AVM.

site of hemorrhage, the initial mortality is significantly less following hemorrhage from an AVM than it is following an aneurysmal hemorrhage. This is due to the presence of venous rather than arterial bleeding and to the usual lack of arterial spasm, even with subarachnoid hemorrhage, in the case of an AVM. In addition, the risk of early rebleeding is significantly less following hemorrhage with an AVM than it is following aneurysmal hemorrhage. Hematomas due to bleeding from AVMs are typically located within the cortex and/or adjacent white

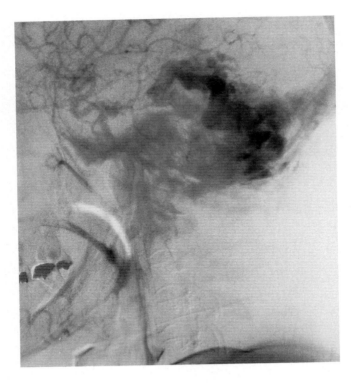

Figure 3-22

matter and occur most commonly in the parietal-occipital regions. This is in contrast to the more centrally located hematomas usually produced by ruptured saccular aneurysms. In addition to a hematoma, CT may also reveal other complications resulting from a ruptured AVM, including hydrocephalus.

Cryptic malformations are those AVMs that are not visualized by angiography. These represent approximately 10% of all AVMs. Nonvisualization with angiography may be the result of thrombosis, destruction secondary to hemorrhage, microvasculature beyond the spatial resolution of angiographic technique, or compression of the feeding vessels by hematoma. In many of these cases, CT can be expected to demonstrate features suggestive of an AVM. However, reliable differentiation from certain neoplasms and acute infarction may not always be possible. The definitive diagnosis of a cryptic AVM is usually made following surgical intervention.

Combined morbidity and mortality rates of up to 50% have been reported for patients with a ruptured AVM. Treatment is aimed at the

complete elimination of the vascular malformation. Catheter embolization has been employed, usually preoperatively, to obliterate both arterial
feeders and vascular channels within the central nidus to reduce the
possibility of subsequent collateral supply to the AVM. As a result of prior
catheter embolization therapy, surgical excision is made technically less
difficult or may in fact be obviated. In addition, embolization has the
added benefit of making the hemodynamic changes involved in the
surgical removal of an AVM more gradual. Surgical excision following
partial embolization must include the entire remaining portion of the
AVM if possible. If the entire vascular malformation is not removed,
collateral vessels will invariably contribute to the vascular supply of the
residual malformation and result in regeneration of the lesion.

Andrew J. Kurman, M.D.
Peter E. Weinberg, M.D.

SUGGESTED READINGS

LEPTOMENINGEAL METASTATIC NEOPLASM

1. Ascherl GF Jr, Hilal SK, Brisman R. Computed tomography of disseminated
   meningeal and ependymal malignant neoplasms. Neurology 1981; 31:567–
   574
2. Brant-Zawadzki M, Enzmann DR. Computed tomographic brain scanning in
   patients with lymphoma. Radiology 1978; 129:67–71
3. Frank J, Girton M, Dwyer A, Wright D, Cohen P, Doppman J. Meningeal
   carcinomatosis in the VX2 rabbit tumor model: detection with Gd-DTPA-
   enhanced MR imaging. Radiology 1988; 167:825–829
4. Glass JP, Melamed M, Chernik NL, Posner JB. Malignant cells in
   cerebrospinal fluid (CSF): the meaning of a positive CSF cytology.
   Neurology 1979; 29:1369–1375
5. Krol G, Sze G, Malkin M, Walker R. MR of cranial and spinal meningeal
   carcinomatosis: comparison with CT and myelography. AJNR 1988;
   9:709–714
6. Lee YY, Glass JP, Geoffray A, Wallace S. Cranial computed tomographic
   abnormalities in leptomeningeal metastasis. AJR 1984; 143:1035–1039
7. Little JR, Dale AJ, Okazaki H. Meningeal carcinomatosis. Clinical manifestations. Arch Neurol 1974; 30:138–143
8. Lukin R, Tomsick TA, Chambers AA. Lymphoma and leukemia of the central
   nervous system. Semin Roentgenol 1980; 15:246–250
9. Morganroth J, Deisseroth A, Winokur S, Schein P. Differentiation of
   carcinomatous and bacterial meningitis. Neurology 1972; 22:1240–1242

10. Pagani JJ, Libshitz HI, Wallace S, Hayman LA. Central nervous system leukemia and lymphoma: computed tomographic manifestations. AJR 1981; 137:1195–1201
11. Wasserstrom WR, Glass JP, Posner JB. Diagnosis and treatment of leptomeningeal metastases from solid tumors: experience with 90 patients. Cancer 1982; 49:759–772
12. Whelan MA, Kricheff II. Intracranial lymphoma. Semin Roentgenol 1984; 19:91–99
13. Yap HY, Yap BS, Tashima CK, DiStefano A, Blumenschein GR. Meningeal carcinomatosis in breast cancer. Cancer 1978; 42:283–286

SUBARACHNOID HEMORRHAGE

14. Bryan RN, Shah CP, Hilal S. Evaluation of subarachnoid hemorrhage and cerebral vasospasm by computed tomography. J Comput Tomogr 1979; 3:144–152
15. Davis KR, Kistler JP, Heros RC, Davis JM. A neuroradiologic approach to the patient with a diagnosis of subarachnoid hemorrhage. Radiol Clin North Am 1982; 20:87–94
16. Drayer BP. Diseases of the cerebral vascular system. In: Rosenberg RN, Heinz ER (eds), The clinical neurosciences, vol 4. Neuroradiology. New York: Churchill Livingstone; 1984:247–360

CEREBELLAR INFARCTION

17. Aoki N. Contrast enhancement of cerebellar infarction on computed tomography. Surg Neurol 1985; 24:141–150
18. Feely MP. Cerebellar infarction. Neurosurgery 1979; 4:7–11
19. Hinshaw DB Jr, Thompson JR, Hasso AN, Casselman ES. Infarctions of the brainstem and cerebellum: a correlation of computed tomography and angiography. Radiology 1980; 137:105–112
20. Ho SU, Kim KS, Berenberg RA, Ho HT. Cerebellar infarction: a clinical and CT study. Surg Neurol 1981; 16:350–352
21. Inoue Y, Takemoto K, Miyamoto T, et al. Sequential computed tomography scans in acute cerebral infarction. Radiology 1980; 135:655–662
22. Masdeu JC. Infarct versus neoplasm on CT: four helpful signs. AJNR 1983; 4:522–524
23. Monajati A, Heggeness L. Patterns of edema in tumors vs. infarcts: visualization of white matter pathways. AJNR 1982; 3:251–255
24. Norton GA, Kishore PR, Lin J. CT contrast enhancement in cerebral infarction. AJR 1978; 131:881–885
25. Rubenstein R, Norman DM, Schindler RA, Kaseff L. Cerebellar infarction—a presentation of vertigo. Laryngoscope 1980; 90:505–514
26. Sypert GW, Alvord EC Jr. Cerebellar infarction. A clinicopathological study. Arch Neurol 1975; 32:357–363
27. Taneda M, Ozaki K, Wakayama A, Yagi K, Kaneda H, Irino T. Cerebellar infarction with obstructive hydrocephalus. J Neurosurg 1982; 57:83–91

28. Wall SD, Brant-Zawadzki M, Jeffrey RB, Barnes B. High-frequency CT findings within 24 hours after cerebral infarction. AJR 1982; 138:307–311
29. Weisberg LA. Cerebellar infarction—clinical and computed tomographic correlations. Comput Radiol 1982; 6:155–160
30. Weisberg LA. Computerized tomographic enhancement patterns in cerebral infarction. Arch Neurol 1980; 37:21–24
31. Woodhurst WB. Cerebellar infarction—review of recent experiences. Can J Sci Neurol 1980; 7:97–99

ARTERIOVENOUS MALFORMATION

32. Bell BA, Kendall BE, Symon L. Angiographically occult arteriovenous malformations of the brain. J Neurol Neurosurg Psychiatry 1978; 41:1057–1064
33. Brunelle FO, Harwood-Nash DC, Fitz CR, Chuang SH. Intracranial vascular malformations in children: computed tomographic and angiographic evaluation. Radiology 1983; 149:455–461
34. Hayman LA, Fox AJ, Evans RA. Effectiveness of contrast regimens in CT detection of vascular malformations of the brain. AJNR 1981; 2:421–425
35. LeBlanc R, Ethier R, Little JR. Computerized tomography findings in arteriovenous malformations of the brain. J Neurosurg 1979; 51:765–772
36. Parkinson D, Bachers G. Arteriovenous malformations. Summary of 100 consecutive supratentorial cases. J Neurosurg 1980; 53:285–299
37. Stein BM, Wolpert SM. Arteriovenous malformations of the brain. Current concepts and treatment. Arch Neurol 1980; 37:1–5, 69–75
38. Terbrugge K, Scotti G, Ethier R, Melancon D, Tchang S, Milner C. Computed tomography in intracranial arteriovenous malformations. Radiology 1977; 122:703–705
39. Weisberg LA. Clinical and computed tomographic findings in thrombosed and cryptic cerebrovascular malformations. Comput Radiol 1982; 6:161–170
40. Weisberg L. Computed tomography in the diagnosis of intracranial vascular malformations. Comput Tomogr 1979; 3:125–132

METASTATIC PARENCHYMAL TUMOR

41. Anand AK, Potts DG. Calcified brain metastases: demonstration by computed tomography. AJNR 1982; 3:527–529
42. Davis JM, Zimmerman RA, Bilaniuk LT. Metastases to the central nervous system. Radiol Clin North Am 1982; 20:417–435
43. Dubois PJ. Brain tumors. In: Rosenberg RN, Heinz ER (eds), The clinical neurosciences, vol 4. Neuroradiology. New York: Churchill Livingstone; 1984:361–455
44. Latchaw RE. Metastases. In: Latchaw RE (ed), Computed tomography of the head, neck, and spine. Chicago: Yearbook Medical Publishers; 1985:265–279

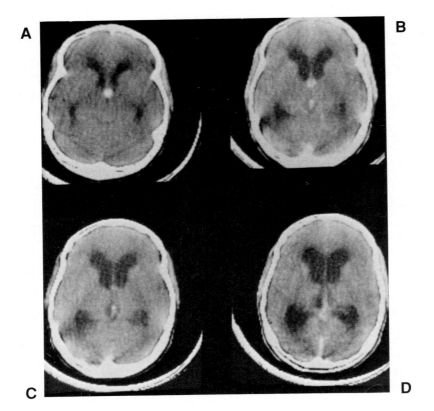

Figure 4-1

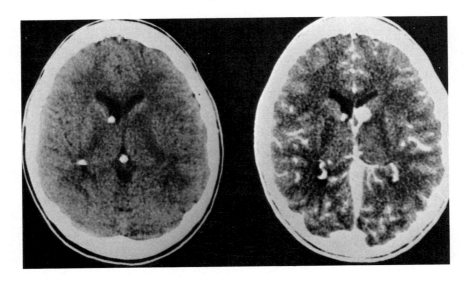

Figure 4-2

Case 4: Congenital Lesions of the Brain

Questions 15 through 19

For each numbered image (Questions 15 through 19) select the *one* lettered diagnosis (A, B, C, D, or E) that is MOST likely. Each lettered diagnosis may be used once, more than once, or not at all.

15. Figure 4-1
16. Figure 4-2
17. Figure 4-3
18. Figure 4-4
19. Figure 4-5

    (A) Tuberous sclerosis
    (B) Lipoma of the corpus callosum
    (C) Agenesis of the corpus callosum
    (D) Sturge-Weber syndrome
    (E) Colloid cyst

Figure 4-1 is an example of a colloid cyst **(Option (E) is the correct answer to Question 15).** Figure 4-1A is a noncontrast computed tomographic (CT) scan that demonstrates a well-demarcated hyperdense mass within the anterior third ventricle (arrow, Figure 4-6). Figure 4-1B, C, and D are contrast-enhanced CT scans that demonstrate no enhancement of the third ventricular mass. There is moderate hydrocephalus due to partial obstruction of the foramina of Monro.

Colloid cysts account for approximately 2% of all intracranial neoplasms. Their incidence is approximately equal in men and women. These neoplasms are histologically benign tumors, most of which are probably of ependymal origin, and are attached to the anterior aspect of the tela choroidea. Their walls consist of a fibrous capsule internally lined with mucus-containing ciliated epithelial cells. Internally, the cysts may contain debris, often including lipid droplets and degenerated leukocytes.

Although colloid cysts are usually congenital in origin, most patients become symptomatic in adulthood. Small colloid cysts in patients that had been asymptomatic are occasionally discovered as an incidental

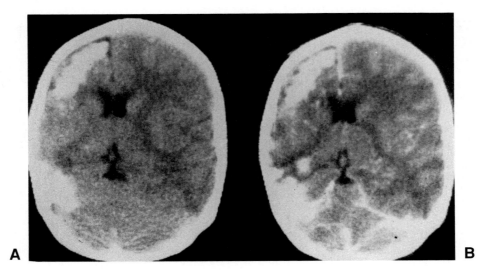

Figure 4-3

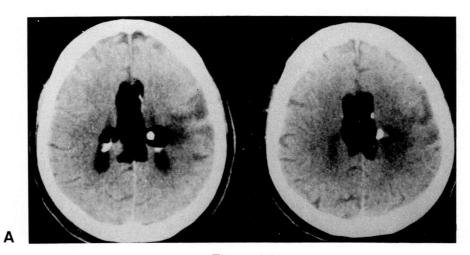

Figure 4-4

88 / *Neuroradiology*

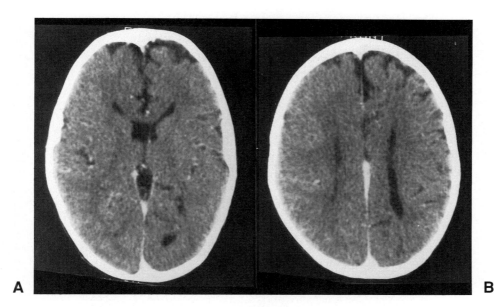

A   B

Figure 4-5

finding at autopsy. Because of their location, these masses commonly extend into the foramina of Monro as they enlarge, causing obstruction and hydrocephalus. This usually occurs when the cysts are still relatively small, although they may occasionally be 3 cm or more in diameter. The most common clinical presentation is headache, which is aggravated by activities, such as coughing and sneezing, that increase intracranial pressure. Since the cysts are frequently mobile to some extent, obstruction and resulting symptoms may be intermittent or affected by changes in head position. In some cases the clinical findings of dementia, ataxia, and urinary incontinence may simulate those of normal-pressure hydrocephalus.

In most cases, colloid cysts can be readily demonstrated by magnetic resonance imaging (MRI) (Figure 4-7). The intraventricular location of these cysts is easy to determine because sagittal, coronal, and axial images can be obtained. These lesions generally have a T1 relaxation time that is less than or equal to that of brain parenchyma, a prolonged T2 relaxation time, and a high spin density. Because of these characteristics, these lesions appear "bright" relative to brain on both T1- and T2-weighted images and have a signal density distinctly different from that of cerebrospinal fluid (CSF). The relatively short relaxation time of colloid cysts probably reflects their high protein content.

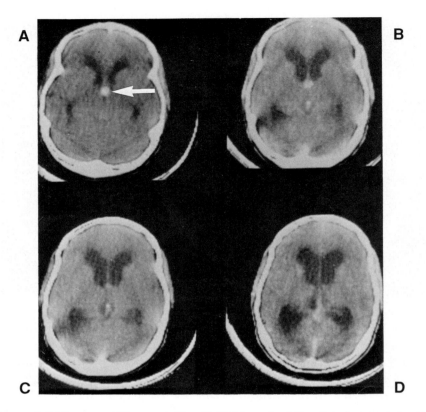

Figure 4-6 (Same as Figure 4-1).   Colloid cyst of the third ventricle. (A) Unenhanced CT demonstrates a discrete hyperdense mass (arrow) within the anterior aspect of the third ventricle. (B through D) Contrast-enhanced CT scans show a moderate degree of hydrocephalus due to partial obstruction of the foramina of Monro.

The CT appearance of colloid cysts is usually characteristic, differentiating them from other third ventricular masses. On noncontrast studies, a colloid cyst most commonly appears as a well-marginated, spherical or ovoid, high-attenuation mass (44 to 76 HU) within the anterior aspect of the third ventricle (Figure 4-8). These masses are occasionally isodense (Figure 4-9) and rarely hypodense centrally. With the administration of contrast material, marked enhancement is uncommon, although there may be a slight increase in attenuation due to capillary blood vessels in the cyst wall or diffusion of contrast into the cyst itself. If significant enhancement is seen, other lesions, such as choroid plexus papilloma, basilar artery aneurysm, intraventricular meningioma, or glioma, must

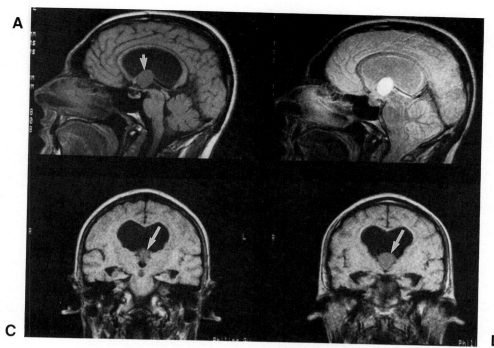

Figure 4-7. Colloid cyst of the third ventricle. (A) T1-weighted midsagittal MRI demonstrates an isodense mass (arrow) in the anterosuperior aspect of the third ventricle. The mass protrudes into the foramina of Monro, and this results in marked enlargement of the lateral ventricles. (B) T2-weighted midsagittal MRI shows the mass to be of high signal intensity. (C and D) T1-weighted coronal MRI with longer TE than in panel A. The mass (arrow) in the anterosuperior aspect of the third ventricle extends through the foramina of Monro and thus produces enlargement of both lateral ventricles.

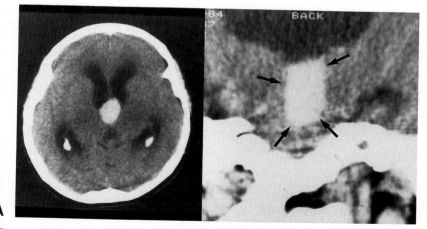

Figure 4-8. Large colloid cyst. (A) Unenhanced transaxial CT demonstrates a large hyperdense mass in the anterior aspect of the third ventricle that obstructs the foramina of Monro. (B) Contrast-enhanced direct coronal scan of the same patient demonstrates the colloid cyst (arrows) filling the anterior third ventricle just inferior to the foramina of Monro.

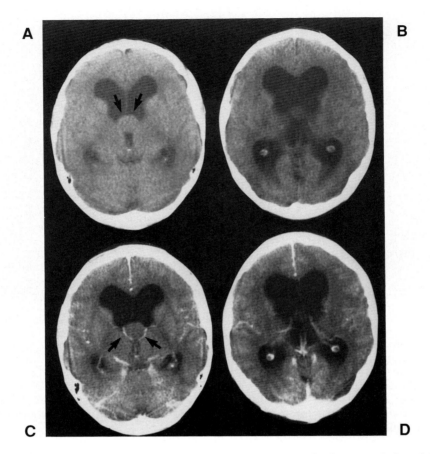

Figure 4-9. Same patient as in Figure 4-7. Colloid cyst of the third ventricle. (A and B) Unenhanced CT scans demonstrate an isodense mass (arrows) in the anterosuperior aspect of the third ventricle. The mass protrudes through the foramina of Monro and causes obstructive hydrocephalus. (C and D) Contrast-enhanced CT scans reveal draping of venous structures around the mass (arrows). There is no enhancement of the mass.

be considered. Calcification in the cyst wall or hemorrhage is rarely seen with colloid cysts.

Figure 4-2 is an example of tuberous sclerosis or Bourneville's disease **(Option (A) is the correct answer to Question 16).** This entity is included as one of the phacomatoses or neurocutaneous diseases along with von Recklinghausen's neurofibromatosis, von Hippel-Lindau disease, Sturge-Weber syndrome, and ataxia telangiectasia or Louis-Bar

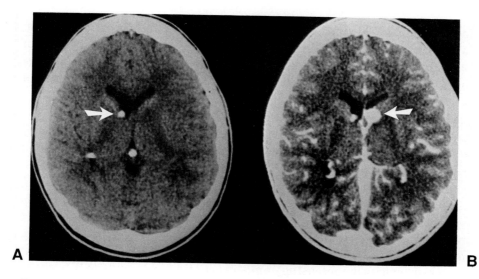

A

B

Figure 4-10. Same patient as in Figure 4-2. Tuberous sclerosis. (A) Unenhanced CT scan demonstrates a small periventricular calcification (arrow) along the margin of the right frontal horn. (B) Contrast-enhanced CT scan shows an enhancing mass (arrow) in the corresponding region adjacent to the left frontal horn. This mass was isodense on the unenhanced CT scan.

disease. This CT scan demonstrates a small periventricular calcification along the margin of the right frontal horn at the level of the foramen of Monro (arrow, Figure 4-10A), with an enhancing mass seen on the postinfusion study in the corresponding region of the opposite frontal horn (arrow, Figure 4-10B).

Tuberous sclerosis is a heredofamilial disease first described by von Recklinghausen and later described in detail by Bourneville in 1880. It is transmitted as an autosomal dominant trait, but sporadic cases are common.

Clinically, the disease is characterized by seizures, mental retardation, and adenoma sebaceum, which primarily involves the skin in a butterfly distribution over the cheeks and forehead. There is also an increased incidence of retinal tumors, optic atrophy, cataracts, syndactylism, spina bifida, and hamartomas of all visceral organs, and especially of the brain. In the brain, hamartomas are most commonly located in the cerebrum along the CSF pathways. However, lesions within the substance of the cerebral hemispheres, cerebellum, and spinal cord may also be found. Hamartomas vary in size, calcifying in increasing numbers with advancing age. Hydrocephalus may result from lesions at the foramen of Monro or elsewhere along the CSF pathway. About 10 to 15% of hamartomas undergo degeneration into giant cell astrocytomas, lesions of low-grade malignancy. This most frequently occurs in lesions located near the foramen of Monro.

Skull radiographs may demonstrate sclerotic patches within the calvarium or intracranial calcifications (arrows, Figure 4-11). Faintly calcified lesions may be difficult or impossible to detect on skull radiographs. The CT findings are characteristic and may be demonstrated prior to the cutaneous manifestations. On noncontrast CT studies, subependymal hamartomas may cause tissue to project into the ventricles, resulting in heterotopias. This accounts for the appearance referred to as "candle gutterings" previously described on pneumoencephalograms. These lesions, along with hamartomas elsewhere in the brain, calcify in increasing numbers over time. Associated CT findings include regions of cerebral atrophy, ventricular enlargement, and thickening of the calvarium. Postinfusion CT demonstrates enhancement only in lesions that have undergone degeneration into gliomas. These lesions usually enlarge over time, sometimes to a marked degree (Figure 4-12).

The periventricular calcifications of tuberous sclerosis in some cases may mimic those seen in intrauterine infections. However, a greater degree of atrophy and the presence of microcephaly usually seen with intrauterine infections allow differentiation in most cases.

Figure 4-3 is a CT scan of a patient with encephalotrigeminal angiomatosis or Sturge-Weber disease, another neurocutaneous syndrome **(Option (D) is the correct answer to Question 17).** Both the nonenhanced CT scan (on the left) and the postinfusion study (on the right) demonstrate areas of calcification involving the cortex of the left hemisphere with associated ipsilateral hemiatrophy, as evidenced by shift of the ventricles toward the side of atrophy and mild ventricular enlargement. There is also gyral enhancement in the left temporal region just anterior to the calcifications adjacent to the inner table of the calvarium (Figure 4-3B).

Sturge-Weber syndrome was first described in 1879. The primary central nervous system lesion consists of a capillary venous angioma, most often in the parietal and occipital regions, involving the meninges of one hemisphere. There is always some degree of atrophy of the underlying hemisphere as well. This is associated with gliosis of the superficial layers of the cerebral cortex. These regions usually calcify enough to be radiologically identifiable after 2 years of age. The

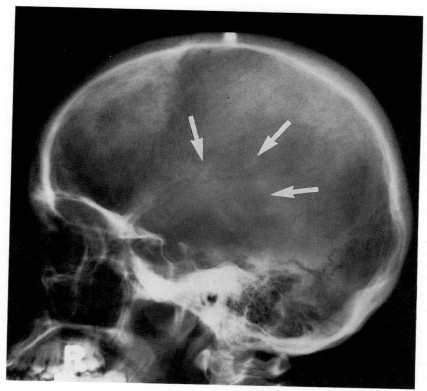

Figure 4-11. Tuberous sclerosis. Lateral skull radiograph demonstrating multiple faint intracranial calcifications (arrows).

A   B   C

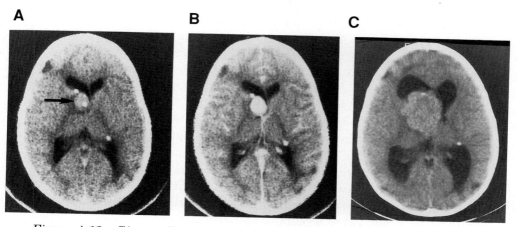

Figure 4-12. Giant cell astrocytoma in a patient with tuberous sclerosis. (A) Unenhanced CT shows multiple periventricular calcifications and a hyperdense periventricular mass adjacent to the foramen of Monro (arrow). (B) Contrast-enhanced CT shows homogeneous enhancement of this mass. (C) Unenhanced CT approximately 1 year later shows marked enlargement of the mass, a surgically confirmed giant cell astrocytoma.

above-described changes are accompanied by a facial angioma or a "port-wine nevus" in the distribution of the ophthalmic division of the trigeminal nerve. This facial lesion usually, but not invariably, occurs on the same side as the leptomeningeal angiomatosis. Other clinical findings include seizures, hemiatrophy, hemiparesis, glaucoma, and a variable degree of mental retardation.

The radiographic findings are virtually pathognomonic of this entity. Skull radiographs obtained after 2 years of age will frequently demonstrate the cortical calcifications, which typically have a curvilinear gyral configuration sometimes referred to as a "tram-track" pattern (Figure 4-13). Long-standing cortical atrophy may result in reduced size of the involved hemicranium (Davidoff-Dyke-Masson syndrome). Noncontrast CT demonstrates the same findings seen in skull radiographs but with greater sensitivity (Figure 4-14). The cortical calcifications are usually limited to the parietal and occipital regions but may be more extensive and occur in other lobes of the brain. Calcifications may sometimes involve even the cerebellum. The hemiatrophy is usually indicated by a shift of the ventricles toward the involved hemisphere, prominence of the cortical sulci, thickening of the ipsilateral calvarium, and increased aeration of the corresponding mastoid air cells. Postcontrast CT studies may demonstrate a faint diffuse enhancement of the involved cortex, sometimes accompanied by prominent vessels corresponding to dilated deep venous structures.

In most cases the combination of the clinical findings and the above-described radiographic and CT findings are sufficiently characteristic to allow definitive diagnosis. In cases where angiography is performed, there may be a diffuse stain over the involved cortex corresponding to the increased enhancement seen on CT studies. An abnormal venous pattern with diversion of blood from cortical veins into the dilated deep venous system may also be evident. Brain scintigraphy may also demonstrate a nonspecific increased uptake over the involved hemisphere.

Figure 4-4 demonstrates a lipoma of the corpus callosum **(Option (B) is the correct answer to Question 18).** These two CT sections demonstrate a mass of fat density with small peripheral calcifications in the midline region at the level of the corpus callosum.

Lipomas of the corpus callosum result from maldevelopment occurring during the third to fifth week of gestation, when mesodermal adipose tissue is incorporated into the neural tube. When these lesions involve the corpus callosum, they are most frequently positioned anteriorly and may be associated with partial agenesis of the corpus callosum. Lipomas

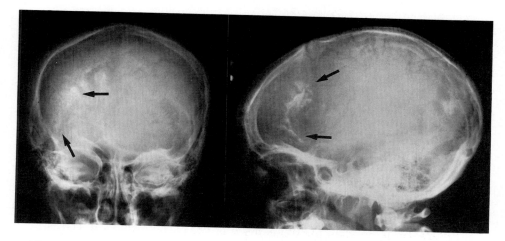

Figure 4-13. Sturge-Weber disease. Anteroposterior and lateral skull radiographs show typical "tram-track" calcifications over the right frontal lobe (arrows). These more frequently occur in the parietal or occipital region.

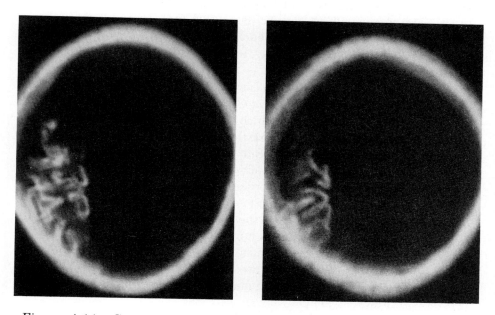

Figure 4-14. Sturge-Weber disease. Unenhanced CT scans at bone-window settings demonstrate characteristic curvilinear gyrus-like calcification.

may occur elsewhere and have been identified in the suprasellar region, quadrigeminal cistern, cerebellopontine angle cistern, and spinal canal. Seizures are the most common associated clinical abnormality, although in some cases corpus callosal lipomas represent an incidental CT finding.

CT demonstrates a fat-density mass in the region of the corpus callosum, causing separation of the lateral ventricles. The density of lipomas is typically less than that of CSF. The low density of the lipoma or calcifications occurring along the margins of the lesion may also be visible on skull radiographs (arrows, Figure 4-15). Large lipomas may incorporate the anterior cerebral artery, which may be mildly dilated. This finding is best demonstrated by cerebral angiography.

Figure 4-5 is an example of agenesis of the corpus callosum **(Option (C) is the correct answer to Question 19).** These CT sections demonstrate elevation of the third ventricle with increased separation of the lateral ventricles.

Agenesis of the corpus callosum is a developmental anomaly occurring in the period from the 12th to the 20th week of gestation. The corpus callosum may be completely absent or partially developed. It may occur as an isolated anomaly or may be associated with other craniocerebral anomalies, including craniofacial encephaloceles, absence of the septum pellucidum and cingulate gyrus, interhemispheric arachnoid cysts, lipomas, and Dandy-Walker cysts.

CT readily demonstrates agenesis of the corpus callosum and any associated anomaly. Characteristic CT findings in these cases include elevation of the third ventricle, which lies between the separated lateral ventricles. These findings are particularly helpful in differentiating absence of the corpus callosum from cavum septi pellucidi and cavum vergae. The lateral ventricles, particularly in the frontal region, are widely separated. Their medial borders are usually straightened or even concave laterally. Frequently, there is enlargement of the occipital horns of the lateral ventricles relative to the body and frontal horns. On coronal CT sections, the lateral ventricles may have a pointed or beaked lateral margin and the frontal horns may have a C-shaped configuration. These findings are also readily demonstrated by MRI (Figure 4-16). In addition, the absence of the corpus callosum may be directly visualized on sagittal MR images (Figure 4-17).

With the advent of CT, and more recently MRI, angiography is rarely needed to confirm the diagnosis of agenesis of the corpus callosum. Angiographic findings, however, are usually fairly typical also. The pericallosal artery is commonly seen to have a stretched, vertically oriented course instead of its usual superiorly bowed configuration. The

Notes

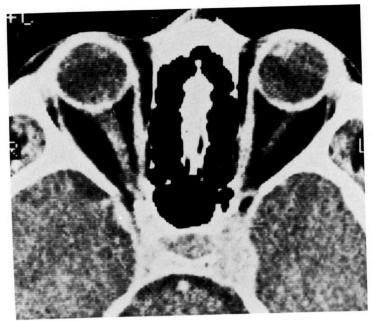

Figure 5-1

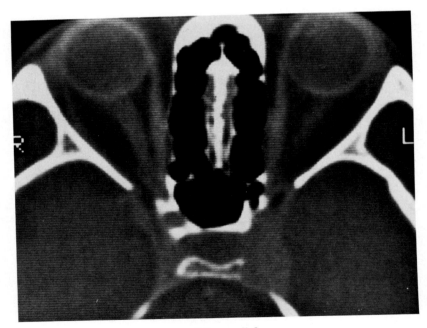

Figure 5-2
Figures 5-1 through 5-3. This 33-year-old man had a left sixth cranial nerve palsy. You are shown postcontrast CT sections of the sellar and parasellar regions obtained by using both soft tissue (Figure 5-1) and bone (Figures 5-2 and 5-3) window settings.

Case 5: Carotid Aneurysm in the Cavernous Sinus

Question 20

Which *one* of the following is the MOST likely diagnosis?

(A) Aneurysm
(B) Pituitary adenoma
(C) Parasellar meningioma
(D) Trigeminal neuroma
(E) Dural arteriovenous malformation

Figure 5-1 depicts a section through the sella, cavernous sinuses, and orbits. The sella is not enlarged, but the left cavernous sinus is enlarged, with its lateral wall being laterally convex (Figure 5-4, arrow). The right cavernous sinus has a normal appearance. The computed tomographic (CT) densities of the two cavernous sinuses appear to be equal. Figure 5-2 is at the same level, but with a bone window setting. The left margin of the dorsum sellae has been eroded (Figure 5-5, arrow). There is no sclerosis. Figure 5-3 is at a lower level. The indentation of the lateral margin of the sphenoid bone (carotid sulcus) is slightly deeper on the left than on the right (Figure 5-6, arrow).

The findings of an enlarged cavernous sinus, widened carotid sulcus, and lack of bone sclerosis make cavernous sinus aneurysm the most likely diagnosis **(Option (A) is correct).** Unilateral bone erosion is also a characteristic feature of parasellar aneurysms and should suggest this diagnosis. The lack of vascular calcification is not inconsistent with aneurysm, since most cavernous sinus aneurysms are not calcified.

The angiographic appearance of the cavernous sinus aneurysm is shown in Figure 5-7. Figure 5-8 shows the opposite carotid artery. It has an enlargement at the same site, indicating that an aneurysm can be expected to develop there also.

Because of the bilaterality of involvement and the relatively young age of the patient, it was decided to attempt to occlude the cavernous carotid

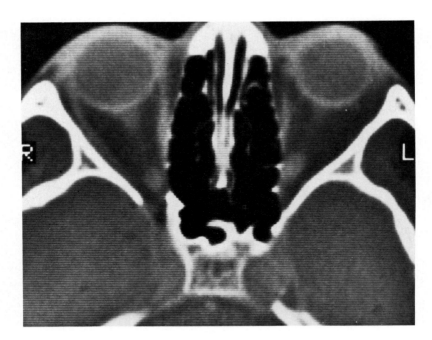

Figure 5-3

aneurysm while preserving carotid flow. Two detachable Hieshima balloons were placed in the aneurysm (Figure 5-9) to produce clotting within its lumen.

Pituitary adenoma (Option (B)) is not a good diagnostic choice in this patient. All pituitary tumors may extend laterally and cause bulging of the lateral wall of the cavernous sinus, but this generally happens only when the tumor is large. Such a tumor should cause considerable sellar enlargement as well, particularly on the side of the displaced cavernous sinus, and suprasellar extension would also be expected in the usual case. The pituitary tumor illustrated in Figures 5-10 and 5-11 is unusual in that there is lateral extension without suprasellar extension. However, note the marked expansion of the right side of the sella, a finding consistent with a large intrasellar tumor that is expanded predominantly inferiorly at the expense of the sphenoid sinus.

Parasellar meningioma (Option (C)) is a major consideration in cases of enlargement of the cavernous sinus. In the test patient, however, there are two main reasons why meningioma is not the most likely diagnosis. Meningiomas generally extend beyond the limits of the cavernous sinus itself, generally onto the tentorium or other structures adjacent to the

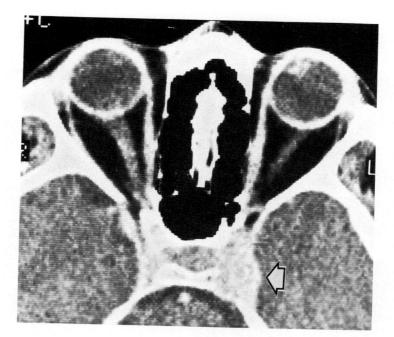

Figure 5-4

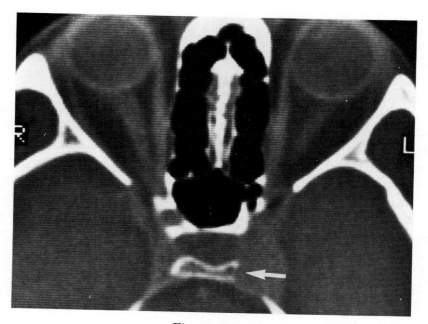

Figure 5-5

Figures 5-4 through 5-6 (Same as Figures 5-1 through 5-3, respectively). The contrast-enhanced axial CT scan (Figure 5-4) demonstrates enlargement of the left cavernous sinus (arrowhead). Bone detail CT images of the sellar and parasellar regions (Figures 5-5 and 5-6) demonstrate erosion of the left lateral margin of the dorsum sellae (arrow, Figure 5-5) and indentation of the lateral margin of the left sphenoid bone (arrow, Figure 5-6).

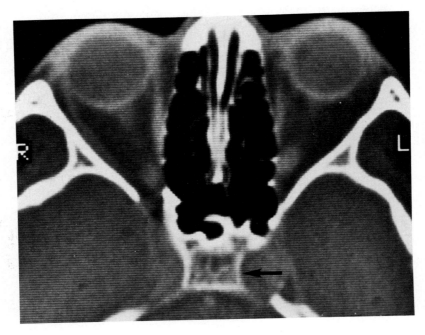

Figure 5-6

cavernous sinus. Also, because there is no bone sclerosis in this case, parasellar meningioma is unlikely.

A trigeminal neuroma (Option (D)) may expand the cavernous sinus, but this would not be a good diagnostic choice in this patient either. Since the trigeminal cistern, which surrounds the gasserian ganglion, is not enlarged but only displaced in this case, we have no evidence supporting the possibility of a trigeminal neuroma. Also, there is no visible extension of mass effect posteriorly along the course of the fifth nerve.

Carotid cavernous fistulae may be of the direct type, with an opening from the carotid artery into the sinus, or of the dural arteriovenous malformation type (Option (E)). The former type of fistula is most often of traumatic origin, while the latter develops spontaneously. In dural arteriovenous fistulae, blood supply is usually derived both from the middle meningeal artery and from small meningeal branches of the cavernous portion of the carotid artery. When a dural arteriovenous malformation involves a cavernous sinus, there is generally no change in the size or density of the sinus on CT scanning. CT demonstrates such a lesion by showing enlargement of ophthalmic veins or other routes of

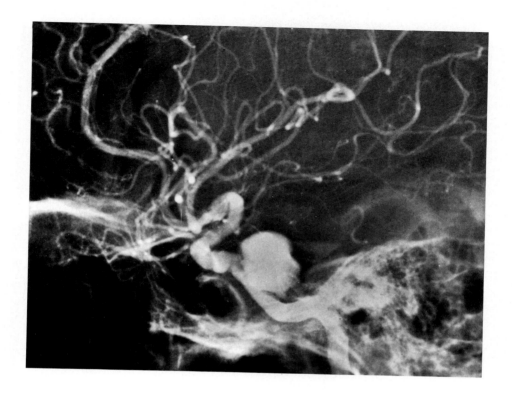

Figure 5-7

Figures 5-7 through 5-9. Same patient as in Figures 5-1 through 5-6. Figure 5-7 is an internal carotid angiogram demonstrating a left cavernous carotid aneurysm. Figure 5-8, the opposite carotid angiogram, shows early aneurysmal dilatation of the right cavernous carotid artery. In Figure 5-9, two detachable balloons have been placed in the left cavernous carotid aneurysm.

drainage, such as the inferior petrosal sinuses. The cavernous sinus may be enlarged in some cases of direct carotid cavernous fistulae with high flow.

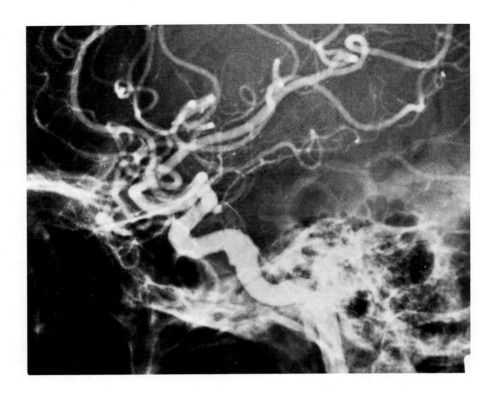

Figure 5-8

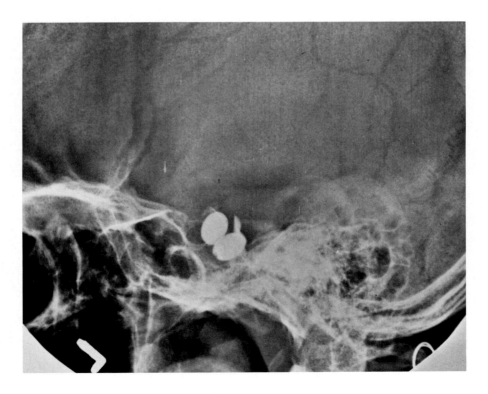

Figure 5-9

110

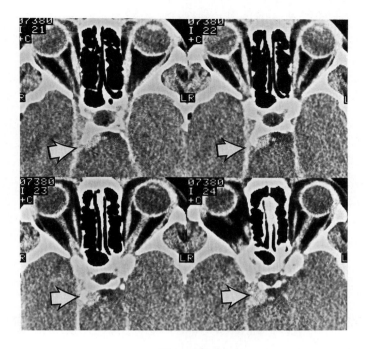

Figure 5-13

in the immediate parasellar region **(Option (D) is false).** Another characteristic angiographic feature that should suggest the diagnosis of parasellar meningioma is narrowing of the cavernous portion of the carotid artery due to encasement by tumor. This feature is seen frequently with parasellar meningiomas but rarely with other tumors, except for carcinoma **(Option (E) is true).**

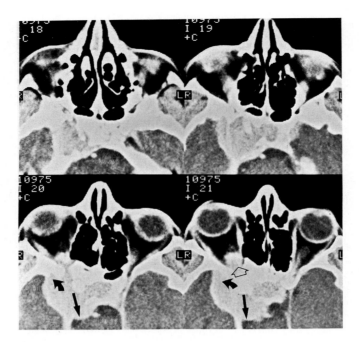

Figure 5-14

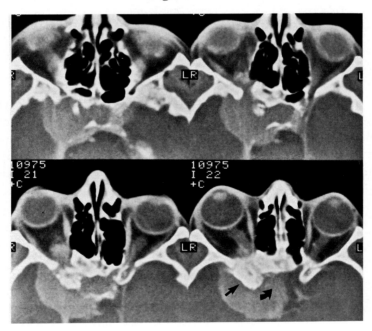

Figure 5-15

Figures 5-14 and 5-15. Postcontrast CT scans, with soft tissue (Figure 5-14) and bone (Figure 5-15) imaging, of a large parasellar meningioma. In Figure 5-14, the tumor extends from the cavernous sinus region posteriorly into the posterior fossa (arrows), anteriorly along the anterior border of the middle fossa (curved arrows), through the superior orbital fissure into the right orbit (arrowhead). In Figure 5-15, note the sclerosis and thickening of bone, particularly the right anterior clinoid (arrow) and the soft tissue mass extending medial to the anterior clinoid process (curved arrow) above the level of the sella.

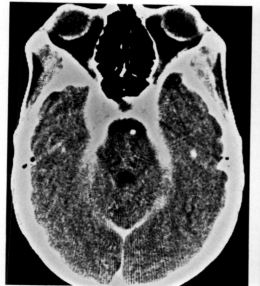 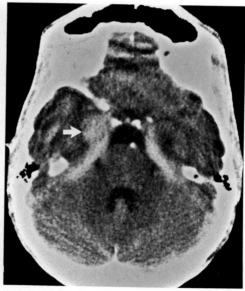

A

B

Figure 5-16. Parasellar and tentorial lymphoma. (A) Contrast-enhanced axial CT section demonstrates a mass involving the right cavernous sinus region, continuous with what appears to be thickening of the adjacent tentorium. However, note that the opposite leaf of the tentorium is also thickened. This finding is consistent with the growth pattern of an infiltrative tumor, such as lymphoma, but would not be typical of meningioma. (B) A more superior section demonstrates the rostral extension of the tumor into the right parasellar region (arrow).

Question 23

Concerning trigeminal neuromas,

(A) they are usually confined to the cavernous sinus region and middle fossa
(B) the pattern of bone erosion is similar to that with other tumors of the cavernous sinus region and middle fossa
(C) they frequently exhibit an intense tumor blush on angiography
(D) the incidence is higher in patients with neurofibromatosis
(E) calcification is rarely seen in them

Trigeminal neuromas are quite rare; less than 5% of intracranial neuromas are trigeminal. In turn, neuromas make up less than 10% of intracranial tumors. All intracranial neuromas, including trigeminal neuromas, occur more frequently in patients with neurofibromatosis **(Option (D) is true).** Trigeminal neuromas arise from the Schwann cell sheath and may originate either in the root of the fifth cranial nerve in the posterior fossa or, more commonly, in the gasserian ganglion. Regardless of the site of origin, most tumors extend along the course of the fifth cranial nerve and are present in both the middle and posterior fossae at the time of diagnosis **(Option (A) is false).** This extension along the fifth nerve may produce an erosion or even amputation of the tip of the petrous pyramid. Erosion of the petrous tip, particularly when accompanied by enlargement of the foramen ovale and/or foramen rotundum, was once a major radiographic indication of trigeminal neuroma, since other parasellar tumors rarely produced similar findings **(Option (B) is false).** These tumors now tend to be diagnosed earlier, and bone erosion is seen less often.

Calcification is rarely present in intracranial neuromas, including trigeminal neuromas **(Option (E) is true).** On the other hand, cystic degeneration of trigeminal neuromas is quite common. It is more frequent in these tumors than in acoustic neuromas, where it occurs in 15% of the cases. The most frequent CT pattern is that of a uniformly enhancing mass in the cavernous sinus region, with extension along the fifth nerve into the posterior fossa (Figure 5-17). With CT scanning, intrathecal metrizamide is sometimes necessary to demonstrate the involvement of the fifth nerve when enlargement is minor and enhancement is not obvious. MRI is now beginning to play an important role in detecting these tumors, since the fifth cranial nerve is generally better identified by MRI than by CT.

Although approximately two-thirds of intracranial neuromas show hypervascularity on selective angiography, neither enlarged vessels nor tumor blush is present in most fifth-nerve tumors, even when visualized by subtraction magnification angiography. The internal carotid artery, which enters the cavernous sinus from below, is displaced only in patients with very large trigeminal neuromas. Vessels in the vicinity of the petrous apex, such as the superior cerebellar artery, may be displaced by large tumors. Even when vascular supply to the tumor is demonstrated, angiographic blush is not too intense **(Option (C) is false)** and certainly not as much as that seen with parasellar meningiomas.

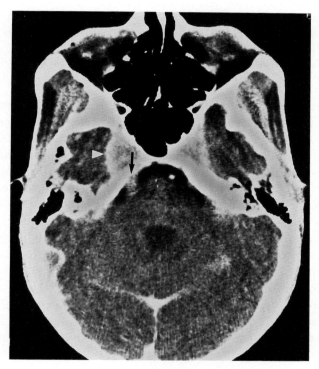

Figure 5-17. Trigeminal neuroma. Postcontrast CT shows a mass at the site of the right cavernous sinus (arrowhead), with characteristic extension posteriorly along the course of the fifth cranial nerve (arrow).

Question 24

Concerning parasellar vascular lesions,

(A) aneurysms of the cavernous portions of the carotid arteries are bilateral in about 5% of patients
(B) dural arteriovenous malformations (AVMs) usually cause enlargement of the cavernous sinus
(C) aneurysms of the cavernous portions of the carotid arteries are more readily treatable than dural AVMs of the cavernous sinus
(D) patients with aneurysms of the cavernous portions of the carotid artery usually present with symptoms caused by rupture
(E) in patients with cavernous sinus AVMs, bilateral eye signs usually indicate bilateral AVMs

Aneurysms are found to be multiple in 15 to 20% of affected patients. Aneurysms of certain locations are likely to be present bilaterally. These include aneurysms in the cavernous portion of the carotid artery as well as those in carotid-ophthalmic, posterior communicating, and middle cerebral trifurcation arterial branches **(Option (A) is false).** The frequency of multiple aneurysms is high enough that selective angiography of all major arteries to the brain is necessary when an aneurysm has been found. Since some aneurysms that cannot be surgically clipped are treated by occlusion therapy, it is obviously necessary to be certain that there is not a mirror aneurysm on the opposite side, the presence of which may necessitate changes in the therapeutic approach.

Carotid cavernous fistulae may be of the direct type, usually of traumatic origin, with an opening in the wall of the artery that allows blood to flow directly into the cavernous sinus, or of the dural AVM type. In the latter, meningeal branches from the internal carotid and middle meningeal arteries supply the blood flow to the fistula. Both the internal and external carotid artery systems are involved in the great majority of cases. The symptoms of carotid cavernous fistulae of either type depend upon the rate of blood flow through the fistula and the routes of blood flow from the cavernous sinus. When the egress of blood is primarily via the ophthalmic veins, primary findings include proptosis, chemosis, ophthalmoplegia, and bruit. When the flow proceeds through the inferior petrosal sinus, the pterygoid plexus, and other posterior routes, the predominant symptoms are annoying bruits and malfunctions of cranial nerves traversing the cavernous sinuses. Since there are connections between the two cavernous sinuses, bilateral eye findings are often present with a unilateral fistula or cavernous sinus AVM **(Option (E) is false).** Because clotting tends to occur within a cavernous sinus or its draining veins involved by a dural AVM, it is common to see eye findings only on the side opposite the fistula. Therapeutic approaches to dural AVM of the cavernous sinus make use of this propensity for clotting. Embolization of the external carotid supply to a dural fistula will usually eliminate the fistula, even though the internal carotid supply is not touched. In other cases, the fistula may be cured by intermittent digital compression, by angiography alone, or even by simply waiting.

The cavernous sinus is generally not enlarged in cases of dural AVM **(Option (B) is false).** On CT these malformations are identified by noting the enlarged size of the superior ophthalmic vein(s) or occasionally by noting an increase in the size of the posterior routes of venous drainage. Direct cavernous carotid fistulae with high flows, on the other hand, may enlarge the cavernous sinus. When a cavernous carotid fistula occurs following the rupture of a cavernous carotid aneurysm, the sinus often appears enlarged.

Rupture of cavernous carotid aneurysms with the production of carotid cavernous fistulae is unusual **(Option (D) is false).** Subarachnoid hemorrhage as a result of rupture is even more unusual; it occurs mainly in cases of carotid-ophthalmic aneurysms that are partially within the cavernous sinus and partially above the sinus. Most patients with cavernous carotid aneurysms present with symptoms referrable to pressure effects within the cavernous sinus, such as diplopia and headache. Over one-third of aneurysms arising from the anterior portion of the sinus, near the ophthalmic artery origin, cause decreased vision. Cavernous carotid aneurysms are difficult to treat, since direct surgery is rarely feasible **(Option (C) is false).** Treatment is generally limited to some form of occlusion therapy. Balloon occlusion techniques are an effective method of therapy in many cases of cavernous carotid aneurysms. The goal may be either to occlude the cavernous artery itself or to occlude the lumen of the aneurysm, depending upon such factors as aneurysm size and shape, the presence of contralateral aneurysms, and the adequacy of collateral circulation.

John R. Bentson, M.D.

SUGGESTED READINGS

CAROTID ANEURYSMS AND FISTULAE

1. Brismar G, Brismar J. Spontaneous carotid-cavernous fistulae. Clinical symptomatology. Acta Ophthalmol 1976; 54:542–552
2. Macpherson P, Anderson DE. Radiological differentiation of intrasellar aneurysms from pituitary tumours. Neuroradiology 1981; 21:177–183
3. Newton T, Hoyt J. Dural arteriovenous shunts in the region of the cavernous sinus. Neuroradiology 1970; 1:71–81
4. Seeger JF, Gabrielsen TO, Giannotta SL, Lotz PR. Carotid-cavernous sinus fistulas and venous thrombosis. AJNR 1980; 1:141–148
5. Seltzer J, Hurtean E. Bilateral symmetrical aneurysms of the internal carotid artery within the cavernous sinus. J Neurosurg 1957; 14:448–451
6. White J, Ballantyne H. Intrasellar aneurysms simulating hypophyseal tumors. J Neurosurg 1961; 18:34–50

PITUITARY ADENOMAS

7. Daniels DL, Williams AL, Thornton RS, Meyer GA, Cusick JF, Haughton VM. Differential diagnosis of intrasellar tumors by computed tomography. Radiology 1981; 141:697–701
8. Glydensted C, Karle A. Computed tomography of intra- and juxtasellar lesions. A radiological study of 108 cases. Neuroradiology 1977; 14:5–13

PARASELLAR MENINGIOMAS

9. Post MJ, Glaser JS, Trobe JD. The radiographic diagnosis of cavernous meningiomas and aneurysms with a review of the neurovascular anatomy of the cavernous sinus. CRC Crit Rev Diagn Imaging 1979; 12:1–34

TRIGEMINAL NEUROMAS

10. Goldberg R, Byrd S, Winter J, Takahashi M, Joyce P. Varied appearance of trigeminal neuroma on CT. AJR 1980; 134:57–60
11. Levinthal R, Benston JR. Detection of small trigeminal neurinomas. J Neurosurg 1976; 45:568–575
12. Moscow NP, Newton TH. Angiographic features of hypervascular neurinomas of the head and neck. Radiology 1975; 114:635–640
13. Schisano G, Olivecrona H. Neurinomas of the gasserian ganglion and trigeminal root. J Neurosurg 1960; 17:306–322

Notes

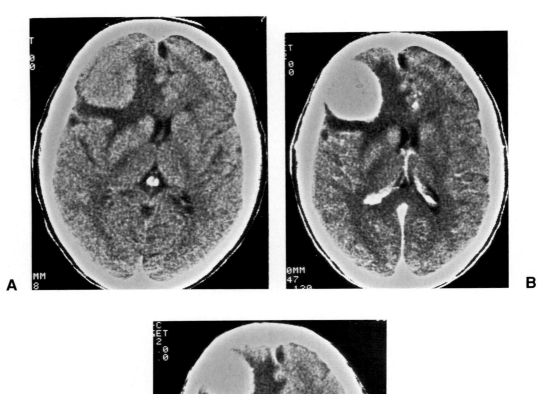

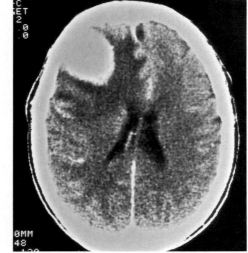

Figure 6-1. This 46-year-old woman presented with a 1-month history of headaches and mild hemiparesis. You are shown pre- and postcontrast computed tomographic scans.

Case 6: Frontal Meningioma

Question 25

Which *one* of the following is the MOST likely diagnosis?

  (A) Cerebral hematoma
  (B) Glioma
  (C) Meningioma
  (D) Metastasis
  (E) Abscess

In this patient's precontrast CT scan (Figure 6-1A), the right frontal mass has a density similar to that of brain. There is adjacent edema and ventricular displacement. The mass does not appear to be calcified, and no thickening of the skull is apparent.

In Figures 6-1B and 6-1C, there is uniform enhancement of the mass on postcontrast CT. The mass is in contact with the skull. Meningioma is thus the most likely diagnosis **(Option (C) is correct).** The peripheral location of the tumor, the large size it has attained without central cavitation, and the high degree of uniform enhancement are all points that favor meningioma. While the amount of surrounding edema might seem unusually marked for a benign tumor, this finding is not unusual in meningiomas. That amount of edema would be very unusual in association with hematomas (Option (A)), and the location would also be unusual. It is not common for gliomas (Option (B)) to have a peripheral location, and it is rare that one attains the size of this tumor without central cavitation unless the glioma is benign, in which case it would be unusual for it to have this intensity of contrast enhancement. A metastasis (Option (D)) can have nearly any appearance, and metastases often do have relatively peripheral locations. However, most metastases are smaller than the tumor demonstrated, and it is unusual for metastatic tumors to reach such a large size without central necrosis. An abscess (Option (E)) is characterized by one or more regions of central lucency, but this finding is not present in the test patient. In the early cerebritis stage, there may be uniform enhancement, but the borders of the lesion would not be as discrete as those in the illustrated case. Cerebritis also normally affects a smaller volume of tissue, and there is little associated edema at this early stage.

Question 26

Concerning gliomas,

(A) calcification of gliomas tends to be diffuse rather than focal
(B) bilateral cerebral hypodensity on computed tomography (CT) suggests infiltration of the corpus callosum
(C) the presence of multiple cavities within a cerebral mass lesion is a reliable sign favoring glioma or other neoplasm over cerebral abscess
(D) an enhancing cerebral mass without surrounding edema seen on CT scanning is more likely to be a glioma than a metastasis
(E) they are less likely than metastases to occur at the corticomedullary junction

Gliomas vary considerably in their CT appearances. In general, the malignant gliomas (grades III and IV, glioblastomas) are large tumors with irregular borders and with marked enhancement on postcontrast CT. These malignant tumors usually have irregular areas of central lucency, which usually represent regions of necrosis. They are usually surrounded by edema, but the area of edema is often small relative to tumor size, particularly by comparison with the peritumoral edema about metastatic tumors. It is not unusual for malignant gliomas to have no apparent associated edema on CT **(Option (D) is true).** However, the majority of cases do exhibit CT evidence of edema. Malignant gliomas are seldom calcified but may show areas of increased density related to hemorrhage.

Gliomas that are more benign (grades I and II) often show no contrast enhancement. This is particularly true of grade I gliomas, which are usually seen as areas of decreased density with ill-defined borders and relatively little mass effect. Grade II gliomas vary considerably, some showing enhancement and even central cavitation, while more commonly there is little if any enhancement. Calcifications are seen more often in low-grade gliomas and tend to be discrete focal aggregates rather than diffuse calcifications, such as those seen in meningiomas **(Option (A) is false).** Oligodendrogliomas calcify more often and more extensively than do astrocytomas, but astrocytomas are more common.

All gliomas tend to occur relatively deep in the brain, involving the frontal and temporal lobes most often. Therefore, a tumor seen at the corticomedullary junction is more likely to be a metastasis than a glioma **(Option (E) is true).** Since malignant gliomas so often have central areas of low density, generally consisting of necrotic material, there is sometimes a problem in differentiating such gliomas from abscesses. In general, the wall of a malignant glioma is thicker and more irregular than that of an abscess, and there is frequently a nodular area projecting into the cavity (Figure 6-2A). This is in contrast to the usual appearance of an abscess, which has a smooth, regular wall of uniform thickness without focal nodularity. Gliomas also are more likely to have multiple cavities than are abscesses. However, some abscesses have multiple cavities; therefore, multiple cavities cannot be relied upon as a sign to differentiate glioma or other neoplasm from abscess (Figure 6-3A) **(Option (C) is false).**

Gliomas have some unusual growth patterns that must be kept in mind. They tend to infiltrate the corpus callosum and present as a contralateral mass that may appear separate on a CT scan. In some cases of low-grade gliomas, all that one may see on a CT scan is nonenhancing zones of hypodensity bilaterally at the level of the corpus callosum. This sign suggests infiltration of the corpus callosum by a tumor, which most often is a glioma, since edema from a unilateral cerebral lesion tends not to cross the corpus callosum **(Option (B) is true).** A glioma may grow by extension in two directions, and some CT sections may appear to demonstrate more than one lesion; in such cases, one should look carefully for signs of joining at another level (Figure 6-4). Tumors may also infiltrate along fiber tracts and present in an apparently isolated portion of the brain. They may also spread by subependymal routes. Pathologic studies show that the infiltration of a glioblastoma passes beyond the apparent limits of the tumor on CT scans. For these reasons, it is likely that the frequency of the multiplicity of origin of gliomatous tumors has been overestimated.

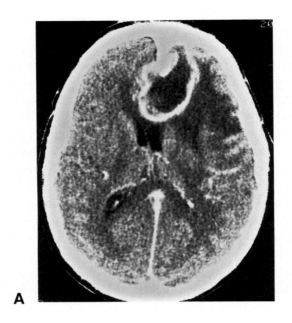

A

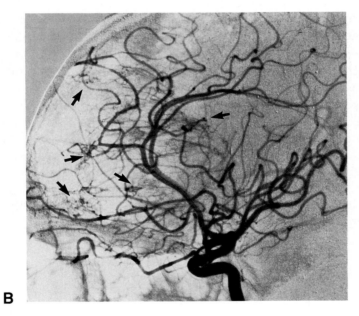

B

Figure 6-2. Frontal lobe glioblastoma. (A) The postcontrast axial CT scan demonstrates a typical appearance, with necrotic center, thick, irregular and nodular wall, adjacent edema, and extension across the midline. (B) The internal carotid angiogram of the same patient shows the hypervascularity (arrows) that is also typical of glioblastomas. Many enlarged vessels in the frontal area appear to parallel each other. Enlargement of deep medullary veins is the other typical angiographic feature of glioblastomas.

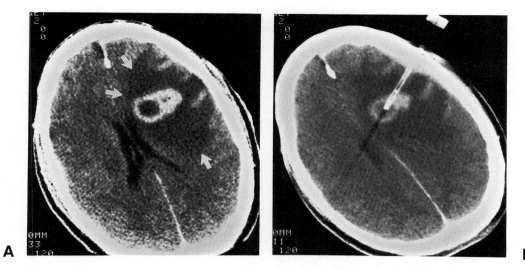

A   B

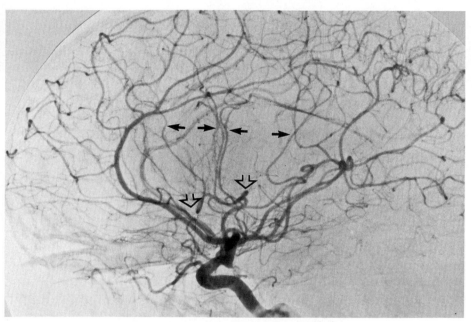

C

Figure 6-3. Cerebral abscess. (A) The postcontrast axial CT scan reveals that this abscess is unusual with regard to the lack of uniformity of wall thickness. However, note the smaller cavities that are beginning to appear in the lateral wall of the abscess. The extensive edema (outlined by arrows) is typical of an abscess. (B) The nature of the lesion was confirmed by CT-guided biopsy, which has been a major improvement in the management of cerebral lesions. (C) The internal carotid angiogram shows stretching and separation of vessels in the suprasylvian region (arrows), along with inferior displacement of the sylvian triangle (arrowheads). There is little hypervascularity. Compare this with the angiogram of the glioblastoma in Figure 6-2.

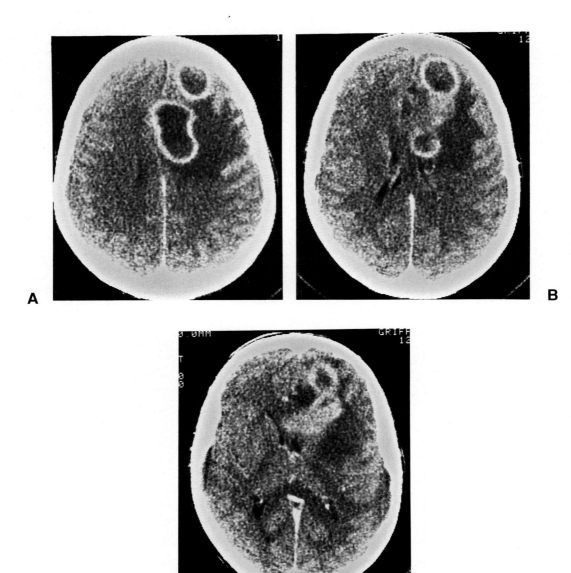

Figure 6-4. Glioblastoma. Three postcontrast CT sections through a frontal lobe glioblastoma. The top section (A) appears to show two distinct masses. However, the lower two sections (B and C) demonstrate a joining of these lesions and a typical extension of the tumor across the genu of the corpus callosum.

tosis 2), but exactly how many patients is difficult to determine, since the usual cutaneous stigmata of this disease are usually not present. Multiple meningiomas vary widely in size and appearance and may be of the same histological type or of different types in the same patient **(Option (E) is true)**. They tend to present clinically at a younger age than do single meningiomas and are often relatively aggressive, rapidly growing tumors.

Question 29

Concerning cerebral hematomas,

(A) contrast enhancement is usually of the ring type
(B) the edema adjacent to them is usually maximal on the day of the bleed
(C) the hematocrit has little effect on their CT density
(D) in the absence of trauma, the presence of multiple high-density lesions on CT suggests bleeding diathesis
(E) in the absence of hypertension, the cause of most hemorrhages will be apparent on CT provided that both pre- and postcontrast scans are performed

Cerebral hemorrhage most often occurs in the basal ganglia and is most commonly a consequence of hypertension. Hematomas not associated with trauma that occur in other locations should always be regarded as potentially signaling an underlying vascular malformation, neoplasm, or aneurysm. Unfortunately, the hematoma often masks the underlying cause; hence, pre- and postcontrast CT will not demonstrate the cause of bleeding in the majority of acute hematomas **(Option (E) is false)**. Cerebral hematomas are obvious lesions on CT because of their high density. This initial high density gradually diminishes, first at the periphery of the hematoma. This decrease in CT attenuation values correlates with the breakdown of erythrocytes, which begins at the periphery of the hematoma. The ruptured erythrocytes release their hemoglobin, which contributes most of the CT density, and this hemoglobin is converted into hemosiderin and ingested by macrophages. It may take 2 to 4 weeks for the hematoma to lose its increased density, with larger hematomas remaining dense longer than smaller ones. The initial density of a cerebral hematoma may vary, depending upon the hemoglobin concentration and hematocrit of the patient's blood **(Option (C) is false)**. Anemic patients may have isodense acute hematomas.

Edema soon appears around the periphery of a cerebral hematoma. This is usually visible as a thin surrounding zone of hypodensity on the

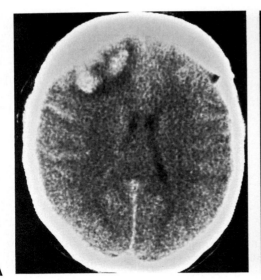
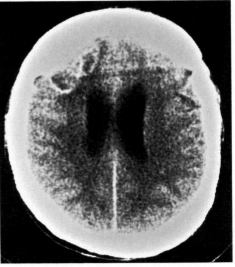

A

B

Figure 6-6. Post-traumatic cerebral hematomas. (A) Noncontrast scan soon after injury shows two adjacent areas of bleeding in the frontal lobe, with surrounding edema. (B) Scan obtained 2 weeks later with contrast infusion demonstrates areas of ring enhancement around the hematomas. The hematomas themselves now have densities lower than that of brain tissue. Without the preceding scan (panel A), such an appearance could be confusing.

first day, but it generally increases over the next few days, and usually is maximal in degree in the middle of the first week following the bleed **(Option (B) is false).** The increase in edema produces an increasing displacement of brain structures, and symptoms often worsen for several days following a bleed. Contrast enhancement occurs in the majority of hematomas, beginning near the end of the first week. Its appearance correlates with the formation of a collagenous capsule about the hematoma. This ring enhancement may last for several weeks. Since the density of the hematoma is decreasing at the same time, a CT scan performed a few weeks after a hematoma may yield a CT pattern that resembles the pattern of other ring-shaped lesions such as neoplasms or abscesses **(Option (A) is true).** This is a particular problem when there has been no preceding scan and no definite history of an acute event some weeks before (Figure 6-6). Another confusing pattern is that of multiple simultaneous cerebral bleeds. These are most commonly seen with severe head trauma. In the absence of a history of head trauma, bleeding diatheses and metastases with a tendency to bleed (such as those from melanoma or choriocarcinoma) are also diagnostic possibilities **(Option (D) is true).**

John R. Bentson, M.D.

SUGGESTED READINGS

MENINGIOMA

1. Martuza RL, Eldridge R. Neurofibromatosis 2. N Engl J Med 1988; 318:684–688
2. Nahser HC, Grote W, Lohr E, Gerhard L. Multiple meningiomas. Clinical and computer tomographic observations. Neuroradiology 1981; 21:259–263
3. New PF, Aronow S, Hesselink JR. National Cancer Institute study: evaluation of computed tomography in the diagnosis of intracranial neoplasms. IV. Meningiomas. Radiology 1980; 136:665–675
4. Russell EJ, George AE, Kricheff II, Budzilovich G. Atypical computed tomography features of intracranial meningioma: radiological-pathological correlation in a series of 131 consecutive cases. Radiology 1980; 135:673–682
5. Smith HP, Challa VR, Moody DM, Kelly DL Jr. Biological features of meningiomas that determine the production of cerebral edema. Neurosurgery 1981; 8:428–433
6. Stevens JM, Ruiz JS, Kendall BE. Observations on peritumoral oedema in meningioma. Part II: mechanisms of oedema production. Neuroradiology 1983; 25:125–131

CEREBRAL EDEMA

7. Cowley AR. Dyke award. Influence of fiber tracts on the CT appearance of cerebral edema: anatomic-pathologic correlation. AJNR 1983; 4:915–925
8. Monajati A, Heggeness L. Patterns of edema in tumors vs. infarcts: visualization of white matter pathways. AJNR 1982; 3:251–255
9. Rieth KG, Fujiwara K, Di Chiro G, et al. Serial measurements of CT attenuation and specific gravity in experimental cerebral edema. Radiology 1980; 135:343–348

HEMATOMA

10. Enzmann DR, Britt RH, Lyons BE, Buxton JL, Wilson DA. Natural history of experimental intracerebral hemorrhage: sonography, computed tomography and neuropathology. AJNR 1981; 2:517–526

11. Kendall BE, Radue EW. Computed tomography in spontaneous intracerebral haematomas. Br J Radiol 1978; 51:563–573
12. Laster DW, Moody DM, Ball MR. Resolving intracerebral hematoma: alteration of the {ring sign} with steroids. AJR 1978; 130:935–939

GLIOMA

13. Burger PC, Dubois PJ, Schold SC Jr, et al. Computerized tomographic and pathologic studies of the untreated, quiescent, and recurrent glioblastoma multiforme. J Neurosurg 1983; 58:159–169

ABSCESS

14. Enzmann DR, Britt RH, Placone R. Staging of human brain abscess by computed tomography. Radiology 1983; 146:703–708
15. Enzmann DR, Britt RH, Yeager AS. Experimental brain abscess evolution: computed tomographic and neuropathologic correlation. Radiology 1979; 133:113–122
16. Whelan MA, Hilal SK. Computed tomography as a guide in the diagnosis and follow-up of brain abscesses. Radiology 1980; 135:663–671

Notes

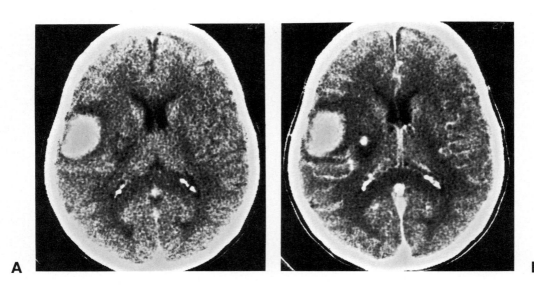

Figure 7-1. This 35-year-old man presented with recent onset of left hemiparesis. You are shown pre- and postcontrast computed tomographic scans.

A

B

Case 7: Cerebral Metastases

Question 30

Which *one* of the following is the MOST likely diagnosis?

(A) Hypertensive hemorrhage
(B) Arteriovenous malformation
(C) Metastatic disease
(D) Mycotic aneurysm
(E) Cavernous hemangioma

Figures 7-1A and 7-2A show a precontrast computed tomographic (CT) scan in which there is a high-density lesion in the right frontoparietal region. A high-density lesion of this size and shape must be considered an acute hematoma, although CT attenuation values should be checked to confirm this. Just medial to the hematoma, a small round area of decreased intensity is seen just lateral to the posterior limb of the internal capsule (Figure 7-2A, arrow). Figures 7-1B and 7-2B show the appearance of the brain following contrast infusion. The hematoma has not changed, as expected, but there is now enhancement of a small lesion near the internal capsule (Figure 7-2B, arrow). The edema adjacent to the small lesion suggests that it is growing rapidly. The most likely diagnosis is metastatic disease, with hemorrhage related to a second metastatic focus that is obscured by the hematoma **(Option (C) is correct).** Hypertensive hemorrhages (Option (A)) usually occur more medially, in the basal ganglia, and the smaller enhancing lesion could not be explained on that basis. There are no enlarged vessels in the vicinity of the bleed; thus, arteriovenous malformation (AVM) (Option (B)) is unlikely. Mycotic aneurysm (Option (D)) is a possible explanation, but the region of the internal capsule would be a very unusual site for a mycotic aneurysm, which does occur in peripheral locations but tends to involve vessels larger than those present in the basal ganglia. Cavernous hemangiomas (Option (E)) may bleed and may be multiple. However, if the smaller lesion were a second cavernous hemangioma, it would be difficult to

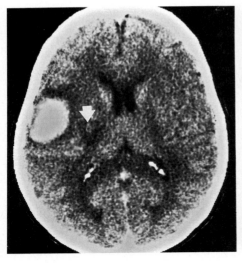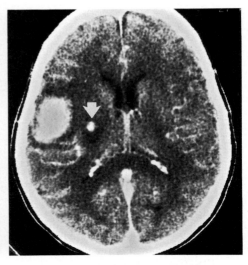

A   **B**

Figure 7-2 (Same as Figure 7-1). (A) The precontrast CT scan shows a high-density lesion in the right frontoparietal region representing an acute hematoma. Just medial to the hematoma there is a small round area of decreased intensity representing edema (arrow). (B) The contrast-enhanced CT scan reveals a small round enhancing lesion (arrow) within the area of edema that represents a metastatic lesion. There has been no change in the appearance of the hematoma.

explain why there is edema around it, since cavernous hemangiomas characteristically have no surrounding edema.

Question 31

Concerning cerebral arteriovenous malformations (AVMs),

(A) their likelihood of rupture increases with increasing lesion size
(B) they usually derive their blood supply from only one major artery
(C) large AVMs and neoplasms of similar size produce similar degrees of ventricular shift
(D) a single draining vein is more typically associated with venous angiomas than with AVMs
(E) aneurysms associated with them rarely bleed

AVMs are the most common of the vascular malformations or hamartomas involving the brain, the others being cavernous hemangiomas, venous angiomas, and telangiectasias. AVMs are more important than these other lesions, not only because of their higher incidence but also because of their greater tendency to bleed and to produce other manifestations such as epilepsy, headache, and neurological deficits related to ischemia of adjacent brain tissue. Bleeding occurs in approximately one-half of the known AVMs, and the occurrence of one bleed makes it more likely that a second one will occur. Curiously, small AVMs have been reported to rupture with a higher frequency than have large ones **(Option (A) is false).** This may be related to the fact that small AVMs may be clinically inapparent until they rupture, whereas large AVMs are more likely to make their presence known by other symptoms such as epilepsy and neurological deficits. Nevertheless, one should be aware of the hazardous nature of AVMs of all sizes, even cryptic lesions that can only be recognized by careful pathologic examination of the margins of hematomas. It is also recognized that bleeding results not infrequently from a small residual portion of an incompletely resected AVM.

The CT appearance of AVMs is usually easily recognizable. Precontrast CT may show the enlarged vessels to have a slightly increased density relative to that of the brain, because of the circulating blood within them. Other possible findings are adjacent areas of low density, related to either brain atrophy or edema, and occasionally calcifications. Calcifications are reported to occur in approximately 20% of AVMs, but this value is probably artificially high. When calcifications are seen, they are most often visible as short curvilinear or even punctate densities along the walls of vessels. Following contrast infusion, AVMs generally have a typical pattern on CT (Figure 7-3). Individual enlarged vessels are often visible within the densely staining nidus of the malformation. Enlargement of arterial feeders may be seen at some distance from the lesion. Most AVMs have more than one feeding artery, and it is not unusual for all the major vessels of a hemisphere to be involved **(Option (B) is false).** Most AVMs have several enlarged draining veins, which often run in diverse directions. The only vascular malformation that typically has a single draining vein is the venous angioma **(Option (D) is true).** There is seldom a problem differentiating between venous angiomas and AVMs on CT, since the former do not have associated enlarged arteries and often make their presence known only by the single enlarged draining vein. About one-half of venous angiomas have a rounded area of high density on CT, usually deep within the cerebral or cerebellar white matter. Cavernous hemangiomas sometimes have an associated draining vein but are more commonly seen as rounded areas of high density on

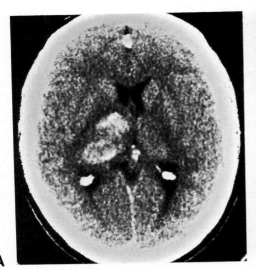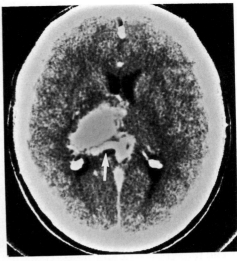

Figure 7-3. AVM with hemorrhage. (A) The precontrast CT scan shows an area of recent bleeding into the right thalamus. (B) The postcontrast CT section demonstrates a very large vessel just posterior to the area of bleeding (arrow); this presumably is a draining vein running toward the vein of Galen. There are other enlarged vessels medial to the bleed, and the density of the thalamic region is more intense, indicating a large AVM nidus in the same region as the hematoma.

precontrast CT, with some degree of contrast enhancement and no surrounding edema or associated enlarged vessels (Figures 7-4 and 7-5).

AVMs characteristically produce no apparent displacement of cerebral structures, such as ventricles. This is helpful in differentiating them from cerebral neoplasms **(Option (C) is false).** This lack of displacement is believed to be related to the gradual atrophy of adjacent brain tissue that accompanies the growth of AVMs. Very large AVMs may produce displacement, particularly when they have giant venous elements.

Aneurysms are associated with approximately 10% of AVMs. These aneurysms most often form at junction points of arteries that are enlarged because they supply the AVMs. It was once thought that these aneurysms had little tendency to bleed and that they were incidental findings of little interest. If a malformation can be resected, these aneurysms may involute as the feeding artery decreases in caliber. However, it is now recognized that aneurysms associated with AVMs may bleed **(Option (E) is false)** and that they should be dealt with before attempting to treat the malformation itself by surgery or embolization. An acute change in

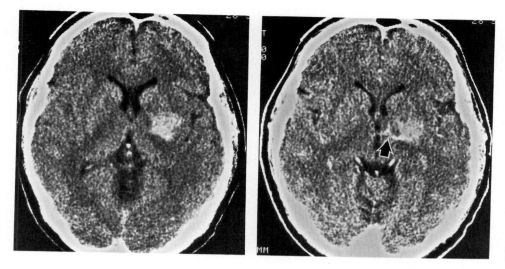

Figure 7-4. Cavernous hemangioma. (A) The precontrast CT scan shows a dense round lesion in the left basal ganglia. (B) On this postcontrast section, the linear density of an enlarged vessel (arrow) can be seen medial to the round lesion.

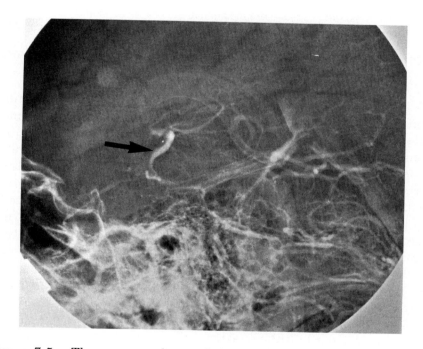

Figure 7-5. The venous phase of a vertebral angiogram shows an abnormal vein of nearly vertical course, just posterior and superior to the sella (arrow). A single vein with this appearance may be associated with a cavernous hemangioma, but it is not certain whether it should be considered a venous angioma associated with a cavernous hemangioma or simply an enlarged draining vein.

pressure within the feeding artery following its distal closure by surgery or embolization has been known to cause rupture of an aneurysm.

While CT will demonstrate most cerebral AVMs, selective angiography remains an essential procedure. Stereoscopic views are particularly helpful in these cases in analyzing the course of feeding vessels. A recent hematoma may mask the presence of an AVM, either by destroying part or all of the malformation or by compressing it so that its vascular elements are not evident. Because of this problem it is often necessary to repeat angiography later in search of a small AVM when dealing with a cerebral hematoma of suspicious origin.

Question 32

Concerning cerebral metastases,

(A) they can involve all intracranial structures, including the pituitary and pineal glands
(B) those most likely to bleed are melanoma and choriocarcinoma
(C) hemorrhage from metastases is less likely to spread to the subarachnoid or ventricular spaces than hemorrhage related to hypertension or AVMs
(D) when there is associated hemorrhage, the tumor itself is usually recognizable on CT by performing postcontrast scans

Metastases have been found involving all intracranial structures **(Option (A) is true).** The most common sites of origin of tumors metastatic to the brain are lung, breast, skin, genitourinary tract, and colon-rectum. While metastases may be found anywhere, they tend to occur at or near the junction of white matter and cortex. They are multiple in the majority of cases but, when single, may be mistaken for primary brain tumors or abscesses, which they often resemble morphologically. The precontrast CT density of metastatic tumors may be more than, less than, or the same as that of normal brain tissue. Lucent centers are common in metastases, since nearly 90% have some degree of central necrosis. While metastases may show uniform contrast enhancement on CT, ring-like stains are more common, particularly in larger tumors. Nearly all large metastases have surrounding edema. Small lesions may or may not have associated edema. The area of edema tends to be greater relative to lesion size with metastases than with primary brain tumors or abscesses. It is important to look for skull lesions in anyone suspected of having metastatic disease. Since precontrast scans do not usually demonstrate metastases that are not visible after contrast infusion,

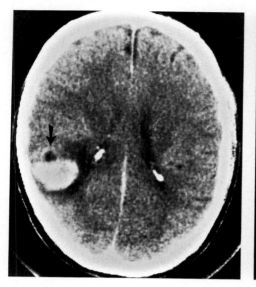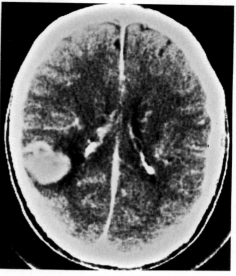

A   B

Figure 7-6. Bleeding from a cerebral metastasis. The metastasis, from a renal cell carcinoma in this case, can be seen as a small, ring-shaped density anterior to the parietal hematoma in both the precontrast (arrow, panel A) and postcontrast (B) axial CT scans. (Case courtesy of Peter E. Weinberg, M.D.)

postcontrast scans alone are frequently used when metastases are suspected. While these will demonstrate the lesions, areas of hemorrhage within the tumors may go undetected.

Bleeding may occur into many different types of intracranial tumors, including glioblastoma, pituitary adenoma, meningioma, hemangioblastoma, reticulum cell sarcoma, neuroblastoma, and metastases. Of metastases, melanoma and choriocarcinoma have a particularly high tendency to bleed **(Option (B) is true).** Melanomas make up approximately 15% of cerebral metastases but make up over 50% of the metastases that bleed. Hemorrhage may also be seen with carcinomas of the kidney, lung, and thyroid. On CT, one generally sees a hematoma without seeing the metastatic tumor that is the underlying cause **(Option (D) is false).** Occasionally, a portion of the neoplasm may be visible adjacent to the hematoma (Figures 7-6 and 7-7). Some bleeds are confined to the interior of the metastasis, giving it an irregularly increased density. A curious finding in some cases of melanoma is the simultaneous appearance of several high-density lesions, probably representing multiple bleeds into metastases (Figure 7-8). Hemorrhages

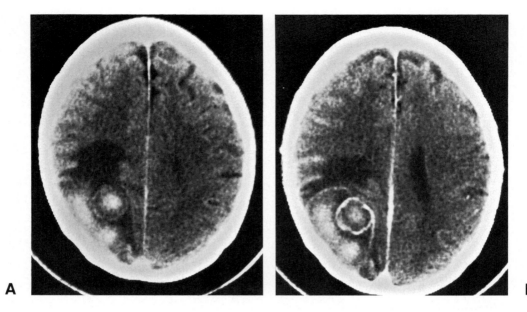

A

B

Figure 7-7. Another renal cell carcinoma metastasis with associated bleeding. Precontrast (A) and postcontrast (B) axial CT scans. In this case, there is visible blood both within and adjacent to the tumor, as seen on the precontrast scan. The wall of the tumor is better visualized after contrast infusion. (Case courtesy of Peter E. Weinberg, M.D.)

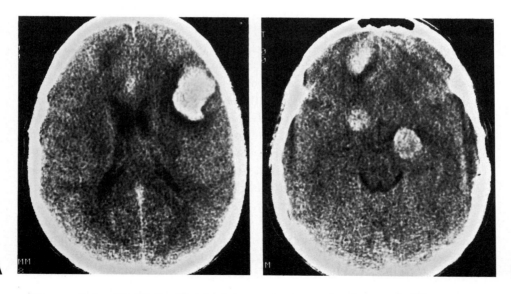

A

B

Figure 7-8. Multiple bleeds into metastases (melanoma). These two sections are from a noncontrast CT scan. The scan had been performed because of acute symptoms produced by the large left frontal lobe bleed (A). However, a lower section (B) showed three more tumors that also had high attenuation values, a finding consistent with recent hemorrhages.

from metastases tend to be smaller than those related to AVMs or hypertension and less often spread to the subarachnoid space or extend into the ventricular system **(Option (C) is true)**. Even when the responsible tumor is not visible, small areas of peripheral brain hemorrhage in the older population should prompt a search for other evidence of metastatic disease.

Question 33

Concerning mycotic aneurysms,

(A) the territory of the middle cerebral artery is most commonly involved
(B) they are usually larger than congenital aneurysms when first detected
(C) medical treatment is frequently successful, obviating surgical therapy
(D) an unusual location is generally the main CT or angiographic finding suggesting that an aneurysm may be mycotic
(E) cerebrovascular accidents due to fungal diseases, such as aspergillosis and mucormycosis, are usually due to rupture of mycotic aneurysms

Mycotic aneurysms are quite rare. They made up less than 10% of the aneurysms encountered in the preantibiotic era and are even less common now. However, these aneurysms are very dangerous and must be kept in mind, especially when a patient with bacterial endocarditis who has some other systemic infection or who is immunosuppressed suddenly develops neurological signs and symptoms. The most common pathogenetic organisms are streptococci, especially alpha-streptococci, and *Staphylococcus aureus*. Mycotic aneurysms probably occur secondary to infected emboli that lodge in cerebral arteries. Bleeding may occur into brain tissue or the subarachnoid space or both. When it occurs, bleeding is often catastrophic.

CT scanning generally will show the hemorrhage that results from mycotic aneurysms but cannot be relied upon to demonstrate the aneurysms. Angiography is indicated when mycotic aneurysms are suspected. The main characteristic feature differentiating mycotic aneurysms from other aneurysms is their more peripheral location, since they generally occur beyond the first branching point of the parent vessel **(Option (D) is true)**. The middle cerebral artery is by far the most often affected cerebral vessel **(Option (A) is true)**. These aneurysms vary in size, but most are relatively small when detected **(Option (B) is false)**.

Therapy of mycotic aneurysms is somewhat controversial. The majority of these aneurysms will heal with appropriate antibiotic therapy alone, and some clinicians advocate this together with periodic angiography to demonstrate continued shrinking of the aneurysms **(Option (C) is true)**. Any increase in aneurysm size during a course of antibiotic therapy must be considered ominous. However, the mortality rate remains sufficiently high that surgery plus antibiotic therapy is sometimes advocated when the aneurysms are first discovered, particularly if they are readily accessible.

Certain fungal diseases, such as mucormycosis and aspergillosis, are notorious for their tendency to cause cerebrovascular accidents. These infections most commonly occur in patients who have poorly controlled diabetes or are immunosuppressed. Involvement of the paranasal sinuses is common, and the infection may extend into the intracranial space through venous pathways. The cavernous sinus is frequently involved. The hyphae of the fungi invade the walls of arteries of the brain, usually near the base, causing thrombosis and subsequent cerebral infarction. The fungi may cause erosion of vessel walls and result in mycotic aneurysm formation, but this is a less common cause of cerebrovascular accidents than the thrombosis mentioned above **(Option (E) is false)**. CT scanning generally shows the presence of one or more infarcts and may also demonstrate an area of cerebritis about the site of the involved vessel.

John R. Bentson, M.D.

SUGGESTED READINGS

METASTATIC DISEASE

1. Gildersleeve N Jr, Koo AH, McDonald CJ. Metastatic tumor presenting as intracerebral hemorrhage. Report of 6 cases examined by computed tomography. Radiology 1977; 124:109–112
2. Holtas S, Cronqvist S. Cranial computed tomography of patients with malignant melanoma. Neuroradiology 1981; 22:123–127
3. Mandybur TI. Intracranial hemorrhage caused by metastatic tumors. Neurology 1977; 27:650–655
4. Potts DG, Abbott GF, von Sneidern JV. National Cancer Institute study: evaluation of computed tomography in the diagnosis of intracranial neoplasms. III. Metastatic tumors. Radiology 1980; 136:657–664
5. Zimmerman RA, Bilaniuk LT. Computed tomography of acute intratumoral hemorrhage. Radiology 1980; 135:355–359

ARTERIOVENOUS MALFORMATIONS

6. Margolis G, Odom G, Woodhall B. Further experiences with small vascular malformations as a cause of massive intracerebral bleeding. J Neuropathol Exp Neurol 1961; 20:161–167
7. Perret G, Nishioka H. Report on the cooperative study of intracranial aneurysms and subarachnoid hemorrhage. Section VI. Arteriovenous malformations. An analysis of 545 cases of cranio-cerebral arteriovenous malformations and fistulae reported to the cooperative study. J Neurosurg 1966; 25:467–490
8. Stein BM, Wolpert SM. Arteriovenous malformations of the brain. II: current concepts and treatment. Arch Neurol 1980; 37:69–75

MYCOTIC ANEURYSMS

9. Frazee JG, Cahan LD, Winter J. Bacterial intracranial aneurysms. J Neurosurg 1980; 53:633–641
10. Whelan MA, Stern J, deNapoli RA. The computed tomographic spectrum of intracranial mycosis: correlation with histopathology. Radiology 1981; 141:703–707

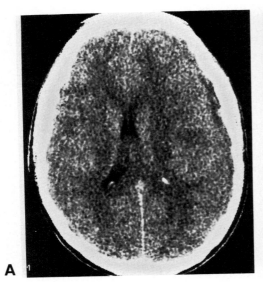 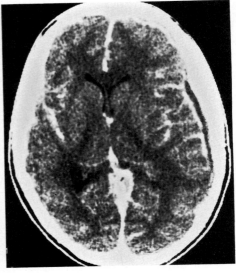

A   B

Figure 8-1

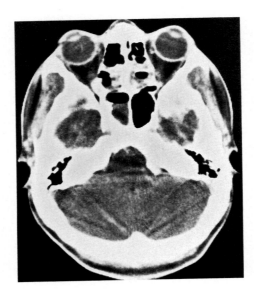

Figure 8-2
Figures 8-1 and 8-2. This 16-year-old boy presented with a 1-week history of headache, vomiting, dysarthria, and seizures. You are shown pre- and postcontrast computed tomographic (CT) scans (Figures 8-1 and 8-2).

Case 8: Subdural Empyema

Question 34

Which *one* of the following is the MOST likely diagnosis?

(A) Subdural hematoma
(B) Subdural hygroma
(C) Subdural empyema
(D) Epidural abscess
(E) Malignant subdural effusion

The precontrast CT scan (Figure 8-1A) shows a thin zone of slightly decreased density between the left frontal lobe and the skull (Figure 8-3A, arrows). There appears to be some widening of the white matter zone on the left with consequent midline shift. The contrast-enhanced CT scan (Figure 8-1B) demonstrates a line of strong contrast enhancement between the brain and the extracerebral fluid collection (Figure 8-3B, arrows). The ventricles and falx are shifted to the right. The scan through the paranasal sinuses (Figure 8-2) demonstrates partial opacification of ethmoid and sphenoid sinuses, a finding consistent with inflammatory disease (Figure 8-4, arrows). The most likely diagnosis is subdural empyema **(Option (C) is correct)**. The main features of the scan supporting this diagnosis are the presence of a source of infection in the paranasal sinuses, the rim of contrast enhancement medial to the subdural fluid collection, and the ventricular displacement that seems out of proportion to such a small amount of subdural fluid.

A subdural hematoma (Option (A)) may have the appearance of the fluid collection on the precontrast scan shown here, but marginal enhancement would be unusual, and a subdural hematoma of such little thickness would not be expected to produce displacement of the ventricles and falx.

Subdural hygroma (Option (B)) is not likely for the same reasons as those outlined above for a subdural hematoma. An epidural abscess (Option (D)) would seldom spread so widely, due to the normal resistance afforded by the attachment of the dura to the bone. In other respects,

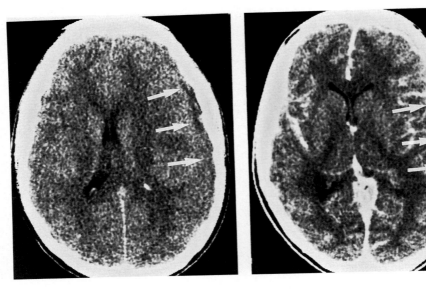

Figure 8-3 (Same as Figure 8-1). (A) The precontrast CT scan shows a thin zone of decreased density between the left frontal lobe and inner table of the skull (arrows). (B) The contrast-enhanced CT scan demonstrates a line of enhancement between the brain and the extracerebral fluid collection (arrows).

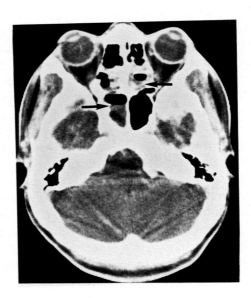

Figure 8-4 (Same as Figure 8-2). CT scan through the paranasal sinuses demonstrates partial opacification of the ethmoid and sphenoid sinuses (arrows). This finding is consistent with inflammatory disease.

this diagnosis would be a reasonable choice. Malignant subdural effusions (Option (E)) are rare, and strong enhancement at the margin of these fluid collections or a ventricular shift that is disproportionate to the size of the collection itself would be unusual.

Question 35

Concerning subdural hematomas,

(A) less than 50% are associated with skull fractures
(B) when acute they are similar in shape to chronic epidural hematomas
(C) they are more often bilateral in young children than in adults
(D) contrast enhancement around their margins indicates a superimposed infection
(E) different densities within them are usually due to either settling or rebleeding

Subdural hematomas typically are of traumatic origin, but the trauma may be relatively mild and may have been overlooked or forgotten. Most subdural hematomas are believed to occur following tearing of bridging veins. However, it should be remembered that these hematomas may also result from injury to arteries on the surface of the brain or from cortical tears. The arachnoid is often torn in such injuries. Another mechanism is partial tear of the inner surface of a dural sinus. Rarely, subdural hematomas may result from rupture of an aneurysm or arteriovenous malformation of the brain.

At one time, skull radiographs were used extensively in the workup of patients with head trauma. The finding of simple skull fractures was considered a warning sign that other post-traumatic sequelae, such as subdural hematomas, might be present. However, less than 50% of patients with subdural hematomas have identifiable skull fractures **(Option (A) is true).** Indeed, less than 25% of patients who have significant intracranial sequelae from head injuries have demonstrable fractures. Because of such findings, the efficacy of skull radiography in the evaluation of head trauma has been strongly questioned in recent years. The evolving practice seems to be more liberal use of CT scanning alone in patients suspected of having significant intracranial trauma. CT scans are not as sensitive as skull radiographs for detecting simple linear fractures, but they will disclose most of the more significant depressed fractures and show signs indicating the existence of basilar skull fractures.

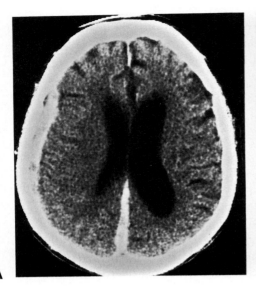
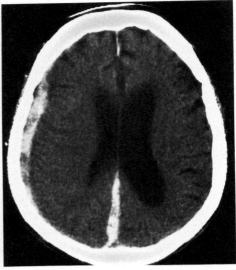

A

B

Figure 8-5. Typical subdural hematoma. Noncontrast axial CT scans. (A) The hematoma extends along the right frontal and parietal bones and also extends along the right side of the falx. (B) Bone window CT settings often help to distinguish a hematoma from the adjacent skull.

Subdural hematomas, since they meet little resistance, tend to spread quite diffusely over the surface of the brain. Therefore, the outer border of subdural hematomas is convex, while the inner border is concave (Figure 8-5). This shape is in contrast to the shape of epidural hematomas, which are biconvex, reflecting the resistance of the dura to being dissected away from the inner table **(Option (B) is false)** (Figure 8-6). Chronic subdural hematomas may have a biconvex shape resembling that of acute epidural hematomas. Subdural hematomas are bilateral in approximately one-third of cases. Bilateral subdural hematomas are much more common in young children than in adults **(Option (C) is true).** Subdural hematomas frequently extend along the surface of the falx or tentorium. Subdural hematomas that are most prominent adjacent to the posterior falx in young children should raise concern about the possibility of a shaking injury.

There is some relationship between the age of a hematoma and its CT density. Acute hematomas have a very high density, due to the high hemoglobin concentration of a retracted clot. With time, rupture of erythrocytes occurs, hemoglobin is released and degraded, and the density of the hematoma drops. At some time, usually between 2 to 6

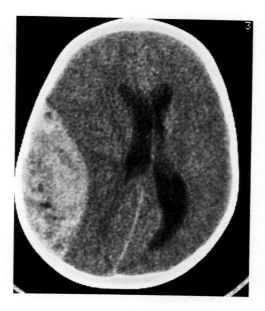

Figure 8-6. Large epidural hematoma. This noncontrast axial CT scan demonstrates the typical biconvex shape of the hematoma.

weeks following injury, the hematoma will be isodense relative to the brain on CT scans, sometimes making it difficult to demonstrate the lesion. This difference in CT density is sometimes used to categorize subdural hematomas into the acute and chronic categories. Some physicians use the term "subacute hematoma" to describe isodense subdural hematomas. One must remember that the correlation between age and density is not exact. Anemic patients may have isodense acute subdural hematomas. In others, an acute subdural collection may have low density on CT scans. This is thought to be related to an arachnoid tear that allows cerebrospinal fluid, possibly mixed with blood, to enter the subdural space. Different densities are commonly noted within a single subdural hematoma. Typically, the more posterior portion of the subdural hematoma has a higher density than that of the anterior portion in a recumbent patient (Figure 8-7). This is believed to be due either to settling of red blood cells within the hematoma or to rebleeding **(Option (E) is true).** Rebleeding appears to be relatively common in subdural hematomas. CT scans frequently demonstrate an increase in the density of a hematoma along with an increase in its size. Rebleeding rather than high osmotic pressure is probably a better explanation for the increase in size often seen with chronic hematomas. Rebleeding does not always

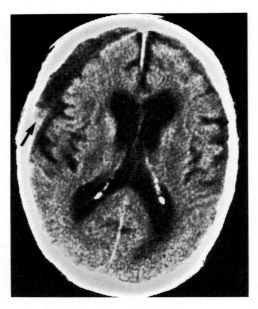

Figure 8-7. Chronic right frontal subdural hematoma. This noncontrast axial CT scan demonstrates higher-density material in the posterior portion of the hematoma (arrow) due to either settling or rebleeding.

result in vertically oriented differences in density. In some cases, a stripe of high density related to rebleeding may be seen parallel to the skull, adjacent to a low-density region of a more chronic subdural hematoma.

Isodense subdural hematomas not recognized by CT scanning once constituted a major diagnostic problem. This problem diminished as the resolution of CT scanners improved. Even in the case of the perfectly isodense hematoma, which is rare, the CT scan demonstrates obliteration of normal sulcal patterns and often some shift of the ventricles. Posterior displacement of a frontal horn and anterior displacement of an occipital horn are unlikely to occur in any condition other than a subdural fluid collection. In most cases, the density of the subdural hematoma is not entirely homogeneous. Contrast infusion also helps to demonstrate the boundary between the brain and the hematoma (Figure 8-8). While neomembranes do form around chronic subdural hematomas, it is not clear whether the thin line of enhancement seen at the junction of the brain and the hematoma reflects the presence of a neomembrane or whether it is related to some loss of integrity of the blood-brain barrier of the compressed cerebral cortex. In most cases, marginal enhancement around a subdural hematoma does not indicate a superimposed infection,

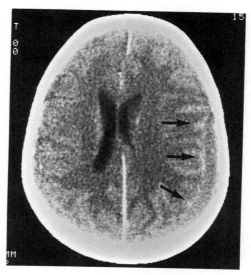

Figure 8-8. Isodense left subdural hematoma. On this contrast-enhanced scan, the surface of the brain is obvious (arrows), and there is more contrast enhancement of sulci adjacent to the left subdural hematoma.

although this possibility should be kept in mind when enhancement is unusually dense **(Option (D) is false).**

Recent experience has shown that magnetic resonance imaging (MRI) is very efficient in detecting subdural hematomas, which are seen as zones of high intensity because of their short T1 and long T2 values. Hematomas that are isodense on CT scans are readily detected by MRI.

Question 36

Concerning subdural hygromas,

  (A) most are considered sequelae of subdural hematomas
  (B) they show marginal contrast enhancement less often than do subdural hematomas
  (C) they are more common in children than in adults
  (D) they infrequently form immediately after head trauma
  (E) when associated with meningitis, the most common organism responsible is *Hemophilus influenzae*

Subdural hygromas are collections of xanthochromic, watery fluid in the subdural space, usually occurring some weeks or months following head trauma. Most are considered to be sequelae of subdural hematomas **(Option (A) is true).** However, it is not unusual to find subdural hygromas in children without known head trauma. A common presentation in infants and young children is enlargement of the head and some additional sign of increased intracranial pressure. Subdural hygromas are more common in children than in adults **(Option (C) is true)** and are frequently bilateral, particularly in children. No skull fracture is present in most cases. The distinction between subdural hygromas and chronic subdural hematomas is blurred, which is to be expected since most subdural hygromas are believed to originate as subdural hematomas. Occasionally, subdural hygromas appear just after head trauma. These are probably the result of a tear in the arachnoid, with subsequent accumulation of cerebrospinal fluid in the subdural space **(Option (D) is true).**

On CT scans, subdural hygromas have a density that is the same or nearly the same as that of cerebrospinal fluid. Marginal enhancement following contrast infusion is seen rarely, even less often than with subdural hematomas **(Option (B) is true).** This lack of enhancement and the frequently bilateral nature of the fluid collections sometimes make it difficult to identify subdural hygromas. This is particularly true in infants, in whom there is often enlargement of ventricles and sulci in addition to widening of the interhemispheric fissure and an increased fluid space between the brain and the skull. These characteristics give the brain an appearance that suggests cerebral atrophy, but this condition is not consistent with the clinical findings of increased intracranial pressure and enlarged head size. The ventricular enlargement is somewhat difficult to explain but may be related to hydrocephalus caused by the interference of subdural hygromas with the passage of cerebrospinal fluid over the cerebral convexities toward the superior sagittal sinus, where absorption takes place. In such cases, the diagnosis of subdural fluid collection can be confirmed by CT scanning following intrathecal injection of a small amount of contrast agent, such as metrizamide.

Meningitis is a relatively common cause of subdural hygromas, also called subdural effusions, in children. The organism most frequently responsible is *Hemophilus influenzae* **(Option (E) is true).** These fluid collections may be seen as early as a few days after the onset of meningitis and may continue to enlarge for some time. The margins of the subdural hygromas found in association with meningitis generally show little or no enhancement. The cause of these effusions is not clear. Inflammation of subdural veins may lead to a loss of fluid into the subdural space.

Tearing of damaged arachnoid would be another possible source of effusions. Fluid loss from newly formed vessels could also produce such collections.

Question 37

Concerning subdural empyemas,

  (A) most cases are related to acute sinusitis
  (B) CT usually shows marginal contrast enhancement
  (C) no angiographically recognizable abnormalities are seen in adjacent cerebral vessels
  (D) surgical drainage is usually not necessary if the responsible organism is known
  (E) clinical signs and symptoms are usually much more marked than those associated with subdural hematomas of similar size

Subdural empyema is a very serious purulent infection of the subdural space that is generally fatal if not treated. Even in the postantibiotic era, mortality rates of 20 to 40% have been reported. Over one-half of the survivors of the disease suffer epileptic seizures. Because of the rapid progression of the disease, it is imperative that an early diagnosis be made. A high degree of suspicion is necessary, since early recognition may be difficult.

Most cases of subdural empyema are related to acute sinusitis, particularly involving the frontal sinuses **(Option (A) is true).** The usual route of access of the infection to the subdural space is through thrombophlebitis of emissary veins. Once the infection has reached the subdural space, it tends to spread rapidly and widely. Although most collections of pus are found over the convexities, interhemispheric collections are common, either alone or in association with convexity collections. Common causative organisms are non-beta-hemolytic streptococci, staphylococci, pneumococci, and enterobacteria. Other sources of subdural empyema are mastoiditis, penetrating wounds, operative procedures, suppurative processes elsewhere in the body, and meningitis. Subdural empyemas secondary to meningitis are found mainly in infants and young children and are usually due to *Hemophilus influenzae, Neisseria meningitidis,* and *Streptococcus pneumoniae.*

The arachnoid membrane constitutes a temporary barrier to the spread of infection; cerebrospinal fluid cultures early in the disease are usually negative, and pleocytosis may be mild. However, a severe aseptic inflammatory reaction generally occurs in the arachnoid and the superficial cerebral cortex. Microscopically, thrombosis of small cortical veins is a prominent feature. This reaction in the cortex is responsible for the cerebral swelling that occurs and also for the impressive clinical findings. In general, the clinical signs and symptoms are much more marked than those associated with other subdural fluid collections of a similar size **(Option (E) is true).** A characteristic clinical triad consists of fever, increasing intracranial pressure, and focal neurologic signs. Seizures are frequent, and coma is not unusual. Headache is an early prominent symptom and is intensified relative to that initially caused by the sinusitis. Meningeal signs are usually early findings also.

Prior to the arrival of CT scanning, cerebral angiography was the most definitive test for identifying subdural empyemas. Angiography demonstrated displacement of cortical vessels away from the inner table, similar to that seen in other subdural fluid collections. Interhemispheric fluid collections could also be identified by angiography. Adjacent to the subdural collections, angiography sometimes revealed spasms of cortical arteries, prolonged flow patterns, and areas without filling of cortical veins **(Option (C) is false).** Superior sagittal sinus thrombosis, also related to the process of retrograde thrombophlebitis, was occasionally found.

CT scanning has been very useful in the detection of subdural empyemas. The typical appearance is that of a fluid collection adjacent to the skull, with intense contrast enhancement of its medial margin **(Option (B) is true).** When the lesion is adjacent to the falx, contrast enhancement of the falx may also be seen. The shape of the abnormality varies. In some cases, a relatively small biconvex fluid collection is seen (Figure 8-9). In others, large crescentic or biconvex fluid collections are present. Inflammatory membranes do form adjacent to subdural empyemas, but failure to demonstrate any membrane in a case in which postcontrast CT has demonstrated marginal enhancement is common. The marginal enhancement in these cases is probably due to blood-brain barrier breakdown in the superficial portion of the cerebral cortex and is related to the aseptic inflammatory reaction. In early cases, the subdural fluid collection may be difficult to recognize because it is so thin. Swelling of the cerebral hemisphere may then be the predominant CT feature, and patients have been known to develop herniation from subdural empyemas without CT having demonstrated an easily recognizable subdural fluid collection. In these early cases, it is essential to pay particular attention to the postcontrast appearance of the superficial portion of the cerebral cortex, since enhancement adjacent to the empyema may also be faint. CT demonstration of sinusitis is a valuable clue in such cases. Rarely,

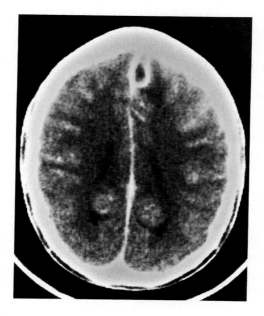

Figure 8-9. Small subdural empyema adjacent to the falx. This contrast-enhanced axial CT scan demonstrates a low-density fluid collection surrounded by intense enhancement. This lesion has a biconvex shape, but its location next to the falx indicates its subdural nature.

CT may demonstrate a cerebral abscess that forms subsequent to the subdural empyema.

Subdural empyemas must be considered as surgical emergencies and should not be treated with antibiotics alone, even if the offending organism is known **(Option (D) is false).** As much of the pus as possible should be evacuated, and intensive antibiotic therapy is indicated. The infected sinuses should also be drained. Follow-up CT scans are generally required to check for the development of pockets of subdural empyemas that were not drained by the initial operative procedure.

Question 38

Concerning epidural abscesses,

(A) they have the same shape on CT scans as subdural empyemas
(B) they are more common than subdural infections following neurosurgical procedures
(C) they are more commonly associated with abnormalities of the cranial vault than are subdural empyemas
(D) their presence is indicated by the separation of a dural venous sinus from the skull
(E) separation of the dura from the skull is readily apparent on CT scans, especially after contrast infusion

Epidural abscesses and subdural empyemas are the main forms of extracerebral intracranial suppuration. Epidural abscesses are less common and also less devastating than subdural empyemas. The dura is a sufficiently good barrier to the spread of infection that focal neurologic signs are rare in conjunction with epidural abscesses. Headache and fever are the most common initial symptoms but are often not recognizable as separate from the symptoms of predisposing sinusitis. If rupture of an epidural abscess occurs, a subdural empyema or even a brain abscess may develop.

Like subdural empyemas, the majority of epidural abscesses occur secondary to paranasal sinusitis or mastoiditis. The mucosal veins of the paranasal sinuses communicate with the diploic veins, which in turn communicate with the venous plexuses related to the dura. Osteomyelitis of the posterior wall of the frontal sinus is often present in cases of epidural abscess. Many cases of epidural abscess arise from infected operative sites, penetrating wounds, osteomyelitis of the skull, and skull fractures. Epidural abscesses are somewhat more common than subdural infections following surgery, although either may occur **(Option (B) is true)**. In general, skull radiographs are positive in a high proportion of epidural abscesses (over 80%) somewhat more often than is noted with subdural empyemas **(Option (C) is true)**.

CT scanning has proved to be an effective means of identifying epidural abscesses (Figure 8-10). A localized intracranial fluid collection with biconvex borders is seen adjacent to the skull. The medial border is enhanced strongly with contrast infusion. Because a displaced dura is readily apparent on postcontrast CT scans, even when there is no infection, the border of an epidural abscess may be apparent relatively earlier than a subdural empyema **(Option (E) is true)**. There are differences in the shapes of the lesions in epidural abscesses and subdural

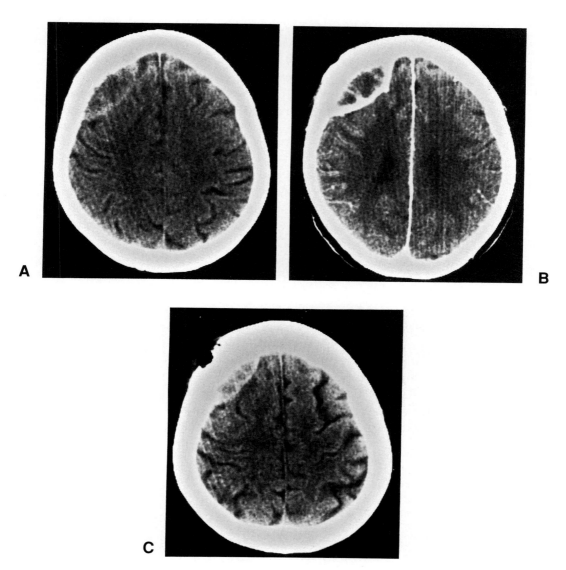

Figure 8-10. Epidural abscesses secondary to tuberculous osteomyelitis of the skull. (A) Even without contrast infusion, the density of the displaced dura is obvious. (B) With contrast infusion, there is marked enhancement of the margin of the abscess. (C) This higher section shows a skull defect related to osteomyelitis.

empyemas **(Option (A) is false).** The strong adherence of the dura to the skull limits the degree of dural dissection by pus, and thus epidural abscesses, like epidural hematomas, have a biconvex shape. It is true that subdural empyemas also have such a shape. However, some subdural empyemas spread diffusely along the inner surface of the skull, and these have a crescent shape. In other cases, subdural empyemas may have biconvex forms, but more than one of these collections is frequently seen in the same patient, a finding unlikely to occur with epidural abscesses. Another distinguishing feature relates to the degree of involvement of the brain. Epidural abscesses induce little edema of adjacent brain, and the degree of brain displacement is proportional to the size of the abscess. In the case of subdural empyemas, there is frequently a striking degree of shift of the ventricles and other brain structures relative to the size of the subdural collection; this is due to the widespread aseptic inflammatory response of brain tissue. Another distinguishing feature that is occasionally helpful is displacement of a venous sinus from the skull in association with an epidural abscess that crosses the midline **(Option (D) is true).** This displacement cannot occur in cases of subdural empyema. Occlusion of a venous sinus, most often the superior sagittal sinus, is possible with both epidural abscesses and subdural empyemas.

Like subdural empyemas, epidural abscesses should be treated surgically as well as with intensive antibiotic therapy. Because of the more benign clinical course of epidural abscesses, institution of therapy is not quite as urgent as it is for subdural empyemas. However, it is important to diagnose and treat these epidural lesions before extension and serious complications develop. Resection of areas of osteomyelitis is often necessary.

John R. Bentson, M.D.

SUGGESTED READINGS

SUBDURAL AND EPIDURAL INFECTIONS

1. Bergstrom M, Ericson K, Levander B, Svendsen P. Computed tomography of cranial subdural and epidural hematomas: variation of attenuation related to time and clinical events such as rebleeding. J Comput Assist Tomogr 1977; 1:449–455
2. Blaquiere RM. The computed tomographic appearances of intra- and extracerebral abscesses. Br J Radiol 1983; 56:171–181

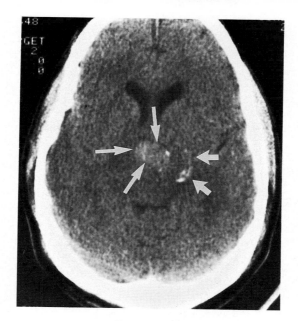

Figure 9-5

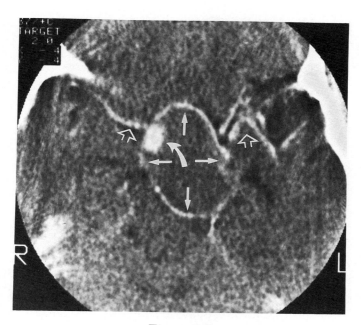

Figure 9-6

Figures 9-5 through 9-8 (Same as Figures 9-1 through 9-4). Figure 9-5
is a precontrast CT scan demonstrating an ill-defined area of high density
in the midline and to the right of the midline (long arrows). There is also
a peripheral curvilinear density along the left side of the mass (short
arrows). Figure 9-6 is a contrast-enhanced CT scan demonstrating the
entire periphery of the lesion (arrows). There is a discrete round area of
enhancement along the anterolateral wall of the mass on the right side
(curved arrow). The visualized short segments of the middle cerebral
arteries are of normal caliber (arrowheads). Figure 9-7 shows a
parasagittal reformatted section through the plane indicated by the
dotted line. An elongated zone of high density (arrows) was seen near the
right lateral margin of the lesion. Figure 9-8 shows a coronal reformatted
image through the plane indicated by the dotted line. A curvilinear area
of high density (arrows) is seen along the right lateral margin of the lesion.

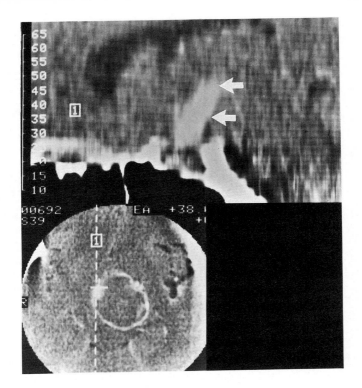

Figure 9-7

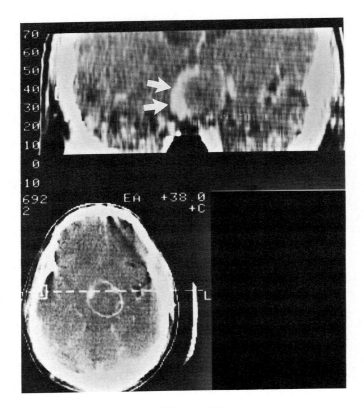

Figure 9-8

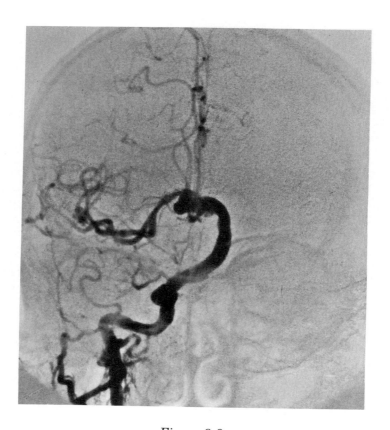

Figure 9-9
Figures 9-9 and 9-10. Same patient as in Figures 9-1 through 9-8. Giant suprasellar aneurysm. Anteroposterior and lateral carotid angiograms show the lumen of the giant aneurysm. Note that the lumen is elongated, irregular, and curved.

The other diagnostic possibilities listed are unlikely. Hypothalamic gliomas, tuberculum meningiomas, and pituitary tumors (Options (A), (B), and (E), respectively) all generally show uniform contrast enhancement on CT scanning. Tuberculum meningiomas are almost never cystic, probably because they come to clinical attention by causing severe visual abnormalities before they become large enough to be necrotic. Hypothalamic gliomas and pituitary tumors are occasionally cystic, but the cystic areas should be visible as low-density regions on precontrast CT scanning. In addition, they rarely calcify. Craniopharyngioma (Option (C)) is probably the most difficult of the choices to eliminate. It is common to see a combination of cyst, calcification, and areas of enhancing tumor

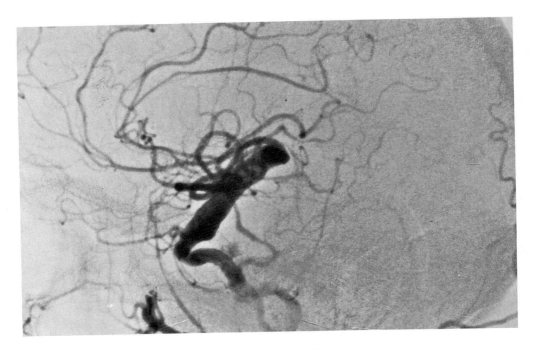

Figure 9-10

within craniopharyngiomas. However, the cystic portion of the tumor is rarely isodense relative to brain. Another feature in the test patient that suggests aneurysm rather than craniopharyngioma is the considerable vertical height and oblong shape of the enhancing region. A tumor nodule with such an oblong shape would be quite unusual.

Question 40

Concerning suprasellar masses,

(A) they all produce similar changes in the sella

(B) craniopharyngiomas and giant aneurysms are the two suprasellar masses most likely to be calcified

(C) a tuberculum meningioma is less likely to present with visual field changes than are other suprasellar tumors

(D) hypothalamic gliomas are more likely to receive major arterial feeders from the ophthalmic arteries than are other suprasellar tumors

(E) bleeding from a pituitary tumor may mimic curvilinear calcification

The suprasellar area is a particularly interesting region in terms of the differential diagnosis of abnormalities. A considerable variety of masses may be present in this region, due to the variety of tissues found there and to the high incidence of abnormalities arising from inclusions of embryonic rests. While these masses may sometimes mimic each other in any single study, a specific diagnosis is usually possible when the results of different diagnostic tests are considered together with the clinical findings.

Careful evaluation of the appearance of the sella is still important in the differential diagnosis of suprasellar masses. While CT and magnetic resonance imaging (MRI) may tend to de-emphasize the importance of the art of interpreting sellar changes, it remains true that much important information can still be gained by careful examination of the sella. Suprasellar masses do not all produce the same changes in the sella **(Option (A) is false).**

A pituitary tumor that extends into the suprasellar space will nearly always cause enlargement of the sella. Because these tumors develop slowly, the sella first enlarges with preservation of its cortical bone. Destruction of the dorsum sellae follows later. The floor of the sella is generally depressed, frequently more markedly on one side than on the other. Craniopharyngiomas may extend into the sella and enlarge it, but this is seen in a minority of cases. The most typical finding of craniopharyngiomas, which occur in a posterior suprasellar location, is a decrease in the height and a flattening of the upper surface of the dorsum sellae. Hypothalamic gliomas often extend into the optic nerves and produce a characteristic appearance of the sella, in which there is enlargement of the chiasmatic sulcus and erosion of the undersurfaces of the anterior clinoid processes, producing a "J-shaped" or "omega" sella. Aneurysms produce various types of sellar enlargement or erosion, depending upon their locations. Occasionally, a cavernous carotid aneurysm will grow directly into the sella and produce a symmetrical enlargement that mimics that of a pituitary tumor. More commonly, unilateral erosion of the sella is seen.

Any of the suprasellar masses may calcify. However, the frequency varies considerably. The highest rate of calcification (variously reported to be 70 to 85%) has been found to occur with craniopharyngiomas in children. Only 25 to 50% of craniopharyngiomas in adults are calcified. Giant aneurysms are the suprasellar masses next most likely to be calcified **(Option (B) is true).** Calcification is apparent by CT in approximately 75% of partially thrombosed giant aneurysms. Giant aneurysms without thrombosis are usually not calcified but are not as common. CT demonstrates calcification in sphenoid and parasellar meningiomas in approximately 25% of cases. Less than 5% of pituitary tumors are calcified. Calcification is seen infrequently in other suprasellar masses, such as hypothalamic and optic gliomas, ectopic pinealomas, metastatic tumors, and sarcoidosis.

Meningiomas that arise from the tuberculum sellae and from the adjacent planum sphenoidale are usually considered together under the category of tuberculum meningiomas. These tumors are generally silent until they have extended posteriorly into the suprasellar area to such an extent that they compress the optic nerves or chiasm, resulting in impaired vision **(Option (C) is false).**

In cases of hypothalamic glioma, carotid angiography often demonstrates displacement and enlargement of anterior thalamoperforate branches of the posterior communicating arteries. The tuberculum or planum sphenoidale meningioma is the suprasellar tumor most likely to receive blood supply from branches of the ophthalmic arteries **(Option (D) is false).**

When pituitary tumors bleed or undergo infarction, the syndrome of pituitary apoplexy may occur. This is characterized by the sudden onset of headache, mental changes, vomiting, and vision loss or diplopia. Bleeding is more common than infarction, and the most common type of bleeding is a solid hematoma within the tumor. Blood is often seen at the periphery of the tumor, mimicking the curvilinear calcification seen with large suprasellar aneurysms **(Option (E) is true).** Angiography is frequently necessary for differential diagnosis in these patients.

Question 41

Concerning tuberculum meningiomas,

   (A) calcification is less common than in craniopharyngiomas
   (B) blood supply is mainly from the middle meningeal artery
   (C) the adjacent planum sphenoidale is commonly eroded
   (D) the pattern of displacement of the internal carotid and anterior cerebral arteries is different from that seen with suprasellar pituitary tumors
   (E) when erosion of the dorsum sellae is seen with this tumor, it usually reflects increased intracranial pressure rather than the effect of adjacent mass

    Meningiomas in the suprasellar area may have several points of origin. Many arise from the dura of the tuberculum. Those arising from the adjacent planum sphenoidale are often included in the category of tuberculum meningiomas for the sake of convenience. Other tumors arise from the diaphragma sellae or from the anterior clinoids. The majority of meningiomas arising from these locations cause sclerosis of adjacent bone. The irregular sclerosis and upward convexity of the roof of the sphenoid sinus is a classical finding of these tumors and is called "blistering." Bone erosion is very rarely seen **(Option (C) is false).** Although hyperostosis is most commonly associated with meningiomas, it may also occur with craniopharyngiomas, metastatic tumors, chordomas, and rarely other suprasellar lesions. Since there is considerable normal variation in the thickness of the planum sphenoidale and even some variation in its shape, it may be difficult to recognize hyperostosis of this region. This was a frequent problem in the past, when hyperostosis of the planum region was not recognized on skull radiographs that had been taken to look for causes of decreasing vision. This contributed to many tragic cases of blindness with large tuberculum meningiomas. With CT scans, the problem is simplified. The hyperostosis and elevation of the planum sphenoidale may be visible on reformatted coronal and sagittal views or on direct coronal projections, and the mass itself is visible around the planum, tuberculum, and sella (Figures 9-11 and 9-12). Fine sections should be done in any such case since the meningioma may be very subtle if it arises in the region of the anterior clinoid with an early involvement of the optic canal. By the time diagnostic studies are performed in the typical case of tuberculum meningiomas, the tumor has extended posteriorly over the sella and superiorly to the extent that the optic nerves and chiasm are compromised. There is generally some erosion of the dorsum sellae, particularly its tip. This is related to the

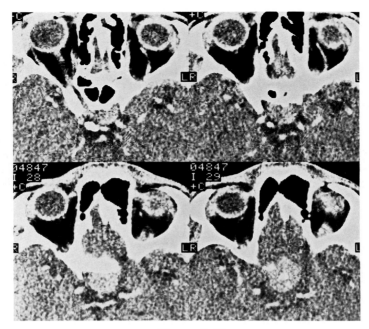

Figure 9-11

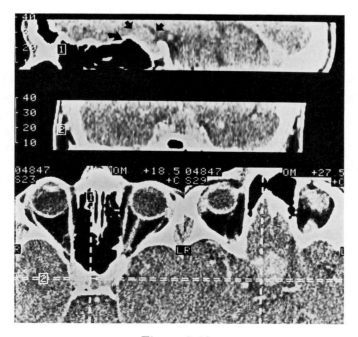

Figure 9-12

Figures 9-11 and 9-12. Tuberculum meningioma. Postcontrast axial CT sections (Figure 9-11) show a suprasellar mass with homogeneous enhancement. The midsagittal reformatted view (Figure 9-12, top) best demonstrates the mass extending over the tuberculum sellae (arrows) and the "blistering" (elevation and sclerosis) of the tuberculum-planum sphenoidale region (curved arrow).

178

effect of the adjacent tumor rather than to a general increase in intracranial pressure **(Option (E) is false).**

Approximately 25% of tuberculum meningiomas are calcified. Calcification is more often diffuse than patchy. The typical tumor in this location is seen as an area of slightly increased density relative to brain on the precontrast scan. Calcification is much more common in craniopharyngiomas, particularly in children **(Option (A) is true).**

Tuberculum meningiomas produce a characteristic pattern of vascular displacement that is easily differentiated from that of pituitary tumors in most cases **(Option (D) is true).** The tumor is more anterior in location than the suprasellar pituitary tumor and displaces the supraclinoid carotid posteriorly. The anterior cerebral artery is displaced posteriorly as well as superiorly; the lateral view of the internal carotid arteriogram will show the A1 segment of the anterior cerebral artery together with the supraclinoid segment of the internal carotid artery forming a reversed-C pattern. Lateral displacement of the cavernous segments of the internal carotid arteries, commonly seen with large pituitary tumors, is not present with tuberculum meningiomas since they do not grow inferiorly into the sella. The majority of tuberculum meningiomas will demonstrate a blush on internal carotid arteriography, but it may be very subtle. By increasing the amount of contrast medium injected and prolonging the injection, nearly all will show a blush. The arterial supply may be from several sources, but the main source is the posterior ethmoidal branch of the ophthalmic artery, which can often be demonstrated by subtraction angiography. Another sign of ophthalmic artery supply, usually apparent on unsubtracted films, is a sudden decrease in the caliber of the ophthalmic artery in the posterior orbit, reflecting the relatively large proportion of ophthalmic artery blood flow that is being channeled to the tumor. The middle meningeal artery does not contribute to the blood supply of the typical tuberculum meningioma **(Option (B) is false).** Besides confirming the diagnosis of tuberculum meningioma, angiography will show whether or not there is significant narrowing of the adjacent internal carotid artery (less often present with tuberculum meningiomas than with cavernous sinus meningiomas) and will rule out suprasellar giant aneurysm, which may mimic tuberculum meningioma on CT.

Question 42

Concerning craniopharyngiomas,

(A) calcification is usually peripheral and curvilinear
(B) they are more often calcified in adults than in children
(C) they are more likely than other suprasellar masses to grow into the posterior fossa
(D) visual changes are less common than endocrine changes
(E) if the solid portion of a partly cystic tumor can be removed, the tumor will rarely recur

Craniopharyngiomas are benign tumors of neuroectodermal origin that arise from remnants of Rathke's pouch. Over 75% of these tumors are found in the suprasellar cistern, and approximately 20% extend into the sella. Occasionally, craniopharyngiomas arise primarily within the third ventricle, more often in adults. It is important to recognize this third ventricular origin, since this affects surgical considerations. Craniopharyngiomas may occur in any age group, but approximately 75% are found in children and adolescents. It is the most common suprasellar mass in childhood, and the second most common, after pituitary adenomas, when the entire population is considered. The most common presenting symptoms are headache and endocrine disturbances, particularly diabetes insipidus. Abnormalities in vision occur later and are often absent, even when the tumors are very large **(Option (D) is true).** This tendency for vision to be spared is probably due to the cystic nature of the majority of craniopharyngiomas, as well as to the typical posterior suprasellar location, which is behind the optic chiasm. The same two factors probably also play a role in the tendency for craniopharyngiomas to grow through the tentorial hiatus into the posterior fossa, which they do more frequently than other suprasellar tumors **(Option (C) is true)** (Figures 9-13 and 9-14).

Calcification is very common in craniopharyngiomas, occurring in about 75% of those cases seen in children and 25 to 50% of those seen in adults **(Option (B) is false).** The calcification is usually coarse and nodular and may be seen in only part of the tumor. Peripheral curvilinear calcification is very rare in craniopharyngiomas, so they tend not to mimic the appearance of suprasellar aneurysms **(Option (A) is false).**

More than 75% of craniopharyngiomas have cystic elements, and more than half are entirely cystic. When a suprasellar mass is partly cystic and partly solid and contains coarse calcifications, the diagnosis is simple. When two of these three findings are present, particularly in children,

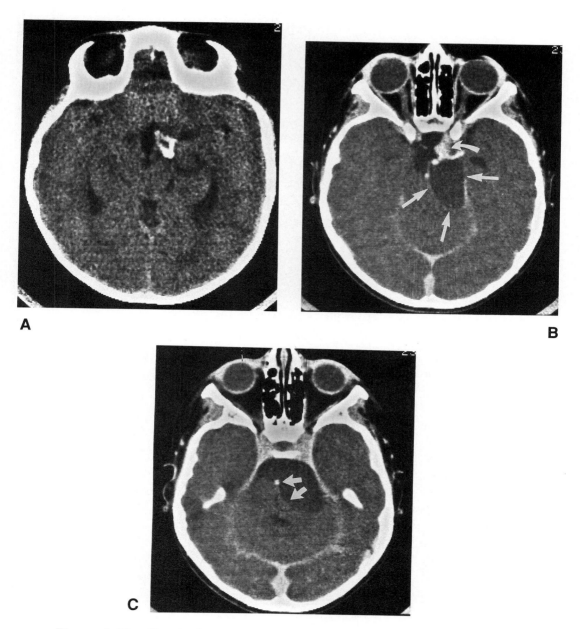

Figure 9-13. Craniopharyngioma in a child. (A) Precontrast section shows dense suprasellar calcification. (B) Postcontrast section immediately above the sella shows the cystic (straight arrows) and the solid (curved arrow) enhancing portions of the tumor. (C) Section at the level of the sella shows extension of the cystic tumor into the posterior fossa, displacing the pons and basilar artery (arrows).

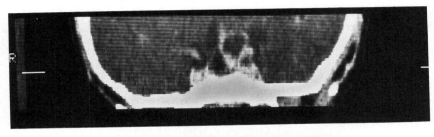

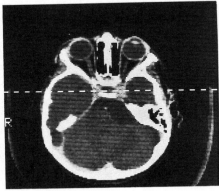

Figure 9-14. Same patient as in Figure 9-13. Reformatted coronal view emphasizes mixed solid and cystic makeup of the tumor.

craniopharyngioma remains the primary choice. When a purely cystic suprasellar mass with an enhancing rim is seen in a child, craniopharyngioma is still the first choice. If the lesion does not have an enhancing rim, differentiation from such lesions as arachnoid cyst and epidermoid tumor is difficult or impossible by CT. Among the suprasellar masses, craniopharyngiomas and hypothalamic gliomas are most likely to cause hydrocephalus. In those unusual cases in which hypothalamic gliomas are partly cystic (Figure 9-15), differentiation from craniopharyngiomas by CT may not be possible. In such cases, it is important to check carefully for an extension of the tumor along the optic nerves or optic tracts, a common feature with hypothalamic gliomas but one not seen with craniopharyngiomas.

Although they are benign, slow-growing tumors, craniopharyngiomas are difficult to treat. They are commonly large by the time they are discovered, and complete surgical excision is often not possible. High rates of recurrence are also common. Since the cysts of craniopharyngiomas are surrounded by a thin wall of tumor tissue, tumors will generally recur if portions of a cyst wall are left in place **(Option (E) is false).**

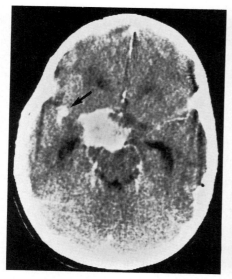
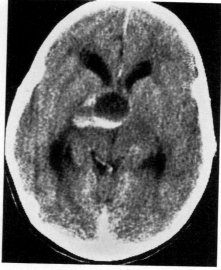

A

B

Figure 9-15. Hypothalamic glioma. Two postcontrast axial CT sections through a large hypothalamic glioma in a child. (A) This level shows a typical large mass with irregular borders. The lateral extension into the right Sylvian fissure (arrow) is unusual. (B) A higher level demonstrates a cyst within the tumor. No optic nerve extension was present in this case.

Postoperative radiation is commonly used in an attempt to decrease the rate of recurrence, even though these tumors are not particularly radiosensitive.

Question 43

Concerning giant aneurysms,

(A) most suprasellar giant aneurysms arise from the internal carotid artery
(B) their CT pattern is most specific when the aneurysm is partially thrombosed
(C) they are usually found in elderly patients with generalized arteriosclerotic disease
(D) following contrast infusion, CT usually shows intense uniform contrast enhancement
(E) when CT shows no calcification within a suprasellar mass, aneurysm is very unlikely

According to the most common definition, a giant aneurysm is one with a diameter of more than 2.5 cm. These aneurysms are quite rare; fewer than 5% of all aneurysms are giant aneurysms. The most common sites of origin include the cavernous portion of the carotid artery, the supraclinoid segment of the carotid artery, and the bifurcation of the internal carotid artery **(Option (A) is true).** Approximately 25% of giant aneurysms arise from the vertebral-basilar system. They may be found in patients of all ages, even in children. The presence of these aneurysms does not correlate well with arteriosclerotic changes in other intracranial arteries **(Option (C) is false).** It is not at all clear why they occur and why they continue to grow, often to very impressive dimensions. Among the possible explanations for continued growth are progressive weakening of the defective wall of the aneurysm and repeated bleeding episodes, with progressive walling-off of these additional bleeds. Giant aneurysms rarely bleed, at least by comparison with other aneurysms. Some surgical series have described bleeding in 25 to 33% of giant aneurysms, but such figures are probably affected by an increased tendency to refer patients with giant aneurysms to specialized surgical centers when there has been subarachnoid or intracerebral bleeding. A wide variety of symptoms result from the growth of these aneurysms, such as headache, visual deficits, ophthalmoplegia, and hydrocephalus. Because of the nature of the symptoms and their superficial resemblance to neoplasms on CT scanning, giant aneurysms are frequently misdiagnosed as brain tumors. It is therefore very important to be aware of the CT signs that suggest the diagnosis of giant aneurysm.

There are three types of giant aneurysms, with three different CT patterns. The most common type of giant aneurysm is the partially thrombosed aneurysm, as seen in the test patient. Nearly 75% of these partially thrombosed aneurysms have some degree of peripheral curvilinear calcification. However, giant aneurysms that are not partially thrombosed are usually not calcified. Therefore, giant aneurysm must always be considered in the diagnosis of suprasellar masses, even when calcification is not present **(Option (E) is false).**

The thrombosed portion of the partially thrombosed aneurysm may be of variable density on a precontrast scan. This does not change with contrast infusion. There is typically good opacification of the wall of the aneurysm; this is presumably related to its rich vascular supply. The lumen of the aneurysm is also strongly enhanced, as expected, but its shape and size vary considerably. It may be serpentine, pursuing an irregular course through the aneurysm. Dynamic CT scanning following bolus injection of contrast agent with graphic data analysis clearly shows the vascular nature of the lumen. The three zones of the aneurysm described above have inspired the use of the term "target sign" to describe

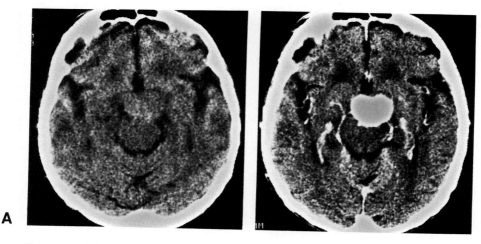

A

B

Figure 9-16. Suprasellar giant globoid aneurysm. (A) The precontrast axial CT scan shows the density of the lesion to be essentially the same as that of adjacent brain, probably due to the patient's anemic state. (B) The postcontrast axial CT scan shows typical uniformly high-density enhancement in an aneurysm without a clot.

this typical CT appearance. Of the three types of giant aneurysm, CT is most specific for the partially thrombosed aneurysm **(Option (B) is true).**

The nonthrombosed giant aneurysm will show intense uniform contrast enhancement on CT. However, these aneurysms are not as common as the partially thrombosed type, and therefore uniform enhancement is not seen in the typical giant aneurysm **(Option (D) is false).** The borders of nonthrombosed giant aneurysms are usually smooth and sharp, and adjacent edema is very unusual. The wall of the aneurysm is seldom calcified. On precontrast CT scans, the aneurysm usually has a higher density than that of adjacent brain. However, this may not be true in anemic patients (Figure 9-16). Meningiomas may closely resemble suprasellar nonthrombosed giant aneurysm. Bone sclerosis is not seen with giant aneurysms and should be looked for in such situations. Angiography is generally advisable in either case.

Completely thrombosed aneurysms are the least common of the three varieties. The appearance of these aneurysms is similar to that of partially thrombosed aneurysms, except that the enhancing aneurysm lumen is not visible. The "target sign" is therefore absent.

John R. Bentson, M.D.

SUGGESTED READINGS

GIANT ANEURYSMS

1. Byrd SE, Bentson JR, Winter J, Wilson GH, Joyce PW, O'Connor L. Giant intracranial aneurysms simulating brain neoplasms on computed tomography. J Comput Assist Tomogr 1978; 2:303–307
2. Ganti SR, Steinberger A, McMurtry JG III, Hilal SK. Computed tomographic demonstration of giant aneurysms of the vertebrobasilar system: report of eight cases. Neurosurgery 1981; 9:261–267
3. Macpherson P, Anderson DE. Radiological differentiation of intrasellar aneurysms from pituitary tumours. Neuroradiology 1981; 21:177–183
4. Pinto RS, Cohen WA, Kricheff II, Redington RW, Berninger WH. Giant intracranial aneurysms: rapid sequential computed tomography. AJR 1982; 139:973–977
5. Post MJ, Glaser JS, Trobe JD. The radiographic diagnosis of cavernous meningiomas and aneurysms with a review of the neurovascular anatomy of the cavernous sinus. CRC Crit Rev Diagn Imaging 1979; 12:1–34
6. Raymond LA, Tew J. Large suprasellar aneurysms imitating pituitary tumour. J Neurol Neurosurg Psychiatry 1978; 41:83–87
7. Schubiger O, Valavanis A, Hayek J. Computed tomography in cerebral aneurysms with special emphasis on giant intracranial aneurysms. J Comput Assist Tomogr 1980; 4:24–32
8. Sonntag VK, Yuan RH, Stein BM. Giant intracranial aneurysms: a review of 13 cases. Surg Neurol 1977; 8:81–84
9. Sundt TM Jr, Piepgras DG. Surgical approach to giant intracranial aneurysms. Operative experience with 80 cases. J Neurosurg 1979; 51:731–742

SELLAR AND PARASELLAR TUMORS

10. Baker HL Jr. The angiographic delineation of sellar and parasellar masses. Radiology 1972; 104:67–78
11. Banna M, Baker HL Jr, Houser OW. Pituitary and parapituitary tumours on computed tomography. A review article based on 230 cases. Br J Radiol 1980; 53:1123–1143
12. Fitz CR, Wortzman G, Harwood-Nash DC, Holgate RC, Barry JF, Boldt DW. Computed tomography in craniopharyngiomas. Radiology 1978; 127:687–691
13. Miller JH, Pena AM, Segall HD. Radiological investigation of sellar region masses in children. Radiology 1980; 134:81–87
14. Naidich TP, Pinto RS, Kushner MJ, et al. Evaluation of sellar and parasellar masses by computed tomography. Radiology 1976; 120:91–99
15. Numaguchi Y, Kishikawa T, Ikeda J, et al. Neuroradiological manifestations of suprasellar pituitary adenomas, meningiomas and craniopharyngiomas. Neuroradiology 1981; 21:67–74

16. Post MJ, David NJ, Glaser JS, Safran A. Pituitary apoplexy: diagnosis by computed tomography. Radiology 1980; 134:665–670

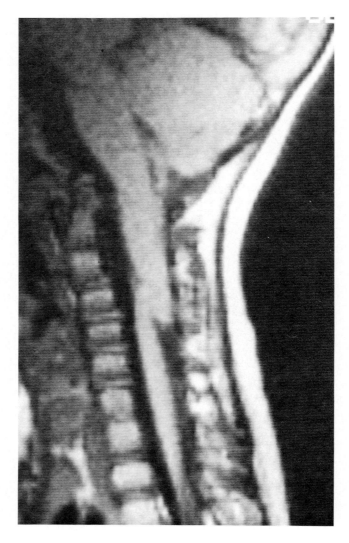

Figure 10-1. This 2-year-old girl presented with weakness of the lower extremities. You are shown a midsagittal magnetic resonance (MR) image of the craniovertebral junction (0.5 T; TR, 500 msec; TE, 30 msec).

Case 10: Chiari II Malformation

Question 44

Which *one* of the following is the MOST likely diagnosis?

(A) Cerebellar tumor with tonsillar herniation
(B) Inferior extraventricular extension of fourth ventricular ependymoma
(C) Chiari II malformation
(D) Spinal cord astrocytoma
(E) Foramen magnum-upper cervical neurinoma

This patient's MR image (Figure 10-1) demonstrates features typical of the Chiari II malformation (see Figure 10-2) **(Option (C) is correct)**. The anatomic features of Chiari II malformation displayed in the image are detailed in the legend to Figure 10-2. Chiari II malformation is characterized by inferior protrusion of the spinal cord, medulla, fourth ventricle, and cerebellum downward through an abnormally large foramen magnum into the upper cervical spinal canal. In many of the cases, the medulla buckles behind the spinal cord, producing a kink at the point of buckling and a spur that corresponds to the actual cervicomedullary junction. The fourth ventricle is tubular and elongate. The signal intensity of all structures corresponds to that of normal brain. These findings are sufficient to permit immediate identification of this abnormality as the Chiari II malformation. As expected for a patient with a Chiari II malformation, this girl also has lumbar spina bifida and repaired myelomeningocele (not shown). Retethering of the spinal cord at the surgical repair site caused the progressive dysfunction of the lower extremities (see Case 14).

Tonsillar herniation from cerebellar tumor (Option (A)) is unlikely, because the structure protruding inferiorly into the spinal canal is the medulla, not the tonsil. The tonsil normally forms part of the posterior inferior wall of the fourth ventricle, whereas the brain stem (pons and medulla) form the anterior wall of the fourth ventricle. The tissue seen extending into the canal lies anterior to the tubular fourth ventricle, and so it is brain stem tissue. Furthermore, there is no evidence of a cerebellar

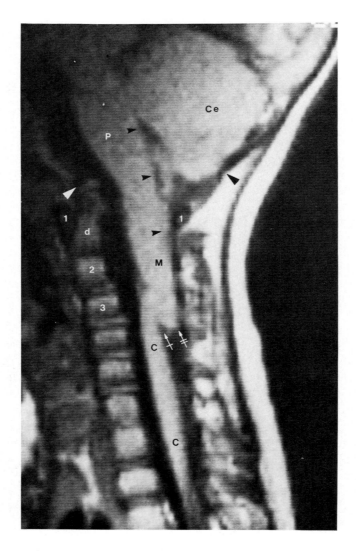

Figure 10-2 (Same as Figure 10-1). The image demonstrates the typical findings of a Chiari II malformation: a wide foramen magnum (between large arrowheads), a narrow C1 ring (1), typical concavity of the posterior borders of C2 and C3 (2 and 3) with a correspondingly widened ventral subarachnoid space, a low position of the spinal cord (C), kinking of the dorsal surface of the cervical spinal cord (crossed white arrow), a spur (doubly crossed white arrow) at the cervicomedullary junction, a low position of the medulla (M), indentation of the ventral surface of the pons (P) by the dens (d), a low position of the cerebellum (Ce), protrusion of the cerebellum inferiorly through the foramen magnum, a low position of the fourth ventricle (small arrowheads), and a virtual absence of the cisterna magna. This case would be classified as group 4 (see Figure 10-13).

tumor. Extraventricular extension of fourth ventricular ependymoma (Option (B)) can be discounted because the fourth ventricle is not expanded and contains no tumor. The tissue protruding into the cervical canal clearly arises in smooth continuity from the floor of the fourth ventricle (i.e., the brain stem) and shows no abnormalities of signal intensity to suggest tumor. Spinal cord astrocytoma (Option (D)) could be considered if the tumor were thought to be exophytic (to account for the kink and spur) and if the tumor were thought to extend directly superiorly into the brain stem. Once again, however, there is no hint of signal abnormality to suggest tumor. Furthermore, a spinal cord astrocytoma could not account for the wide foramen magnum, which is clearly a congenital abnormality. A foramen magnum-upper cervical neurinoma (Option (E)) can be discounted, because the lesion shown is clearly intrinsic to brain parenchyma and does not invaginate into it from the outside.

Diverse lesions may present with clinical evidence of a cervicomedullary lesion and with radiological evidence of "lumps and bumps" within the uppermost spinal canal, just below the foramen magnum. Wickbom and Hanafee analyzed 105 masses presenting immediately below the foramen magnum and documented that the vast majority of these (77%) were the lower poles of cerebellar tonsils that had herniated inferiorly because of either infratentorial tumor (49%) or supratentorial tumor (28%). Eleven percent of masses were the lower poles of intracranial tumors that had grown downward through the foramen magnum into the spinal canal. Eight percent were the deformed hindbrains associated with Chiari malformations. Only 4% were primary tumors of the cervical spine and foramen magnum (Table 10-1). Similarly, in 40 lesions of the foramen magnum, LaMasters et al. found 14 cases of Chiari malformations (8 Chiari I and 6 Chiari II) but only 8 primary benign extramedullary tumors of the foramen magnum (5 meningiomas and 3 neuromas). Therefore, interpretation of images that display upper spinal "masses" must take into account the frequency of tonsillar herniation, the possibility of direct spinal extension of an intracranial mass, and the twofold-greater likelihood of Chiari malformations than of rare primary spinal-foramen magnum masses.

Table 10-1. Differential diagnosis of 105 masses situated immediately
below the foramen magnum*

Diagnosis	No. of cases	%
Tonsillar herniation	81	77.1
Infratentorial tumor	52	
Supratentorial tumor	29	
Direct intraspinal extension of intracranial tumor	12	11.5
Exophytic fourth ventricular tumor	7	
Cerebellar-tonsillar astrocytomas	3	
Cerebellopontine angle tumor	1	
Brain stem glioma	1	
Chiari malformation	8	7.6
Chiari I	6	
Chiari II and III	2	
Primary spinal-foramen magnum tumor	4	3.8
Neuroma	2	
Dermoid	1	
Hemangioendothelioma	1	

*Adapted from Wickbom and Hanafee [32].

Question 45

Tonsillar herniation

  (A) may be diagnosed confidently when the lower poles of the tonsils lie inferior to the lower lip of the foramen magnum

  (B) is the most common mass displacement caused by space-occupying intracranial lesions

  (C) is more common with occipital glioma than with anterior falcine meningioma

  (D) is more common with external obstructive hydrocephalus than with aqueductal stenosis

  (E) is associated with a positive Lhermitte's sign

    The normal position of the tonsil is variable. The precise baseline chosen for determining the tonsillar position is the line drawn between the inferior lip of the clivus at the anterior rim of the foramen magnum (basion) and the *inferior* surface of the posterior rim of the foramen magnum (opisthion). The basion and opisthion are easily delineated on sagittal magnetic resonance imaging (MRI), because the low-signal cortical bone stands out in contrast to the high-signal apical fat pad of

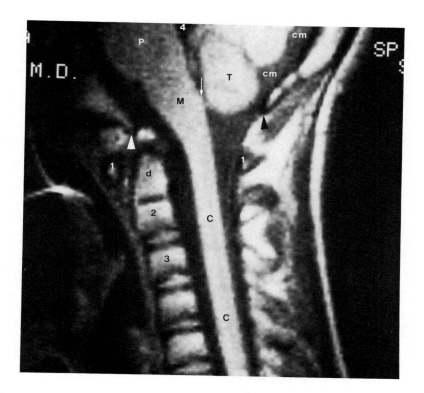

Figure 10-3. Normal cervicomedullary and craniovertebral junctions. Sagittal MR image (0.5 T; TR, 500 msec; TE, 30 msec) in a 12-year-old boy. The plane of the foramen magnum is defined by the line drawn between the basion (large white arrowhead) and the opisthion (large black arrowhead). The pons (P), medulla (M), tonsil (T), fourth ventricle (4), and cervicomedullary junction lie above this line. The cisterna magna (cm) is full and leads to the full subarachnoid space surrounding the spinal cord (C). The clava (white arrow) is the name given to the tubercle of the gracile nucleus at the upper end of the dorsal columns of the spinal cord, i.e., at the cervicomedullary junction. The clava normally forms a slight mound that is convex toward the tonsil and fourth ventricle. The ostium of the central canal of the spinal cord lies just anterior to the clava. Visualized portions of the cervical spine include the anterior and posterior arches of C1 (1), the base of C2 (2), the dens (d), and C3 (3).

the dens and the suboccipital fat behind the foramen magnum (Figures 10-3 and 10-4). Barkovich et al. showed that the lower pole of the tonsil may normally lie anywhere from 8 mm above the foramen magnum to 5 mm below it (mean, 1 mm above the foramen magnum). Fourteen percent of normal patients have tonsils slightly below the foramen magnum.

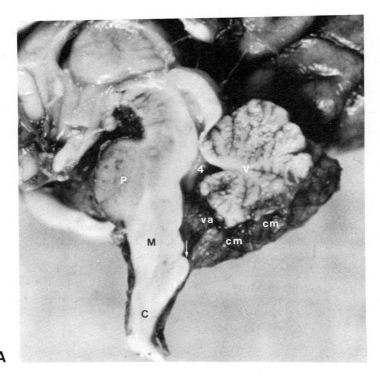

A

Figure 10-4. Normal anatomy of the cervicomedullary junction. (A) Midsagittal specimen of a 10-week-old girl demonstrates the anatomic relationships among the pons (P), medulla (M), spinal cord (C), clava (white arrow), fourth ventricle (4), vallecula (va), cisterna magna (cm) overlying the medial surface of the cerebellar hemisphere, and vermis (V). (B) Paramedian sagittal specimen of a 2-month-old girl demonstrates the ovoid shape and the off-midline, paramedian position of the tonsil (T) between the medulla (M) and the cerebellum (Ce). The part of the cerebellum shown is the lateral portion of the vermis where it merges into the cerebellar hemisphere. P = pons. Note that the folia and fissures of the tonsil are aligned horizontally, perpendicular to the posterior surface of the medulla. The folia and fissures of the vermis are oriented radially, like a starburst centered on the fastigium of the fourth ventricle (4). This difference in orientation is appreciable by MRI and helps in analyzing the site and effects of pathology. (Photographs are modified from Yousefzadeh and Naidich [34]).

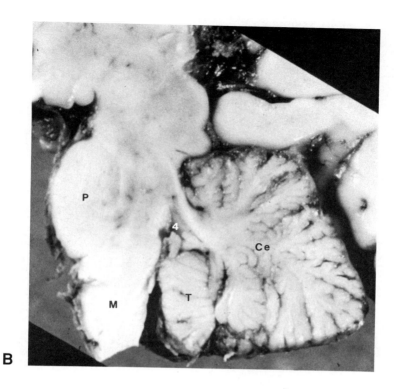

B

Thus, protrusion of the tonsils less than 2 mm below the foramen magnum is probably of no clinical significance. A lower limit of normal set at 2 mm below the foramen magnum discriminates symptomatic abnormal patients from normal subjects with 100% sensitivity and 98.5% specificity. With the lower limit of normal at 3 mm below the foramen magnum, the corresponding values are 96% sensitivity and 99.5% specificity.

Aboulezz et al. similarly found that the lower poles of normal tonsils lay from 20 mm above the foramen magnum to 2.8 mm below the foramen magnum (mean, 2.9 mm above). They concluded that the tonsillar position was normal if the lower pole lay no more than 3 mm below the basion-opisthion line, equivocally abnormal if it lay 3 to 5 mm below this line, and definitely abnormal if it lay more than 5 mm below this line **(Option (A) is false).**

Because of the wide range of normal positions for the tonsil, a tonsil that lies "within normal limits," i.e., only a few millimeters below the foramen magnum, may actually be abnormal and may have been displaced to this position by a mass or malformation. Furthermore, the

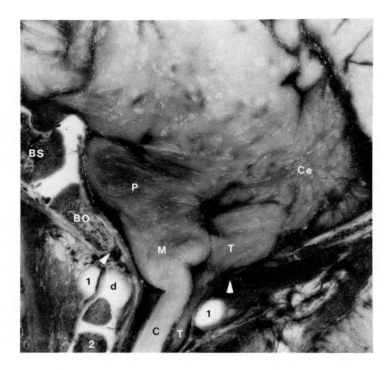

Figure 10-5. Sagittal anatomic specimen of tonsillar herniation in a newborn. Severe cerebral swelling compresses the cerebellum (Ce), pons (P), and medulla (M), displaces them inferiorly, buckles the cervicomedullary junction, and causes marked caudal herniation of the tonsil (T) through the foramen magnum (arrowheads) into the cervical subarachnoid space posterior to the spinal cord (C). Also labeled are the ossification centers for the basisphenoid (BS) and basiocciput (BO) that form the clivus, as well as the anterior and posterior arches of C1 (1), the cartilaginous tip of the dens (d), and the body of C2 (2).

two tonsils may be asymmetrical and may extend inferiorly for different distances.

The term tonsillar herniation signifies caudal protrusion of one or both tonsils into the cervical spinal subarachnoid space posterolateral to the spinal cord. Such herniation may be symmetrical or asymmetrical and mild or very severe. Most frequently the tonsils herniate no further inferiorly than the level of the C1 arch. Rarely, tonsillar tissue may protrude far caudally (Figure 10-5).

Tonsillar herniation is the most common mass displacement caused by space-occupying intracranial lesions **(Option (B) is true).** It is especially pronounced when the vector of forces is aligned along the clivus or other walls of the posterior fossa, thereby driving the tonsils inferiorly into the spinal canal. Thus, tonsillar herniation is especially prominent with posterior fossa tumors, large incisural masses, and large anterior frontal masses such as anterior falcine meningiomas (Figure 10-6). Tonsillar herniation is far less likely to result from occipital masses, since the posterior fossa is then relatively protected from the force of the mass by the rigid posterior falx and tentorium **(Option (C) is false).** Tonsillar herniation may be expected in approximately 8% of *all* supratentorial tumors and 38% of *all* infratentorial tumors. Wickbom and Hanafee reported that, among the latter, it occurs in 65% of tumors of the cerebellar hemispheres and vermis, 56% of tentorial meningiomas, 30% of cerebellopontine angle masses, and 16% of brain stem masses. Tonsillar herniation is also frequent when severe supratentorial hydrocephalus balloons the lateral and third ventricles without creating any balancing force within the posterior fossa. This situation occurs, for example, in patients with aqueductal stenosis or periaqueductal tumors (Figure 10-7). In aqueductal stenosis, the dilated third ventricle also commonly bulges through the incisura to compress the cerebellum directly, crowding the tonsils further inferiorly toward the foramen magnum. Conversely, in external obstructive hydrocephalus (communicating hydrocephalus) the forces are more equally balanced between the supratentorial ventricles above and the enlarged fourth ventricle and basal cisterns below. Moreover, as reported by El Gammal, in communicating hydrocephalus the dilated basal cisterns tend to elevate the tonsils and cerebellum off the floor of the posterior fossa, away from the foramen magnum, reducing the chance of tonsillar herniation **(Option (D) is false).**

Pathologically, tonsillar herniation results in tonsillar edema and swelling. The swollen tonsils usually appear bulbous rather than triangular. The tonsils become molded or "notched" by the round lip of the foramen magnum. Detection of such notching suggests tonsillar herniation, irrespective of the exact position of the lower pole of the tonsil. When tonsillar swelling is severe, it may be followed by necrosis of the subjacent, compressed medulla and spinal cord; superficial cortical hemorrhages where the cerebellar folia are compressed against the edges of the foramen magnum; and even hemorrhagic necrosis of the tonsils themselves.

When the cerebellar tonsils and hemispheres are squeezed into the spinal subarachnoid space, cerebellar tissue may be deposited in the leptomeninges of the more dependent portions of the spinal cord. Such tissues may grossly mimic metastases to the subarachnoid space.

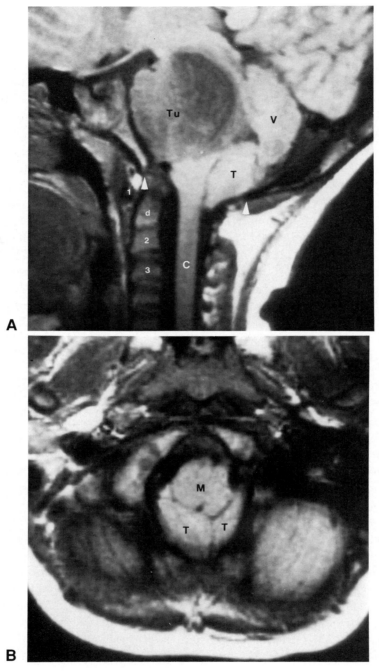

Figure 10-6. Tonsillar herniation from a posterior fossa mass in a 6-year-old boy with a brain stem glioma. (A) Midsagittal MR image (1.5 T; TR, 600 msec; TE, 20 msec). The large tumor (Tu) compresses the tonsil (T), displaces the tonsil posteriorly to obliterate the cisterna magna, and causes the tonsil to herniate downward through the foramen magnum (arrowheads) into the cervical subarachnoid space posterior to the spinal cord (C). V = vermis; 1 = C1; 2 = C2; 3 = C3; d = dens. (B) Axial MR image (same parameters) at and below the foramen magnum. The two tonsils (T) fill the subarachnoid space posterior to the cervicomedullary junction (M).

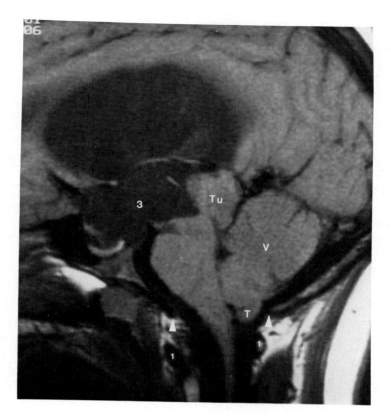

Figure 10-7. Obstruction of the aqueduct by a large tectal tumor in a 13-year-old boy. Sagittal MR image (1.5 T; TR, 600 msec; TE, 25 msec). Hydrocephalic distension of the lateral and third (3) ventricles plus the mass of the tumor (Tu) itself compress the brain stem and vermis (V), obliterate the cisterna magna, and drive the tonsil (T) inferiorly through the foramen magnum (arrowheads). 1 = C1.

Clinically, tonsillar herniation gives rise to painful neck stiffness, aggravated by movement. Passive flexion of the neck can cause an "electric shock" that travels down the trunk. This is a positive Lhermitte's sign **(Option (E) is true).**

Tonsillar herniation may also result in splinting that is interpreted as torticollis, especially when an asymmetrical posterior fossa tumor causes asymmetrical or unilateral tonsillar herniation. Less commonly, such torticollis results from a spinal cord tumor. Patients with torticollis and any suspicious clinical or historical findings should be studied extensively to exclude an underlying tumor.

Question 46

Tumors that grow downward through the foramen magnum into the posterior cervical subarachnoid space include:

(A) ependymoma
(B) medulloblastoma
(C) cerebellar astrocytoma
(D) epidermoid tumor of the fourth ventricle
(E) meningioma

Intracranial tumors may grow directly into the cervical spinal canal, producing anatomic distortions that can mimic the appearance of other conditions. Thus, ependymomas, medulloblastomas, cerebellar astrocytomas, epidermoid tumors of the fourth ventricle, and meningiomas of the posterior fossa may all grow into the spinal subarachnoid space **(Options A through E are all true).** Tonsillar tumors may grow through the foramen magnum as a special type of tonsillar herniation (Figure 10-8). Fourth ventricular ependymomas characteristically expand the fourth ventricle, elevate the vermis, grow exophytically through the foramen of Magendie, fill the vallecula and cisterna magna with a gelatinous mass of tumor, and then grow caudally through the foramen magnum into the cervical subarachnoid space behind or entirely around the entire upper cervical cord (Figure 10-9). Brain stem gliomas may expand the medulla and give rise to exophytic nodules of tumor that extend into and inferior to the foramen magnum (Figure 10-10). A specific analysis of the primary site of origin of tumors that extend directly through the foramen magnum indicates that such growth may be expected with approximately 10% of all infratentorial tumors, 39% of tumors arising within the fourth ventricle, 6% of tumors of the cerebellar hemispheres and vermis, 4% of cerebellopontine angle tumors, and 3% of brain stem tumors. Such growth is not expected with tentorial meningiomas or supratentorial tumors. The "lumps and bumps" associated with direct caudal growth of a tumor (or with tonsillar herniation) should not be misinterpreted as a Chiari I or Chiari II malformation or vice versa.

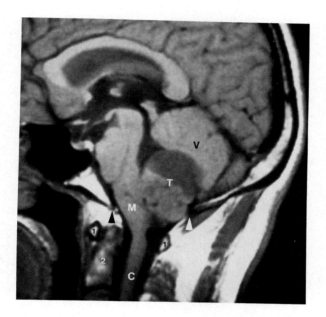

Figure 10-8. Tonsillar hemangioblastoma in a 41-year-old man. Sagittal MR image (1.5 T; TR, 600 msec; TE, 20 msec). A tumor within the tonsil (T) enlarges the tonsil, elevates the vermis (V), compresses the cisterna magna, and grows downward through the foramen magnum (arrowheads) to form a lobulated mass within the cervical spinal canal superior to C1 (1). The mass also compresses the medulla (M) and displaces the cervicomedullary junction inferiorly. 2 = C2; C = spinal cord.

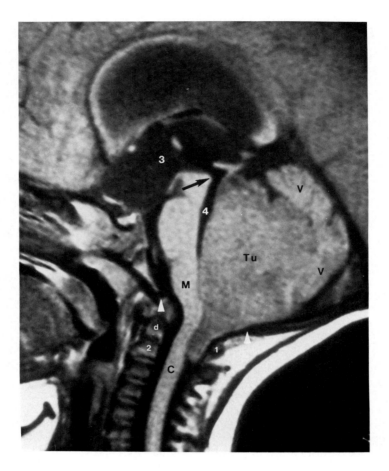

Figure 10-9. Ependymoma in a 1-year-old girl (1.5 T; TR, 600 msec; TE, 25 msec). The slightly inhomogeneous mottled low-signal-intensity tumor (Tu) elevates and compresses the vermis (V), compresses the fourth ventricle, extends through the foramen of Magendie and vallecula to fill the cisterna magna, and grows downward through the foramen magnum (arrowheads) to form a tongue of tissue in the posterior cervical subarachnoid space. The medulla (M) and spinal cord (C) are compressed and displaced anteriorly. The lateral and third (3) ventricles, the aqueduct (black arrow), and the residual proximal fourth ventricle (4) show obstructive dilatation. Note the CSF flow void within the aqueduct and fourth ventricle. d = dens; 1 = C1; 2 = C2.

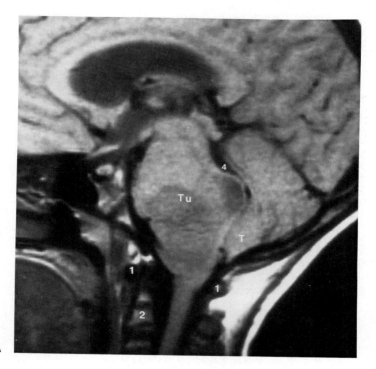

A

Figure 10-10. Brain stem glioma in a 7-year-old boy. (A and B) Sagittal MR images (1.5 T; TR, 600 msec; TE, 25 msec). The inhomogeneous low-signal-intensity tumor (Tu) expands the brain stem and bulges exophytically into the fourth ventricle (4), bowing it posteriorly. The tumor expands the medulla (M), displaces it downward through the foramen magnum (arrowhead), and creates a bulbous cervicomedullary junction that superficially resembles the kink and spur of the Chiari II malformation (see Figures 10-2 and 10-16). The tonsil (T) is compressed, and its tip is driven caudally through the foramen magnum into the cervical spinal canal. 1 = C1; 2 = C2. (C) Axial MR image (same parameters) at and just inferior to the foramen magnum. The inhomogeneous tumor extends into the medulla (M) and expands the restiform body (white arrow) asymmetrically. The two tonsils (T) herniate caudally to different degrees.

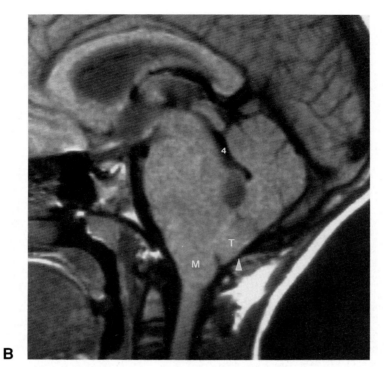

B

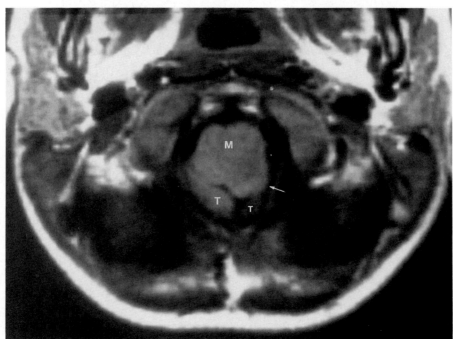

C

Question 47

Concerning the Chiari malformations,

(A) clinically evident myelomeningocele signifies Type II
(B) cervical "spur" and "kink" signify Type I
(C) segmentation anomalies of the cervical spine and skull base are more commonly associated with Type I than with Type II
(D) hydrocephalus occurs more frequently with Type I than with Type II
(E) downbeat nystagmus suggests the presence of Type I

The Chiari II malformation is a specific deformity of the hindbrain that is nearly always associated with myelomeningocele. In brief, this malformation consists of caudal displacement of (i) the cervical spinal cord, (ii) the cervicomedullary junction, (iii) the medulla (and often the pons), (iv) the fourth ventricle, and (v) the cerebellum (Figure 10-2). These structures protrude into the upper cervical spinal canal to a variable degree, producing a spectrum of pathology that is easily identified as the Chiari II malformation. Nearly every case of Chiari II deformity is associated with myelomeningocele **(Option (A) is true).** These conditions are so closely associated that detection of either implies the presence of the other. In any patient with cervicomedullary pathology, the presence of concurrent myelomeningocele strongly suggests that the pathology is related to Chiari II malformation rather than tumor.

In the Chiari II malformation, the bony and dural posterior fossa is abnormally small. The foramen magnum is unusually large, with a long sagittal dimension. Perhaps for these reasons, the neural structures that should grow *within* the posterior fossa instead grow downward through the large foramen magnum into the upper cervical spinal canal. Evidence suggests that the spinal cord descends as much as possible, so that the dorsal cervical roots ascend retrograde from the cord to their exit foramina. The individual segments of the cervical cord become compacted and shortened in their vertical height (Figure 10-11). The extent to which the cervical cord can descend is limited by the attachment of the dentate ligaments to the dura.

The normal dentate ligaments are fibrous bands of pia mater that extend downward along the equator of the spinal cord between the dorsal and ventral pairs of nerve roots on each side. The lateral borders of the dentate ligaments attach to the dura at 21 regularly spaced sites, the highest of which lies between the foramen magnum and the rootlets of the hypoglossal (twelfth cranial) nerve. In normal patients the dentate ligaments are short, so the cord can descend only 3 mm. If the dentate

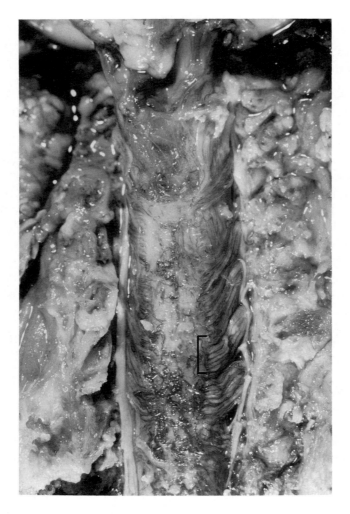

Figure 10-11. Chiari II hindbrain. Upper cervical spinal cord viewed from behind. The dorsal cervical nerve roots C2 to C6 ascend to their exit foramina. The vertical distance (bracket) over which the rootlets arise for each of the seven dorsal cervical nerve roots defines the height of each cervical cord segment. The closer spacing of the C3 to C6 dorsal nerve rootlets indicates shorter cervical cord segments and suggests vertical compression and compaction of these segments. (Reprinted from Naidich et al. [15] with permission.)

ligaments are cut, the cord may descend as much as 10 mm. In patients with Chiari II malformations the dentate ligaments are variable in length, permitting varying degrees of cord descent. The dentate ligaments are also unusually broad and tend to spread out over the dorsal surface of the cord as an "aponeurosis" or "sling" that suspends the cord from the foramen magnum.

The medulla and cervicomedullary junction usually descend into the cervical spinal canal with the cord (Figures 10-12 and 10-13). The degree of descent varies, creating a spectrum of changes (Figure 10-13). In some cases, the medulla stays directly in line with the cord. In more severe cases, the medulla descends further by buckling behind the cervical cord (Figure 10-12). This buckling kinks the dorsal surface of the cervical cord over the upper border of the dentate "sling." The inferior tip of the medulla forms a spur just posterior to the cord. The cervicomedullary junction lies at the apex of the spur. Thus, the kink and spur are characteristic of the Chiari II malformation but do not appear in every case **(Option (B) is false).**

The medullary spur typically lies between C2 and C4 but may lie as low as the upper thoracic region. The length of the spur correlates with the length of the myelomeningocele, i.e., the number of bifid spinal arches. The length of the spur does not correlate with the specific site of the myelomeningocele.

The Chiari II cerebellum also descends into the cervical spinal canal (Figures 10-14 and 10-15). The inferior border of the cerebellum protrudes downward through the large foramen magnum to rest upon the posterior arch of the C1 ring. A pool of cerebrospinal fluid (CSF) may create a cistern beneath this portion of the cerebellum. From that point, a smaller "tongue" or "peg" of cerebellum protrudes further inferiorly through the C1 ring to lie posterior to the medulla. This peg is usually composed of the nodulus, uvula, and pyramis of the vermis. In 75% of cases, the peg is shorter than the medullary spur, and so the tip of the nodulus lies superior to the tip of the spur. In 25% of cases, the peg is longer than the spur, and so the nodulus lies inferior to the spur (Figure 10-16D and E).

The Chiari II fourth ventricle is a narrow, elongated tube that descends through the posterior fossa, exits via the foramen magnum, and then continues inferiorly into the spinal canal, where it lies immediately behind the medulla, between the medulla and the cerebellum (Figure 10-12). The choroid plexus and the roof of the fourth ventricle form a fibrovascular membrane that extends between the tip of the peg and the tip of the spur (Figure 10-15B). The lowest extent of the fourth ventricle is at or inferior to the tip of the spur (i.e., the cervicomedullary junction)

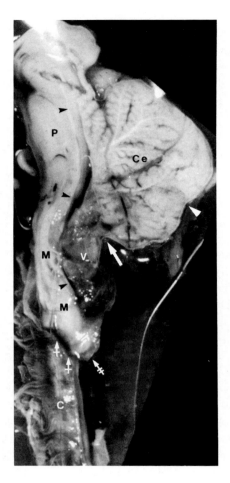

Figure 10-12. Chiari II malformation. Medullary protrusion and cervicomedullary kink. Sagittal anatomic specimen of the brain stem, cerebellum, and fourth ventricle with the plane of section angled to avoid cutting the spinal cord. Anterior is to the left. The large white arrowhead indicates the position of the posterior lip of the foramen magnum. The large white arrow indicates the position of the posterior arch of C1. The Chiari II medulla (M) protrudes below the foramen magnum into the cervical spinal canal. The medulla buckles dorsal to the cervical spinal cord (C), forming a kink (crossed white arrows) and a spur (doubly crossed white arrow). The spur lies dorsal to and overlaps the spinal cord. The cerebellum (Ce) protrudes well below the foramen magnum. The peg (V) protrudes even lower through the C1 ring to lie behind the medulla. The fourth ventricle (small black arrowheads) forms an elongated tube that descends into the cervical spinal canal between the medulla and the cerebellum. The pons (P) and cerebellum are notched at the level of the foramen magnum. The peg is notched at C1. The cascade of hernias within the spinal canal creates multiple "bumps" that should not be misinterpreted as tumors. (Reprinted with permission from Naidich et al. [15]. In this image, the positions given for the foramen magnum and C1 correct an error in the original illustration.)

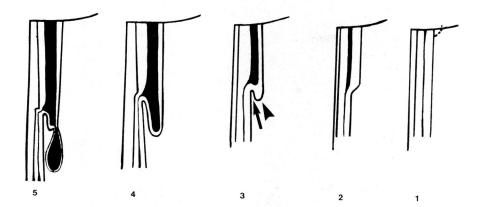

| 5 | 4 | 3 | 2 | 1 |

Figure 10-13. Spectrum of cervicomedullary deformities in the Chiari II malformation. Lateral diagrams of the cervical cord, medulla, and fourth ventricle show a graded series of increasingly more severe deformities. Curved lines at the top indicate the foramen magnum. Black shading indicates the fourth ventricle and the central canal of the spinal cord. (1) Group 1 (4% of cases). The medulla and fourth ventricle do not descend below the foramen magnum. The sole evidence of hindbrain deformity is mild inferior displacement of the spinal canal with ascending cervical nerve roots. (2) Group 2 (26% of cases). The medulla and fourth ventricle descend vertically, in line with and above the displaced cervical cord. The fourth ventricle leads directly inferiorly to the central canal of the cord. (3) Group 3 (26% of cases). The medulla shows mild buckling behind the cord, with less than 5 mm of overlap of the medulla on the cord. This buckling creates the kink (arrow) and spur (arrowhead). Because of the buckling, the fourth ventricle lies partly behind the cord and the central canal arises from the anterior surface of the fourth ventricle. (4) Group 4 (23% of cases). The medulla shows more severe buckling, with more than 5 mm of overlap. (5) Group 5 (21% of cases). Severe buckling is associated with a sac-like process or diverticulum of the dorsal surface of the fourth ventricle that protrudes caudad to the kink and spur. Group 1 cases are found only in patients with sacral, lumbosacral, or lumbar myelomeningocele. The converse is not true; more severe group 2 to 5 deformities are as prevalent among lumbosacral and purely sacral lesions as elsewhere. (Reprinted with permission from Emery and MacKenzie [10].)

(Figure 10-13). When the medulla lies directly in line with the spinal cord, the fourth ventricle forms a vertical tube directly above the central canal of the spinal cord. When the medulla buckles behind the cord, the fourth ventricle descends behind the kink toward or beyond the medullary spur, occasionally forming a tear-drop diverticulum behind the spinal cord. In

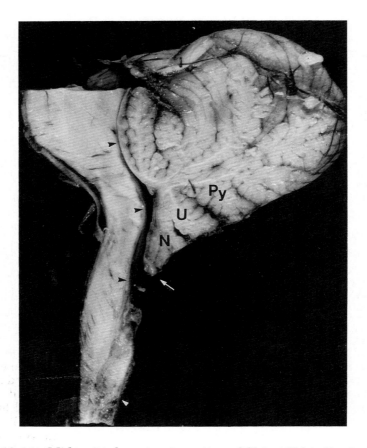

Figure 10-14. Midsagittal anatomic section of Chiari II hindbrain (same patient as in Figure 10-11). The anterior is to the left. The nodulus (N), uvula (U), and pyramis (Py) of the vermis contribute to a cerebellar "peg" or "tail," which protrudes into the cervical subarachnoid space posterior to the fourth ventricle (black arrowheads), medulla, and spinal cord. In this specimen, cerebellar herniation is less extensive than medullary herniation, so the tip of the peg (white arrow) lies above the spur (white arrowhead). (Reprinted with permission from Naidich et al. [15].)

these cases, the central canal of the cord arises from the anterior surface of the fourth ventricle.

The protrusion of cerebellum behind the medulla and of the medulla behind the cord creates a "cascade" of hernias, each of which displaces and compresses all other structures anterior to it. The entire complex is enclosed in the narrow C1 ring that acts like the constricting ostium of a strangulating hernia.

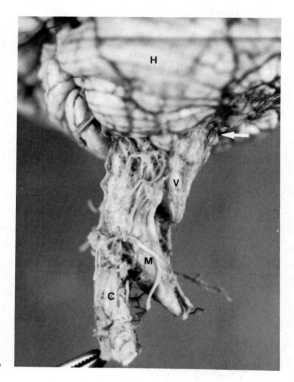

A

Figure 10-15. Lateral views of the Chiari II hindbrain. The anterior is to the left. (A) Uncut anatomic specimen. The overlapping herniations of the medulla (M) on the spinal cord (C) and of the vermian/cerebellar peg (V) on the medulla create a cascade of hernias which impacts in the C1 ring (white arrow). Each new hernia compresses the structure(s) anterior to it, displaces it anteriorly, and narrows its sagittal dimension. Note that the cerebellar hemispheres (H) may extend anteriorly to wrap around the brain stem. (B) Midsagittal section of (A) displays notching of the cerebellum (Ce) at the foramen magnum (large white arrowhead) and at the posterior arch of C1 (large white arrow), extension of the cerebellar hemisphere (H) anterior to the brain stem, marked elongation of the fourth ventricle (small black arrowheads), distal dilatation of the fourth ventricle with the choroid plexus (small white arrow), beaking of the tectum midbrain (MB), and a large massa intermedia (mi). C = spinal cord; M = medulla; P = pons. (Reprinted with permission from Naidich et al. [15].)

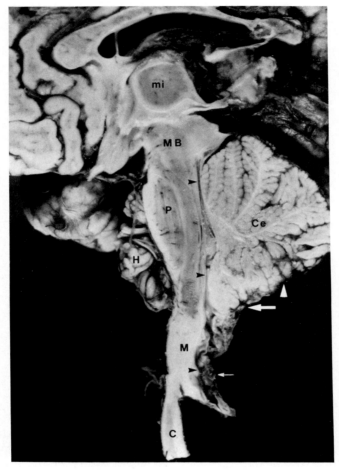

B

The Chiari II deformity has only limited association with segmentation anomalies and other bony anomalies of the cervical spine. In 7% of cases, there is partial fusion of two contiguous neural arches. In 2.5% there is fusion of C2 and C3. Basilar impression and assimilation of C1 to the occiput, which are common in the Chiari I malformation, are not observed in the Chiari II malformation **(Option (C) is true).**

As has been described by Blaauw, the bony posterior arch of C1 is incomplete in 70% of cases of Chiari II malformation. This defect is always filled in by a fibroelastic band, which is distinct from the surrounding tissue and which is firmly attached to the club-shaped free ends of the incomplete arch. C2 is always intact. In 2% of cases, small defects are present in the posterior arches of some of the lower cervical vertebrae. Increased cervical lordosis, concavity of the anterior wall of the spinal canal, and increased size of the ventral subarachnoid space are commonly observed at C2-C3.

Patients with Chiari II malformations have a very high frequency of syringohydromyelia. Cervical cord hydromyelia is present in 40 to 95% of cases and is most marked in the lower cervical segments (Figures 10-16A and B and 10-17). Cervical segments 1 and 2 are typically spared. Cervical cord syringomyelia is present in 4 to 22% of cases and typically occurs dorsal to the central canal of the cord. Syringobulbia is observed in less than 1% of cases (Figure 10-18).

Hydrocephalus is very common in patients with Chiari II malformations. More than 95% show ventricular enlargement (Figure 10-19), and more than 90% require shunt diversion of CSF. In patients with Chiari I deformities (*vide infra*), ventricular dilatation is present in only approximately 20% of cases. Thus, hydrocephalus is more frequent with Chiari II than with Chiari I deformity, although it is common in both **(Option (D) is false).**

Clinically, nearly all patients with Chiari II malformations have at least occasional problems with hindbrain dysfunction. The problems are serious in 32%, and 11% of affected children die of the hindbrain dysfunction. These represent 73% of all deaths in children with myelomeningocele. In the neonatal period, patients suffer prolonged respiratory pauses with hypoxemia, repeated spells of apnea, bilateral vocal cord paralysis, dysphagia with reflux, and repetitive aspirations leading to chronic pulmonary problems. Older children suffer pain in the neck and base of the skull, nystagmus, lower cranial nerve dysfunction, and upper-extremity weakness, hypotonia, or spasticity. A sudden onset of quadriparesis is rare.

The Chiari I malformation consists of downward prolongation of the cerebellar tonsils through the foramen magnum into the cervical subarachnoid space behind the spinal cord (Figure 10-20). In the "classic" Chiari I malformation, the fourth ventricle, medulla, and inferior vermis are not displaced. In actuality, these structures frequently show mild deformity that aggravates the difficulty of distinguishing Chiari I from Chiari II malformations radiologically. Clinically, differentiation is easier. Chiari I malformation is not associated with myelomeningocele. Chiari II malformation is associated with myelomeningocele in nearly every case.

In patients with Chiari I malformations, one or both cerebellar tonsils protrude caudally below the foramen magnum. In studies of Chiari I patients, Barkovich et al. found that the lower pole of the tonsil lay from

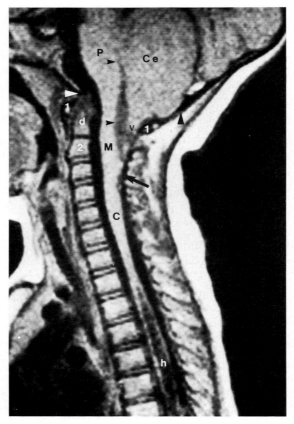

A

Figure 10-16. Spectrum of MR appearances of the Chiari II deformity (0.5 T; TR, 500 to 750 msec; TE, 30 to 35 msec). (A) Group 2. Caudal protrusion of the medulla (M) in line with the spinal cord (C) in a 2-year-old girl. The minimal caliber change indicates the cervicomedullary junction (black arrow). The fourth ventricle (small black arrowheads) is tubular, elongated, and mildly dilated. Dilatation of the intraspinal portion of the fourth ventricle suggests hydromyelia (h) seen distally. The foramen magnum (large arrowheads) is large. The C1 ring (1) is relatively narrow. The cerebellum (Ce) protrudes below the foramen magnum to rest on the posterior arch of C1. The vermian peg (v) descends through the C1 ring behind the fourth ventricle. The dens (d) indents the pons (P). 2 = C2. (B) Groups 3 and 4. Buckling of the medulla (M) behind the spinal cord (C) forming a kink and a spur (black arrow) at C3-C4 (3-4) in a 2-year-old girl. The cerebellum (Ce) protrudes below the posterior lip of the foramen magnum (arrowhead) to rest on the posterior arch of C1 (1). The vermian peg (v) is small and protrudes only slightly through the C1 ring. Concurrent hydromyelia (h) creates a focal, tense, fusiform low-signal-intensity space within the spinal cord at C5-C6 (5-6). This appearance should not be mistaken for a cystic tumor. P = pons; 2 = C2; 7 = C7; d = dens. (C) Group 5. A sac-like diverticulum (4) of the fourth ventricle (small black arrowheads) protrudes far below the kink and spur (black arrow). Tissue within the diverticulum is believed to be choroid plexus. The cerebellum (Ce) protrudes caudally beyond the posterior lip (large black arrowhead) of the foramen magnum to rest on the posterior arch of C1 (1). P = pons; V = vermian peg; M = medulla; C = spinal cord. (D and E) Group 2. A long vermian peg (V, white arrow) protrudes caudally beyond the medulla (M) and cervicomedullary junction in a 5-year-old girl. Arrowheads indicate the tubular fourth ventricle. Ce = cerebellum; C = spinal cord.

214

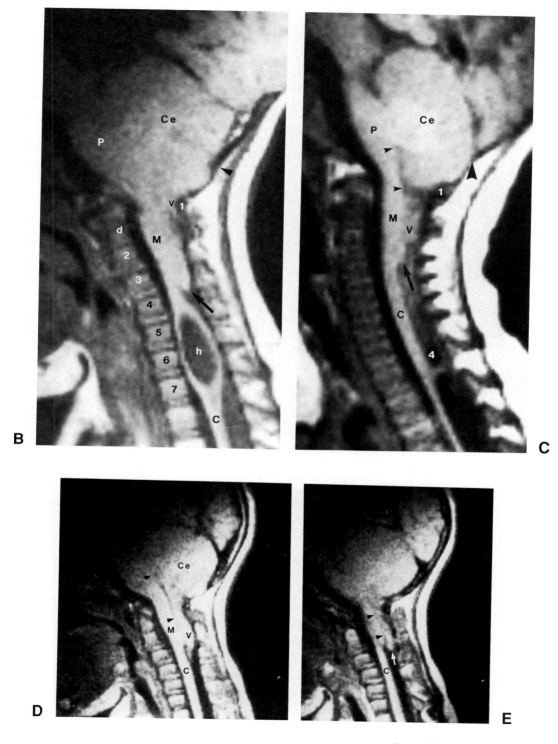

B

C

D

E

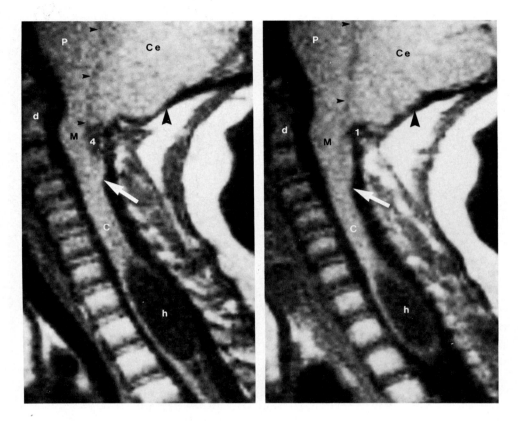

Figure 10-17. Chiari II malformation with tense, fusiform hydromyelia (h). Sagittal MR images (0.5 T; TR, 500 msec; TE, 30 msec) in a 5-year-old girl. Caudal protrusion of the cerebellum (Ce) below the wide foramen magnum (large arrowhead), tubular fourth ventricle (small arrowheads) with distal dilatation (4), low position of the pons (P) with indentation by the dens (d), caliber change at the cervicomedullary junction (white arrow), and characteristic concavity and increased lordosis at C2-C3 signify a Chiari II deformity. With a history of concurrent myelomeningocele, the focal, fusiform, low-signal-intensity lesion (h) that distends the spinal cord and the more caudal low-signal zone almost certainly represent hydromyelia, not a tumor. M = medulla; 1 = C1.

3 to 29 mm below the foramen magnum (mean, 13 mm below). Sherman et al. found that the lower pole of the tonsil lay from 1 to 27 mm below the foramen magnum (mean, 8 to 9 mm below). Operative findings reported by Paul et al. in 71 patients disclosed the lower poles of the tonsils just below the foramen magnum in 4%, at C1 in 62%, at C2 in 25%, and at C3 in 3%. In 6%, the tonsillar position was not specified.

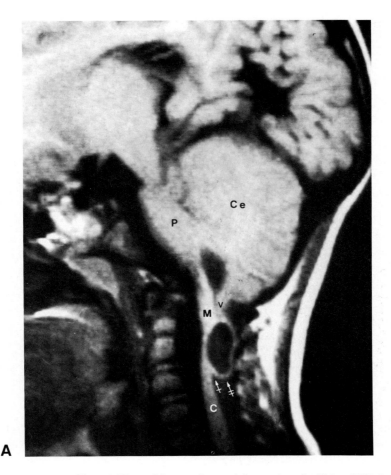

A

Figure 10-18. Chiari II malformation with syringobulbia. MR images (0.5 T; TR, 500 to 550 msec; TE, 30 msec) in a 7-year-old boy. (A) Sagittal MR image. (B and C) Axial MR images at the level of the low posterior fossa (B) and upper cervical spine (C). The typical caudal protrusion of the spinal cord (C), medulla (M), cerebellum (Ce), and peg (v) plus the typical kink (crossed white arrow) and spur (doubly crossed white arrow) signify a Chiari II malformation. The low-intensity cavities represent paramedian syringobulbia within the restiform body (upper space and axial image B) and within the medullary spur (lower space and axial image C). P = pons.

In the Chiari I malformation, the tonsils are typically elongated and pointed, with a triangular shape in sagittal images (Figures 10-21 and 10-22). They are often asymmetrical in size and position. Occasionally only one of a pair of tonsils protrudes inferiorly. The cisterna magna is

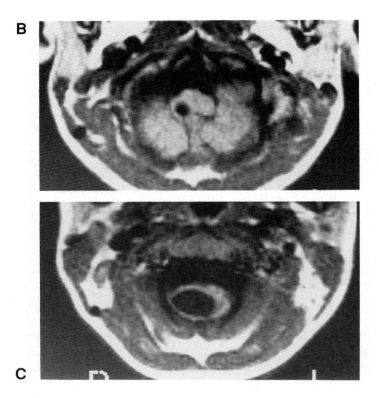

B

C

normal in 16% of cases, appreciably small in 47%, and obliterated in
37%. Identification of a small or absent cisterna magna always should
suggest the possibility of a Chiari I malformation (and a differential
diagnosis of a tumor) (Figures 10-21 through 10-23).

Tonsillar ectopia is associated with variable degrees of fibrosis and
gliosis that appear to influence whether or not there is associated
syringohydromyelia. In some patients the tonsils have nearly normal
color and consistency and have few sites of adhesion to the surrounding
membranes and neural structures. These patients have a low frequency
of syringohydromyelia. In other patients (41 to 63% of Chiari I patients),
the tonsils appear white and firm and are bound down to the dura,
arachnoid, vermis, and spinal cord in an intense mat of scar that also
overlies the foramen of Magendie. These patients exhibit a markedly
increased frequency of syringohydromyelia.

In patients with Chiari I malformations, the overall prevalence of
syringohydromyelia varies from about 33 to 73% (Figure 10-23). The
syrinx cavity is variable in length, spanning 1 to 17 vertebral segments

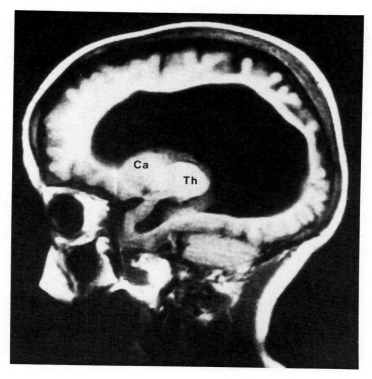

A

Figure 10-19. Chiari II malformation with aqueductal stenosis and unshunted hydrocephalus in a 14-year-old girl. Sagittal MR images (0.5 T; TR, 500 msec; TE, 30 msec). (A) Marked dilatation of the lateral ventricle compresses and thins the cerebral mantle and compresses and displaces the caudate nucleus (Ca) and thalamus (Th) anteriorly and inferiorly. (B) The dilated lateral ventricle compresses, elevates, and bows the corpus callosum (cc). The anterior recesses and the suprapineal recess of the third ventricle (3) are markedly distended. The aqueduct is narrowed and appears to terminate at the black arrow. The fourth ventricle (4) is dilated. Note the characteristic deformity (white arrow) of the hindbrain at C3.

(average, 7 to 8 segments). Large cavities exhibit haustrum-like ridges in their walls (Figure 10-23B). Typically, the cavity spares the C1 segment of the spinal cord. The cavity is associated with cord enlargement in 50% of cases and with cord atrophy in 16%. It is eccentric in 69% of cases and lobulated in 38%. T1-weighted images best display the relationship of the cavity to the cord and the presence of tonsillar ectopia. T2-weighted images may show the increased signal intensity of gliosis at the rostral end of the cavity and at substantial distances away from

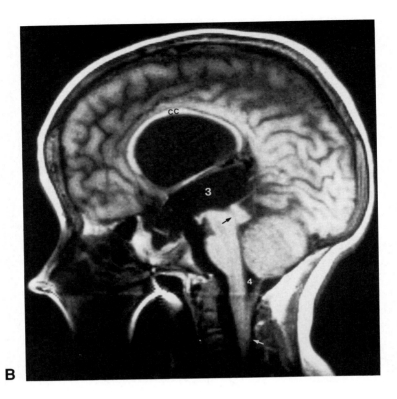

B

the cavity. Such an increased signal may also be observed with spinal cord tumors, leading to potential misdiagnosis.

CSF flow voids are seen in 81% of cord cavities and do not help to differentiate the syringohydromyelia of a Chiari I malformation from a tumor cavity. Tonsillar ectopia is observed in 13% of patients with post-traumatic syrinx cavities and in 40% of patients with tumor cavities. Thus, the simple detection of both a cord cavity and a low position of the tonsils does not establish a definite diagnosis of a Chiari I malformation with syringohydromyelia; a tumor cannot be excluded.

In many ways the Chiari I malformation may be regarded as a malsegmentation of the neural elements of the cervicomedullary junction and of the bony elements of the craniovertebral junction. Basilar impression is found in 23 to 50% of Chiari I patients. Assimilation of C1 to the occiput is observed in 1 to 11% of patients, partial fusion of C2 and C3 is observed in 18%, Klippel-Feil deformity is observed in 8%, cervical spina bifida occulta is observed in 3 to 6%, and widening of the cervical spinal canal (from hydromyelia) is observed in 18%.

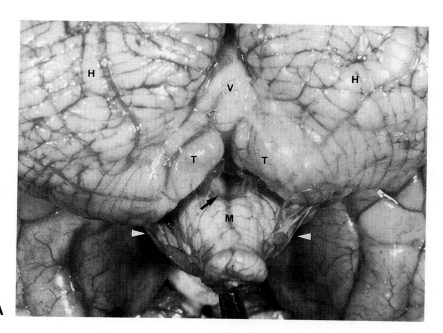

A

Figure 10-20. Anatomic specimens. (A) Fresh anatomic specimen of the normal hindbrain, viewed from below and behind, demonstrates the normal relationships among the cerebellar hemispheres (H), vermis (V), tonsils (T), medulla (M), and foramen of Magendie (black arrow). The approximate level of the foramen magnum is indicated by the arrowheads. (B) Operative exposure of a Chiari I malformation, seen from below and behind, demonstrates low, slightly asymmetrical position of the tonsils (T), well below the foramen magnum (arrowheads). The vermis (V) is also slightly low in position. The cerebellar hemispheres (H) appear normal.

Hydrocephalus is found in approximately 20% of patients with Chiari I malformations and in more than 90% of patients with Chiari II malformations. Patients with Chiari I malformations usually present as adolescents or adults, whereas those with Chiari II malformations usually present in the newborn period. There is a slight female predominance. The concomitant symptoms include pain in about 70% of patients (especially headache in about half of these), numbness in about 50%, weakness of one or more extremities in 18 to 56%, and unsteadiness in 12 to 40%. Most patients have multiple symptoms.

In patients with Chiari I malformations, physical examination reveals three major neurological syndromes: (i) central cord syndrome (20 to 65% of patients), consisting of combined disassociated sensory loss, sometimes

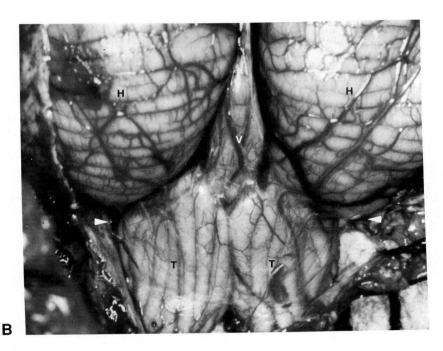

B

with segmental weakness and long tract signs simulating an intramedullary tumor; (ii) foramen magnum compression (22 to 38% of patients), consisting of ataxia, corticospinal and sensory deficits, cerebellar signs, and lower cranial nerve palsies; and (iii) cerebellar syndrome (10 to 11% of patients) with truncal ataxia, nystagmus, and limb ataxia.

Chiari I patients exhibit nystagmus in about 40% of cases. Nystagmus is rotatory or horizontal in about 60% of affected patients and downbeat in the remainder. Nystagmus is an involuntary repetitive movement of the eyeball in a certain direction. Typically the motion has both rapid and slow components: a jerk-like motion in one direction and a slower recovery in the opposite direction. The direction of the conspicuous rapid component is used to designate the type of nystagmus. Thus, downbeat nystagmus characteristically has a fast component in the downward direction, whereas upbeat nystagmus has a fast component in the upward direction. Nystagmus may occur with the eye gazing straight ahead (primary position nystagmus) or only in certain positions of the eye (downgaze nystagmus, lateral gaze nystagmus, etc.).

Primary position downbeat nystagmus is a significant sign of structural pathology in the region of the cervicomedullary junction. Its presence mandates search for a treatable lesion such as a Chiari I malformation or an extramedullary tumor at the foramen magnum. Approximately 31% of patients with downbeat nystagmus have Chiari I

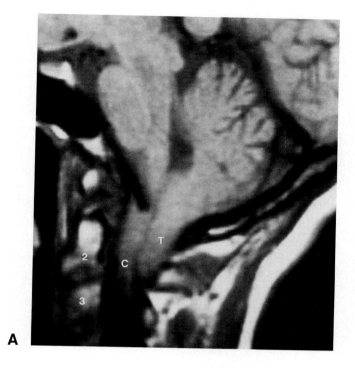

A

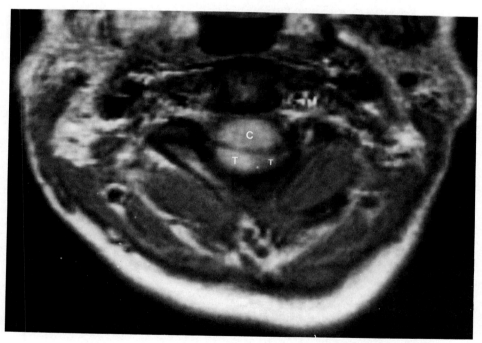

B

Figure 10-21. Chiari I malformation in a 48-year-old woman. (A) Sagittal MR image (1.5 T; TR, 600 msec; TE, 20 msec). Caudal elongation of the tonsil (T) through the foramen magnum to C2-C3 (2-3) causes anterior displacement and compression of the cervical spinal cord (C). The cisterna magna is nearly obliterated. (B) Axial MR image (1.5 T; TR, 2,000 msec; TE, 35 msec). Asymmetrical protrusion of the tonsils (T) flattens the sagittal dimension of the spinal cord (C).

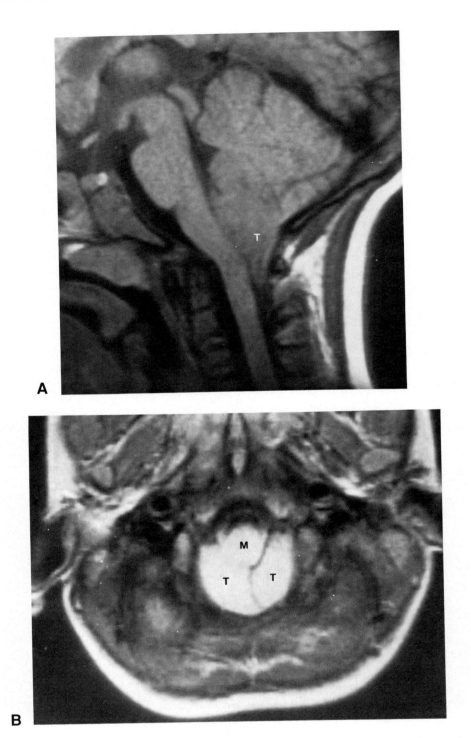

Figure 10-22. Chiari I malformation in a 5-year-old girl. (A) Sagittal MR image (1.5 T; TR, 600 msec; TE, 25 msec). The inferior cerebellum and tonsil (T) exhibit a "pointed" triangular shape where they protrude downward through the foramen magnum and the C1 ring. (B) Axial MR image (1.5 T; TR, 2,000 msec; TE, 35 msec). Two large tonsils (T) fill the cisterna magna behind the cervicomedullary junction (M).

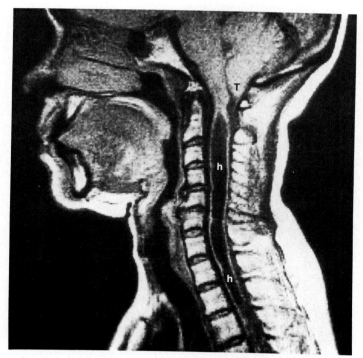

A

Figure 10-23. Chiari I malformation with hydromyelia in a 61-year-old man. Sagittal (A) and coronal (B) MR images (0.5 T; TR, 700 msec; TE, 30 msec) disclose caudal protrusion of triangular tonsils (T) through the foramen magnum and behind the cervical spinal cord to C1, preservation of a narrow segment of the spinal cord at C1, and marked multisegment cylindrical hydromyelia (h). The cisterna magna is small. (Reprinted with permission from Naidich and Zimmerman [17].)

malformations, and about 17% of patients with Chiari I malformations manifest downbeat nystagmus **(Option (E) is true).** However, downbeat nystagmus is not pathognomonic of Chiari I malformations and may also be observed with morphine toxicity, demyelinating disease, cerebellar atrophy, and degenerative encephalopathy.

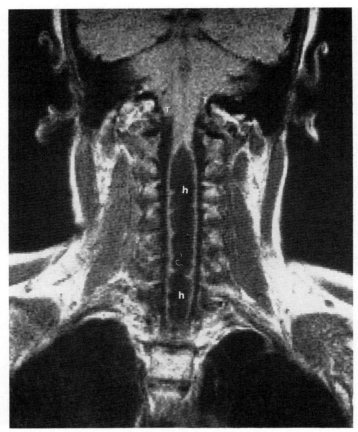

B

Question 48

Spinal cord astrocytomas:

(A) represent hematogenous dissemination of cerebral astrocytomas
(B) extend over several cord segments
(C) remain buried within the substance of the cord and displace relatively normal but compressed cord tissue circumferentially
(D) are associated with intramedullary cysts in more than 25% of cases
(E) generally present clinically with both hydrocephalus and papilledema

Intramedullary tumors of the spinal cord constitute about 4% of central nervous system neoplasms in children, and astrocytomas account for between 30 and 60% of such intramedullary tumors. Ependymomas alone

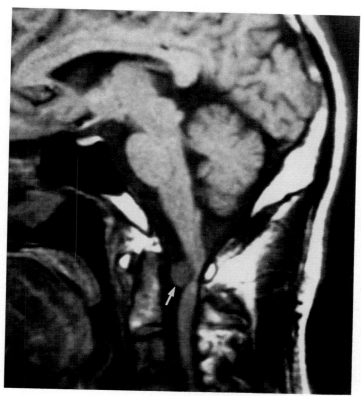

A

Figure 10-25. C1 neurofibroma in a 39-year-old man. MR images (1.5 T; TR, 600 msec; TE, 25 msec). (A) Midsagittal MR image demonstrates an ovoid, well-circumscribed, slightly hypodense anterior spinal mass (white arrow) that compresses the spinal cord and displaces it posteriorly. (B) Paramedian MR image demonstrates that the mass (white arrow) increases in size laterally as it nears the neural foramen.

not) be myelinated. Neurofibromas occur almost exclusively in association with von Recklinghausen's neurofibromatosis. Thus, neurofibromas nearly always imply underlying neurofibromatosis. Grossly, neurofibromas are much less well defined than neurinomas and often form masses that become continuous with thickened nerve roots (Figure 10-25). Plexiform neurofibromas may create masses that involve multiple nerves, fill multiple adjacent neural foramina, and merge into huge confluent paraspinal masses (Figure 10-26).

Neurinomas and neurofibromas account for approximately 15 to 30% of all space-occupying tumors of the spinal canal (Table 10-2). The spinal levels most commonly involved are C2-C3, C5-C6, T3-T4, and T9-T12. Approximately 70% of neurinomas are intradural-extramedullary le-

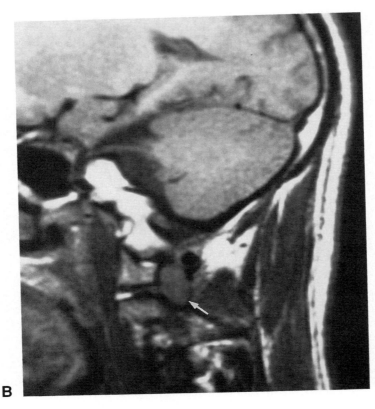

B

sions. The rest are equally frequently extradural and intradural-extradural in location. Intramedullary neurinomas are exceptionally rare.

"Dumbbell" or "hourglass" tumors are lesions that are constricted in the middle by growth through a limiting structure. In the spine, these may be either (i) dumbbell intradural-extradural, constricted by the dura itself, or (ii) dumbbell extradural-extracanalicular, constricted by the walls of the neural foramen. Dumbbell tumors of all histologies account for 10 to 15% of all space-occupying vertebral column lesions.

Approximately 15 to 30% of neurinomas are dumbbell tumors. Indeed, neurinomas are the most common dumbbell tumors of the spine (47% of cases), followed by malignant blastomas (23%) and meningiomas (11%). Dumbbell neurinomas are more commonly cervical (50% of cases) than thoracic (39%) or conus-cauda equina (12%) in location. Dumbbell meningiomas are usually thoracic (75% of cases) and less often cervical (25%).

Dumbbell extradural-extracanalicular neurinomas typically enlarge the neural foramen **(Option (C) is true).** They typically exhibit reduced

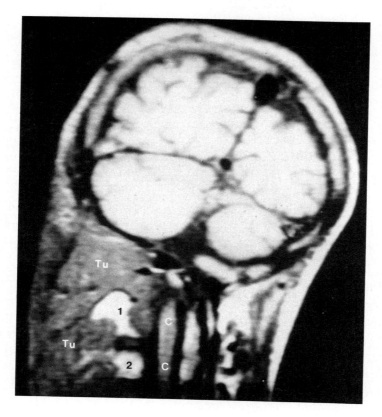

Figure 10-26. Plexiform neurofibroma in an 18-year-old boy with von Recklinghausen's neurofibromatosis. Coronal MR image (1.5 T; TR, 600 msec; TE, 25 msec). The plexiform tumor (Tu) forms an intracanalicular mass at C1 (1), grows through the neural foramina to envelop the lateral masses of C1 (1) and C2 (2), distracts the occiput from C1, causing head tilt, and invades the posterior fossa. The spinal cord (C) is not displaced on this section. (Courtesy of R. A. Zimmerman, M.D., University of Pennsylvania, Philadelphia.)

attenuation on noncontrast computed tomography and stand out in contrast to the higher-density muscles **(Option (D) is false).** They characteristically enhance densely on postcontrast computed tomographic scans **(Option (E) is true).**

On T1-weighted MRI, neurinomas usually exhibit a signal intensity equal to (85% of cases) or less than (15%) that of adjacent neural tissue and greater than (95% of cases) or equal to (5%) that of CSF. The signal is nearly always homogeneous but may occasionally be heterogeneous because of cysts, hemorrhage, or regions containing more fibrous tissue. On T2-weighted MRI, most neurinomas show a signal intensity greater

Table 10-2. Relative frequencies of 4,885 space-occupying spinal lesions

Diagnosis	No. of cases	%
Neurinomas and neurofibromas	1,129	23.1
Meningiomas	1,088	22.4
Gliomas and other intramedullary tumors	644	13.2
Sarcomas	399	8.2
Vascular tumors and angiomas	318	6.5
Metastases	294	6.0
Ependymomas	126	2.5
Others	887	18.1
Total	**4,885**	**100**

*Adapted from Arendt [36].

than that of neural tissue and equal to that of CSF. However, neurinomas may occasionally have signal intensities less than or greater than that of neural tissue. Thus far, no specific MRI characteristics have been found that reliably distinguish spinal neurilemmomas from neurofibromas or meningiomas. Distinction from other tumors is difficult to impossible on the basis of signal intensities alone.

Tumors of the foramen magnum lie high within the cervical spinal canal or cross the foramen magnum as they extend between the intracranial and intraspinal spaces. In some cases these are subdivided into craniospinal lesions (which grow downward) and spinocranial lesions (which grow upward).

Extramedullary tumors of the foramen magnum constitute about 3% of tumors that affect the spinal cord. The most common benign ones are meningiomas (about 70% of cases). Next most common are neurinomas and neurofibromas (about 25% of cases). In 10% of cases, a meningioma or neurinoma of the foramen magnum is merely one of multiple benign intracranial or cervical tumors. Endotheliomas, dermoids, lipomas, and arachnoid cysts are uncommon lesions of the foramen magnum.

Meningiomas of the foramen magnum constitute 3% of all meningiomas of the neural axis and 21% of spinal meningiomas. Approximately two-thirds are spinocranial and one-third are craniospinal. These tumors attach to the dura along the rim of the foramen magnum, especially where the vertebral arteries penetrate the dura (Figure 10-27). They may also attach along the exit zones of the nerve roots as far inferiorly as the C3 roots. Nearly all (96%) of these meningiomas are subarachnoid or subdural in location. In rare cases (4%) they are extradural.

The large majority of foramen magnum meningiomas lie anterior or anterolateral to the medulla and spinal cord, and so they displace the neural tissue dorsally. Stein et al. found that 84% of these meningiomas lay anterolateral to the spinal cord, 4% lay directly anterior to the cord, and 12% lay posterior or posterolateral to the cord. From a slightly different viewpoint, Yasuoka et al. found that 60% were anterior to the cord, 21% were lateral to the cord, and 19% were posterior to the cord. These meningiomas also frequently displace, compress, or encase the vertebral arteries.

Nearly all foramen magnum neuromas (95%) lie at C2, and only a few (5%) lie at C1; all are spinocranial lesions. Unlike neuromas at other sites, approximately 85% of foramen magnum lesions are neurofibromas, and 15% are neurinomas. About 85% of patients with multiple tumors at the foramen magnum have a neurofibroma at C2 as well as other neurofibromas situated between C1 and C5. Spinal neuromas preferentially involve the dorsal (sensory) nerve roots and lie dorsolateral to the spinal cord. Only about 10% lie along the anterior surface of the cord.

Benign extramedullary tumors of the foramen magnum have been notoriously difficult to diagnose clinically or radiologically. Patients present with suboccipital or neck pain (49% of cases), dysesthesias of the extremities (39%), gait disturbance (7%), and weakness of the extremities (5%). However, the initial neurological examination is unremarkable in 50% of patients. The complaints have initially been misdiagnosed as cervical spondylosis (21% of cases), multiple sclerosis of the spinal cord (18%), syringomyelia (16%), intramedullary tumor (14%), Chiari I malformation (5%), and carpal tunnel syndrome (5%). Too often the correct diagnosis was made only when the patient was in extremis.

Now, MRI clearly depicts the entire cervicomedullary junction and displacement of the cord by a foramen magnum tumor. Meningiomas and neurofibromas both commonly appear isointense relative to the spinal cord on T1-weighted images. On T2-weighted images, meningiomas tend to remain more nearly isointense relative to the spinal cord, whereas neurofibromas often exhibit increased signal intensity. Meningiomas also tend to be more homogeneous in their signal intensity, whereas neurinomas, especially large ones, may be quite inhomogeneous secondary to areas of cyst and hemorrhage.

Thomas P. Naidich, M.D.
Scott W. Atlas, M.D.
David G. McLone, M.D., Ph.D.

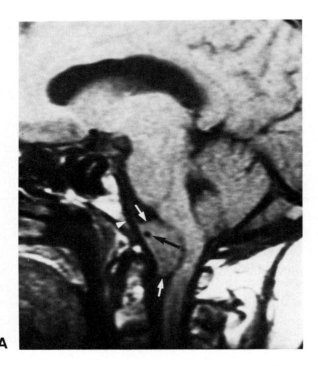

A

Figure 10-27. Foramen magnum meningioma in a 63-year-old woman. (A) Midsagittal section (1.5 T; TR, 600 msec; TE, 20 msec). The well-defined mass (white arrows) has a broad basal attachment along the anterior dura of the craniovertebral junction and a dome that compresses and displaces the medulla and upper cervical spinal cord. With this sequence, the mass is slightly hypointense with respect to the brain. The signal void of cortical bone is thickened (arrowhead) along the base of the mass, suggesting hyperostosis. The vertebral artery (black arrow) is encased. (B) Midsagittal section (1.5 T; TR, 2,500 msec; TE, 30 msec) shows a marked increase in the signal intensity of the tumor relative to the brain stem and spinal cord. (Courtesy of R. A. Zimmerman, M.D., University of Pennsylvania, Philadelphia.)

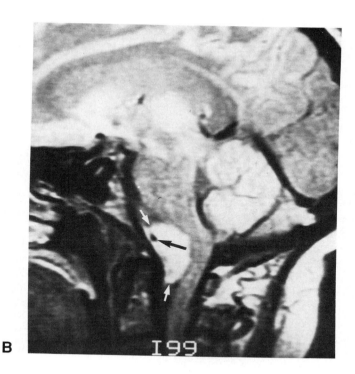

B

SUGGESTED READINGS

CHIARI MALFORMATIONS

1. Aboulezz AO, Sartor K, Geyer CA, Gado MH. Position of cerebellar tonsils in the normal population and in patients with Chiari malformation: a quantitative approach with MR imaging. J Comput Assist Tomogr 1985; 9:1033–1036
2. Banerji NK, Millar JH. Chiari malformation presenting in adult life. Its relationship to syringomyelia. Brain 1974; 97:157–168
3. Batnitzky S, Hall PV, Lindseth RE, Wellman HN. Meningomyelocele and syringohydromyelia. Some radiological aspects. Radiology 1976; 120:351–357
4. Blaauw G. Defect in posterior arch of atlas in myelomeningocele. Dev Med Child Neurol [Suppl] 1971; 25:113–115
5. Cahan LD, Bentson JR. Considerations in the diagnosis and treatment of syringomyelia and the Chiari malformation. J Neurosurg 1982; 57:24–31
6. Cameron AH. The Arnold-Chiari and other neuro-anatomical malformations associated with spina bifida. J Pathol Bacteriol 1957; 73:195–211
7. Cogan DG. Down-beat nystagmus. Arch Ophthalmol 1968; 80:757–768

8. Daniel PM, Strich SJ. Some observations on the congenital deformity of the central nervous system known as the Arnold-Chiari malformation. J Neuropathol Exp Neurol 1958; 17:255–266

9. du Boulay G, Shah SH, Currie JC, Logue V. The mechanism of hydromyelia in Chiari type I malformations. Br J Radiol 1974; 47:579–587

10. Emery JL, MacKenzie N. Medullo-cervical dislocation deformity (Chiari II deformity) related to neurospinal dysraphism (meningomyelocele). Brain 1973; 96:155–162

11. Harwood-Nash DC, Fitz CR. Neuroradiology in infants and children, vol 3. St. Louis: CV Mosby; 1976:1000–1014

12. MacKenzie NG, Emery JL. Deformities of the cervical cord in children with neurospinal dysraphism. Dev Med Child Neurol [Suppl] 1971; 25:58–67

13. McLone DG, Naidich TP. Myelomeningocele. Outcome and late complications. In: Epstein F, Hoffman HJ (eds), Disorders of the developing nervous system: diagnosis and treatment. Boston: Blackwell Scientific; 1986:77–107

14. Naidich TP. The craniovertebral junction: Chiari malformations I and II (abstr). In: CT '82, Internationales Computertomographie Symposium. Germany: Schnetztor-Verlag; 1982:78–84

15. Naidich TP, McLone DG, Fulling KH. The Chiari II malformation: part IV. The hindbrain deformity. Neuroradiology 1983; 25:179–197

16. Naidich TP, Pudlowski RM, Naidich JB, Gornish M, Rodriguez FJ. Computed tomographic signs of the Chiari II malformation. Part I. Skull and dural partitions. Radiology 1980; 134:65–71

17. Naidich TP, Zimmerman RA. Common congenital malformations of the brain. In: Brant-Zawadzki M, Normal D (eds), Magnetic resonance imaging of the central nervous system. New York: Raven Press; 1987:131–150

18. Park TS, Hoffman HJ, Hendrick EB, Humphreys RP. Experience with surgical decompression of the Arnold-Chiari malformation in young infants with myelomeningocele. Neurosurgery 1983; 13:147–152

19. Paul KS, Lye RH, Strang FA, Dutton J. Arnold-Chiari malformation. Review of 71 cases. J Neurosurg 1983; 58:183–187

20. Peach B. The Arnold-Chiari malformation with normal spine. Arch Neurol 1964; 10:497–501

21. Peach B. Arnold-Chiari malformation. Anatomic features of 10 cases. Arch Neurol 1965; 12:613–621

22. Pedersen RA, Troost BT, Abel LA, Zorub D. Intermittent downbeat nystagmus and oscillopsia reversed by suboccipital craniectomy. Neurology 1980; 30:1239–1242

23. Rhoton AL Jr. Microsurgery of Arnold-Chiari malformation in adults with and without hydromyelia. J Neurosurg 1976; 45:473–483

24. Saez RJ, Onofrio BM, Yanagihara T. Experience with Arnold-Chiari malformation, 1960 to 1970. J Neurosurg 1976; 45:416–422

25. Sherman JL, Barkovich AJ, Citrin CM. The MR appearance of syringomyelia: new observations. AJR 1987; 148:381–391

26. Teng P, Papatheodorou C. Arnold-Chiari malformation with normal spine and cranium. Arch Neurol 1965; 12:622–624

CRANIOCERVICAL JUNCTION

27. Barkovich AJ, Wippold FJ, Sherman JL, Citrin CM. Significance of cerebellar tonsillar position on MR. AJNR 1986; 7:795–799
28. El Gammal T. Extra-ventricular (communicating) hydrocephalus: some observations on the midline ventricles. AJR 1969; 106:308–328
29. Emery JL. Kinking of the medulla in children with acute cerebral oedema and hydrocephalus and its relationship to the dentate ligaments. J Neurol Neurosurg Psychiatry 1967; 30:267–275
30. Northfield DW. The surgery of the central nervous system. A textbook for postgraduate students. Oxford: Blackwell Scientific; 1973:31–32
31. Stein BM, Leeds NE, Taveras JM, Pool JL. Meningiomas of the foramen magnum. J Neurosurg 1963; 20:740–751
32. Wickbom I, Hanafee W. Soft tissue masses immediately below the foramen magnum. Acta Radiol [Diagn] 1963; 1:647–658
33. Yasuoka S, Okazaki H, Daube JR, MacCarty CS. Foramen magnum tumors. Analysis of 57 cases of benign extramedullary tumors. J Neurosurg 1978; 49:828–838
34. Yousefzadeh DK, Naidich TP. US anatomy of the posterior fossa in children: correlation with brain sections. Radiology 1985; 156:353–361

VENTRICULAR TUMORS

35. Naidich TP, Tomita T, Pech P, Haughton V. Direct coronal computed tomography for presurgical evaluation of posterior fossa tumors. J Comput Assist Tomogr 1985; 9:1065–1072

SPINAL CORD TUMORS

36. Arendt A. Spinal gliomas. In: Vinken PJ, Bruyn GW (eds), Handbook of clinical neurology, no. 20. Tumours of the spine and spinal cord. Part II. Amsterdam: North-Holland Publishing Company; 1976:323–351
37. Arseni C, Meretsis M. Tumours of the lower spinal cord associated with increased intracranial pressure and papilloedema. J Neurosurg 1967; 27:105–110
38. Britton J, Marsh H, Kendall B, Kingsley D. MRI and hydrocephalus in childhood. Neuroradiology 1988; 30:310–314
39. Cooper PR, Epstein F. Radical resection of intramedullary spinal cord tumors in adults. Recent experience in 29 patients. J Neurosurg 1985; 63:492–499
40. Elsberg CA, Strauss I. Tumors of the spinal cord which project into the posterior cranial fossa. Arch Neurol Psychol 1929; 21:261–273
41. Epstein F, Epstein N. Surgical treatment of spinal cord astrocytomas of childhood. A series of 19 patients. J Neurosurg 1982; 57:685–689
42. Oi S, Raimondi AJ. Hydrocephalus associated with intraspinal neoplasms in childhood. Am J Dis Child 1981; 135:1122–1124
43. Reimer R, Onofrio BM. Astrocytomas of the spinal cord in children and adolescents. J Neurosurg 1985; 63:669–675

44. Scotti G, Scialfa G, Colombo N, Landoni L. Magnetic resonance diagnosis of intramedullary tumors of the spinal cord. Neuroradiology 1987; 29:130–135
45. Slooff JL, Kernohan JW, MacCarty CS. Primary intramedullary tumors of the spinal cord and filum terminale. Philadelphia: WB Saunders; 1964

NEURINOMAS AND NEUROFIBROMAS

46. Braun M, Cosnard G, Cabanis EA, et al. NMR imaging and neuromas. J Neuroradiol 1986; 13:209–225
47. Dodge HW Jr, Love JG, Gottlieb CM. Benign tumors at the foramen magnum. Surgical considerations. J Neurosurg 1956; 13:603–617
48. Dross PE, Raji MR. CT myelography of calcified thoracic neurilemmoma. AJNR 1985; 6:967–968
49. Knitter K. Spinal meningiomas, neurinomas and neurofibromas and hourglass tumours. In: Vinken PJ, Bruyn GW (eds), Handbook of clinical neurology, no. 20. Tumours of the spine and spinal cord. Part II. Amsterdam: North-Holland Publishing Company; 1976:177–322
50. LaMasters DL, Watanabe TJ, Chambers EF, Norman D, Newton TH. Multiplanar metrizamide-enhanced CT imaging of the foramen magnum. AJNR 1982; 3:485–494
51. Rubenstein LJ. Tumors of the central nervous system, atlas of tumor pathology, second series, fascicle 6. Washington, DC: Armed Forces Institute of Pathology; 1970
52. Scotti G, Scialfa G, Colombo N, Landoni L. MR imaging of intradural extramedullary tumors of the cervical spine. J Comput Assist Tomogr 1985; 9:1037–1041
53. Zulch KJ. Brain tumors. Their biology and pathology (transl by Rothballer AB, Olszewski J). New York: Springer; 1965:22–88

Notes

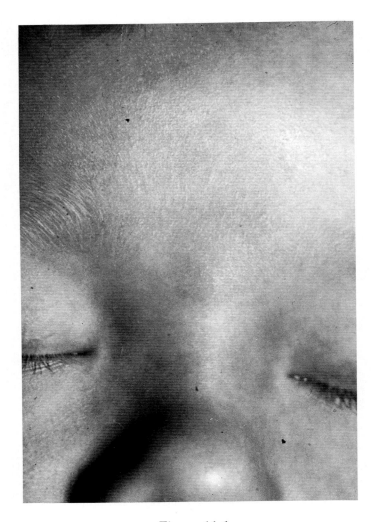

Figure 11-1

Figures 11-1 through 11-4. This 16-month-old boy presented with painful swelling at the glabella. You are shown a photograph of the patient's face (Figure 11-1), direct coronal noncontrast computed tomographic (CT) scans through the glabella (Figure 11-2; soft tissue window) and the nasofrontal junction (Figure 11-3; bone window image), and axial noncontrast CT scans through the nasofrontal junction and glabella (Figure 11-4).

Case 11: Infected Dermal Sinus

Question 50

Which *one* of the following is the MOST likely diagnosis?

(A) Infected dermal sinus/epidermoid cyst
(B) Nasal glioma
(C) Nasofrontal cephalocele
(D) Histiocytosis X
(E) Sinus pericranii

The test images (Figures 11-1 through 11-4) show swelling at the nasal root, edema of the soft tissues, bone destruction with sequestra, a well-defined canal through the nasal processes of the frontal bone just above the nasofrontal suture, widening of the foramen cecum with distortion of the crista galli, and a dense mass at the intracranial end of the bony canal (see Figures 11-5 through 11-7). These findings suggest a congenital malformation with secondary infection: a nasal dermal sinus and cyst with osteomyelitis and cellulitis **(Option (A) is correct).** This boy presented with painful swelling at the glabella and a history of intermittent redness, swelling, and discharge from a "pimple" at the glabella since birth. The initial patient photograph (Figure 11-1) demonstrates fullness at the glabella but no sinus ostium. The site of the ostium becomes evident when pressure at the sides of the nasal root expresses secretions (Figure 11-8).

Nasal glioma and nasofrontal encephalocele (Options (B) and (C)) must be considered in the differential diagnosis. Both occur at this site and both may be associated with a bony canal and deformity of the crista galli. Indeed, the presence of the canal and of the deformed crista requires consideration of a congenital lesion. However, the edema and sequestra clearly indicate the presence of infection, and so we must choose a congenital lesion that has become infected.

Histiocytosis X (Option (D)) would explain the acute inflammatory features of the lesion, but it could not explain well the presence of a

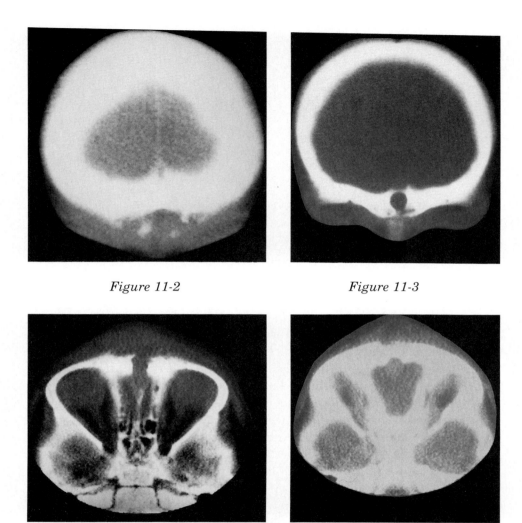

Figure 11-2   Figure 11-3

Figure 11-4

well-corticated canal at a site typically associated with congenital malformations.

Sinus pericranii (Option (E)) is excluded, because sinus pericranii is not typically midline and does not typically become infected. Sinus pericranii usually exhibits increased size with elevated intracranial pressure, a feature not described in the history given for this patient.

The most common frontonasal tumors of children and adults are dermoid cysts and sinuses (32%), hemangiomas (30%), and menin-

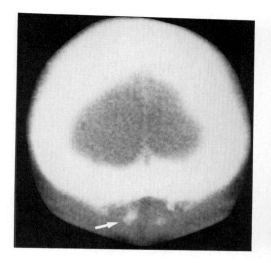

Figure 11-5

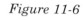

Figure 11-6

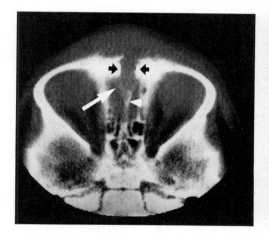

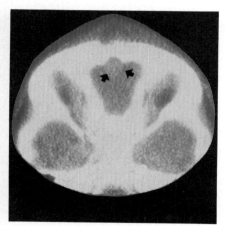

Figure 11-7

Figures 11-5 through 11-7 (Same as Figures 11-2 through 11-4). Coronal noncontrast CT scan (Figure 11-5) shows loss of normal fat planes and multiple sequestra (arrow), indicating cellulitis and osteomyelitis at the glabella. Coronal noncontrast CT scan (Figure 11-6) shows the well-defined midline canal (black arrow), which extends through the frontal bone just superior to the frontonasal suture. Axial noncontrast CT scans (Figure 11-7) show soft tissue that extends from the glabella through the canal (black arrows) to form a midline intracranial extradural mass (white arrow) just anterior to the crista galli (white arrowhead) and (b) an interdural mass (black arrows) between the leaves of the falx. Histologic examination of the excised specimen revealed an epidermoid cyst. (Reprinted with permission from Naidich et al. [5].)

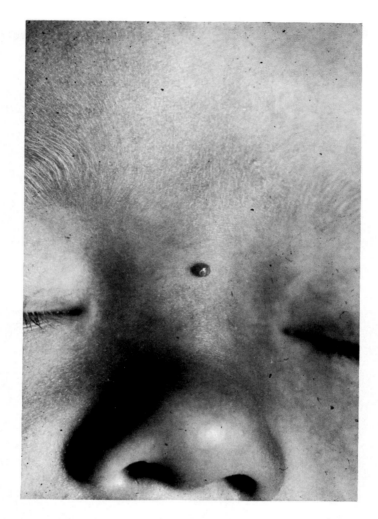

Figure 11-8. Digital compression at the sides of the glabella expresses pus from the pinpoint, otherwise undetectable ostium.

goencephaloceles and nasal gliomas (19%). Neurofibromas (6%), lymphangiomas (4%), and lipomas (4%) are uncommon. Fibromas, teratomas, and granulomas are unusual (2% each). The hemangiomas and lymphangiomas at this site are identical to those found elsewhere and require no further discussion. The dermal sinuses, nasal gliomas, and meningoencephaloceles form a spectrum of pathology with a common embryologic basis. An understanding of that embryology makes it easy to remember the diverse manifestations of these diseases.

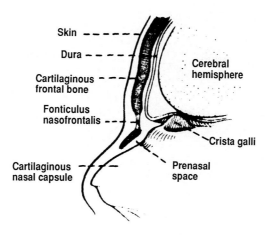

Figure 11-9. Diagram of the anatomic relationships of the fonticulus nasofrontalis and the prenasal space to the dura, the ossified nasal and frontal bones, and the cartilaginous nasal capsule. (Adapted with permission from Sessions [10].)

Developmental Bases for Nasofrontal Lesions. In the early embryo, the embryonic frontal bones are separated from the embryonic nasal bones by a small fontanelle, the fonticulus nasofrontalis. The nasal bones are separated from the subjacent cartilaginous nasal capsule by the prenasal space (Figure 11-9). This space extends from the base of the brain to the nasal tip. Midline diverticula of dura normally project anteriorly into the fonticulus nasofrontalis and anteroinferiorly into the prenasal space. These diverticula touch the ectoderm. Normally, the diverticula regress and the bone plates of the skull close together. The fonticulus nasofrontalis is closed by the nasal processes of the frontal bone to make the frontonasal suture. The cartilaginous nasal capsule develops into the upper lateral nasal cartilages and the ethmoid bone, including the crista galli, cribriform plates, and perpendicular plate of the septum. The two leaves of the falx insert into the crista galli, one leaf passing to each side of the crista.

At the skull base, the frontal and ethmoid bones close together around a strand of dura, creating the foramen cecum. This foramen is easily seen at the bottom of a small depression that lies just in front of the crista galli. It is not certain whether the foramen is situated exactly at the frontoethmoidal junction or between the nasal processes of the frontal bones.

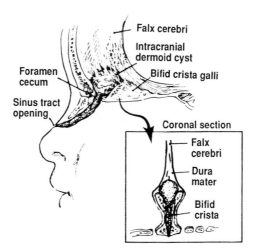

Labels in figure:
- Falx cerebri
- Intracranial dermoid cyst
- Bifid crista galli
- Foramen cecum
- Sinus tract opening
- Coronal section
- Falx cerebri
- Dura mater
- Bifid crista

Figure 11-10. Diagram of a "typical" nasal dermal sinus and cyst traversing the prenasal space and the enlarged foramen cecum to form a mass anterior to and within a grooved, "bifid" crista galli. (Inset) The anatomic relationships of the leaves of the falx to the sides of the crista galli direct upward extension of the mass into the interdural space between the leaves of the falx. (Reprinted with permission from Gorenstein et al. [13].)

If the diverticula of dura become adherent to the superficial ectoderm, they may not regress normally. Instead, they may pull ectoderm with them as they retreat, creating an ectodermal tract that extends from the glabella through a canal at the nasofrontal suture to the crista galli or beyond the crista to the interdural space between the two leaves of the falx. A similar persistent tract may pass from the external surface of the nose, under or through the nasal bones, and ascend through the prenasal space to enter the cranial cavity at the foramen cecum just anterior to the crista galli (Figure 11-10). Such a tract would be associated with a widened foramen cecum, distortion and grooving of the crista galli, and extension into the interdural space between the two leaves of the falx. Depending on the precise histology of the portions of the tract that persist, these tracts could develop into superficial glabellar and nasal pits, fully patent glabellar and nasal dermal sinuses, and/or one or several (epi)dermoid cysts and/or fibrous cords—exactly as do the analogous remnants of the vitelline duct and neurenteric canal. Rarely, the sinus tract cysts and cords may extend into or become adherent to the brain itself.

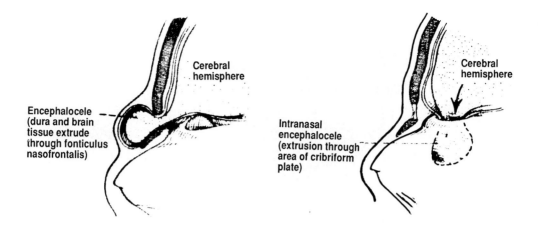

Figure 11-11. Schematic representation of the origin of the extranasal (glabellar) cephaloceles (left) and the intranasal transethmoidal cephaloceles (right). (Reprinted with permission from Gorenstein et al. [13].)

Nasal cephaloceles and gliomas may arise by an analogous mechanism. If the same dural diverticula were to persist as patent communications that contained leptomeninges, cerebrospinal fluid (CSF), and neural tissue, they would constitute glabellar and nasal meningoencephaloceles (Figure 11-11). Were such developing meningoencephaloceles to become "pinched" off and (nearly) isolated from the cranial cavity by subsequent constriction of the dura and bone, they would then constitute heterotopic foci of meninges and neural tissue at the glabella and nose. These benign, non-neoplastic heterotopias are given the dreadful name of glabellar and nasal gliomas (Figure 11-12).

Normal Development of the Nasal Septum. The normal nasal septum and skull base form in a predictable fashion. Knowledge of this pattern, which has been well described by Scott, is necessary for interpreting imaging studies of this region without serious error. In brief, the cartilage of the nasal capsule is the foundation of the upper part of the face (Figure 11-13). The bony elements of the facial skeleton appear around it and replace it, in part. The lateral masses of the ethmoid form in part by enchondral ossification of the nasal capsule. The frontal processes of the maxillary bones, the premaxillary bone, the nasal bones, the lacrimal bones, and the palatine bones all form in membrane in close relationship with the roof and lateral walls of the cartilaginous nasal capsule. The vomer develops within the perichondrium of the septal process. Eventually, nearly all the nasal capsule becomes ossified or atrophied.

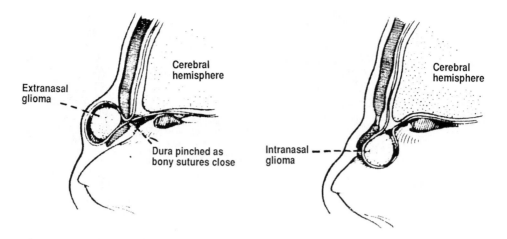

Figure 11-12. Diagram of the origins of extranasal gliomas (left) and nasal gliomas (right). (Reprinted with permission from Gorenstein et al. [13].)

All that remains of the cartilage of the nasal capsule in adults is the anterior part of the nasal septum and the alar cartilages that surround the nostrils.

The midline septal cartilage is directly continuous with the cartilaginous skull base (Figure 11-13). At birth, the skull base has three major ossification centers. These are the basioccipital center, the basisphenoid center, and the presphenoid center. The septal cartilage has not yet ossified. The lateral masses of the ethmoid have ossified, forming paired paramedian bones, but the cribriform plate is still cartilaginous or fibrous. At birth, therefore, the entire midline of the face may be a lucent stripe of cartilage situated between the paired ossifications in the lateral masses of the ethmoids. This lucent midline can simulate a midline cleft on imaging studies.

The septal cartilage extends along the midline from the nares to the presphenoid bone. Anteriorly and inferiorly, the septal cartilage attaches to the premaxillary bone by fibrous tissue. Posteriorly, the septal cartilage is continuous with the cartilage of the cranial base. Inferiorly, the lower edge of the septal cartilage is slotted into a U- or V-shaped groove that runs along the entire upper edge of the vomer (Figure 11-14). This groove is designated the vomerine groove. It should not be mistaken for a midline cleft in the septum.

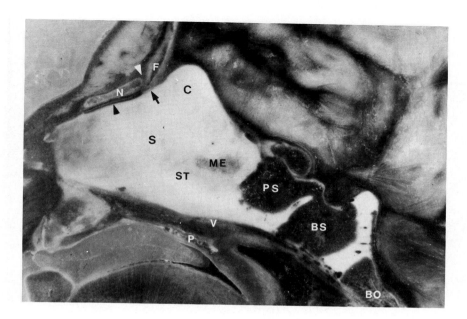

Figure 11-13. Midsagittal cryomicrotome section of a full-term neonate demonstrates the normal relationships—at birth—among the ossified frontal bone (F), the ossified nasal bone (N), the nasofrontal suture (white arrowhead), and the cartilaginous nasal capsule (large white structure) that forms the yet unossified nasal septum (S) and crista galli (C). The ossified hard palate (P) and ossified vomer (V) lie below the septal cartilage. Note the direct line from the prenasal space (black arrowhead) through the foramen cecum (arrow) to the normal depression or "fossa" just anterior to the crista galli. The midline septal cartilage is directly continuous with the cartilaginous skull base. The basioccipital (BO), basisphenoidal (BS), and presphenoidal (PS) ossification centers are well formed. The mesethmoidal (ME) ossification center is just beginning to form. When the vomer and mesethmoid enlarge, the residual cartilage between them will be designated the sphenoidal tail (ST).

At about the time of birth or during the first year, a fourth, mesethmoid center appears in the septal cartilage anterior to the cranial base. This center will form the perpendicular plate of the ethmoid. The residual portion of septal cartilage that extends posterosuperiorly toward the cranial base between the perpendicular plate and the vomer is designated the sphenoidal tail of the septal cartilage.

Initially, the ossifying perpendicular plate is separated from the rest of the facial skeleton by (i) the unossified cartilage or fibrous tissue of the cribriform plates and (ii) the sphenoidal tail (Figure 11-15). At about the

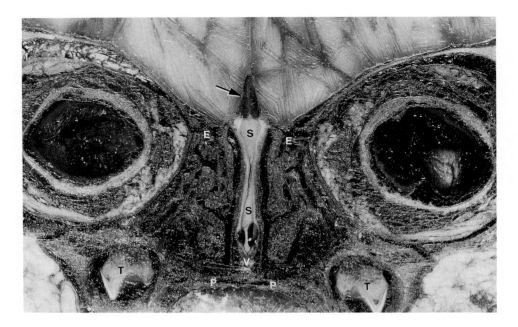

Figure 11-14. Coronal cryomicrotome section through the nasal cavity of a full-term stillborn infant at the level of the optic globes. The lateral ethmoid centers (E), the midline vomer (V), and the palatal shelves (P) of the maxillae are well ossified. The unossified septal cartilage (S) slots into the vomerine groove in the upper surface of the Y-shaped vomer. The crista galli (arrow) is beginning to ossify, forming a pointed "cap." The cribriform plates have not ossified. Note the normal position of the floor of the anterior fossa with respect to the two orbits and optic globes. T = unerupted teeth.

third to the sixth year, the lateral masses of the ethmoid and the perpendicular plate of the ethmoid become united across the roof of the nasal cavity by ossification of the cribriform plate. Somewhat later, the perpendicular plate unites with the vomer below. As the two bones approach, the vomerine groove may become converted into a vomerine tunnel. This should not be mistaken for a bony canal around a dermal sinus or cephalocele. Growth of the septal cartilage continues for a short period after craniofacial union is complete. This probably explains the common deflection of the nasal septum away from the midline. Because the appearance of the nasal septum varies with patient age, one must interpret computed tomographic "evidence" of midline defects and sinus tracts carefully.

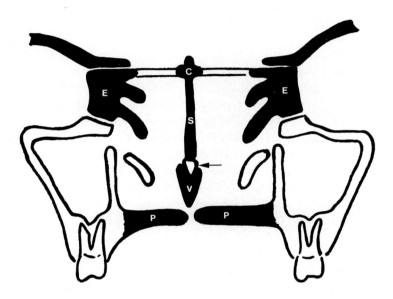

Figure 11-15. Diagram of the pattern of ossification around the nasal cavity. The ossified crista (C) and septal cartilage (S) form a bony cross that is isolated from the lateral ethmoid centers (E) by the unossified cribriform plates and from the vomer (V) by the sphenoidal tail (arrow). Although the maxillae are ossified, only the palatal shelves (P) have been inked in to emphasize their relationships to the vomer. (Modified from Scott [9].)

Question 51

Nasal dermal sinuses:

(A) lie in the true midline of the body
(B) present as sinus ostia or as cysts with nearly equal frequency
(C) extend intracranially in 80% of cases
(D) progress to squamous cell carcinoma in approximately 2% of cases
(E) are associated with a widened foramen cecum and distorted crista galli only when the dermoid elements enter the cranial cavity

A nasal dermal sinus is a thin epithelium-lined tube that arises at an external ostium situated along the midline of the nose and that extends deeply for a variable distance, sometimes reaching the intradural intracranial space **(Option (A) is true).** A nasal dermal cyst is a midline epithelium-lined cyst that arises along the expected course of the dermal sinus. It may exist as an isolated mass or it may co-exist with a dermal sinus (Figure 11-16). Histologically, nasal dermal sinuses may be true dermoids containing skin adnexae or may be pure epidermoids devoid of such adnexae. Dermoids and epidermoids are equally common. However, dermoid cysts and sinuses are found more commonly along the bridge of the nose. Pure epidermoids are more common at the glabella-nasion border and have a sevenfold-increased incidence of associated infection.

Nasal dermal sinuses and cysts constitute 3.7 to 12.6% of all dermal cysts of the head and neck and 1.1% of all such cysts throughout the body. They may be detected at any age, but most present early (mean age, 3 years). There is no sex predilection. Most cases arise sporadically, though kindreds with nasal dermal sinus have been reported.

The lesions may appear at any site from the glabella downward along the bridge (dorsum) of the nose to the base of the columella. Approximately 56% of lesions present as midline cysts; the remaining 44% present as midline sinus ostia **(Option (B) is true).** The external ostium of the sinus lies at the glabella-nasion border in 29%, the bridge of the nose in 21%, the nasal tip in 21%, and the base of the columella in 29%. Rarely, multiple sinus ostia are present, or sinuses and cysts coexist at both the glabella and the nasal bridge.

Nasal (epi)dermoid cysts are usually found in one of three areas: (i) the midline just superior to the nasal tip, (ii) the junction of the upper and lower lateral cartilages, or (iii) the medial canthal area. Glabellar cysts external to the frontal bone are less common. The cysts may be soft and discrete or indurated. They may erode through the overlying skin to form secondary pits.

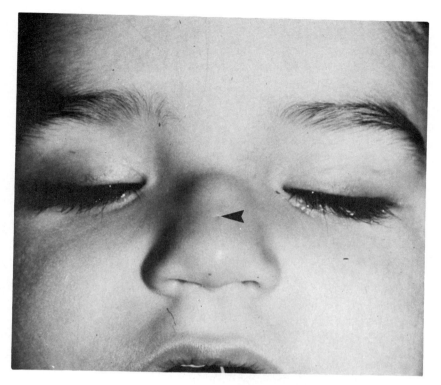

A

Figure 11-16. Nasal dermal sinus in a 10-month-old boy with increasing swelling of the nose. (A) Photograph of the face demonstrates a pinpoint ostium (arrowhead) on the dorsum of the nose. (B) Surgical dissection traces the sinus tract (black arrow) inward to a well-defined ovoid dermoid cyst (white arrow) within the septum. The cyst reached just to the cribriform plate. (C) Operative specimen demonstrates the proportions and contours of the dermal sinus and cyst. Arrowhead indicates the superficial cutaneous end of the tract.

Clinically, these lesions present as midline pits or fenestrae, occasionally containing sparse wiry hairs (Figure 11-17); as intermittent discharge of sebaceous material and/or pus (Figures 11-1 and 11-8); as intermittent inflammation; as a mass of increasing size with variable broadening of the nasal root and bridge; as intermittent episodes of meningitis; or as a behavioral change secondary to frontal lobe abscesses (Figure 11-18). At times, the ostium is tiny and undetectable until pressure is applied against the adjacent tissue to express cheesy material from the ostium (Figure 11-8).

The deep extensions of nasal dermal sinuses and cysts are variable. They can be shallow pits that end blindly in the superficial tissues. They

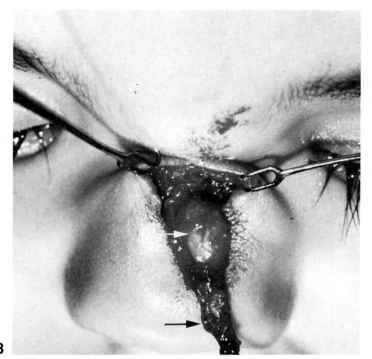

B

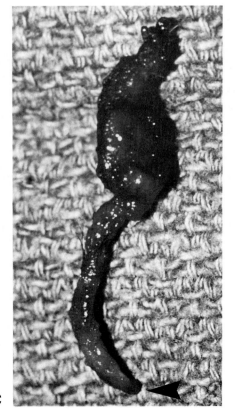

C

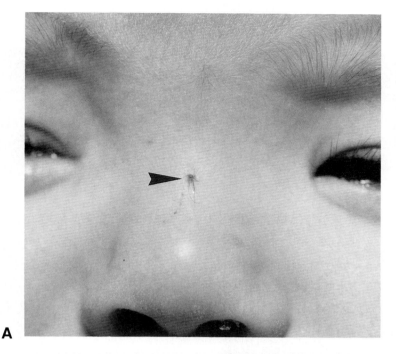

A

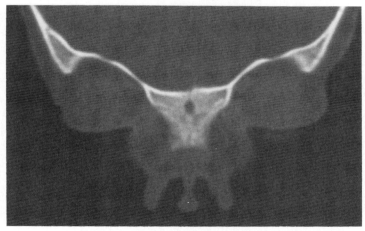

B

Figure 11-17. Nasal dermal sinus with intracranial extension in a 1-year-old girl with a clinically evident sinus. (A) Patient photograph. A small tuft of hairs protrudes from a midline dermal sinus on the dorsum of the nose. (B) Direct coronal CT scan. A well-marginated canal penetrates between the nasal process of the frontal bones. (C to F) Axial CT scans reveal a soft tissue mass (C, white arrow) deep to the widened nasal bridge, the bony canal (D, black arrow) leading to the widened nasal septum, and the large foramen cecum (E, black arrows), and bifid crista galli (F, white arrow). At surgery, the dermal sinus tract and extranasal dermoid were traced upward through the foramen cecum into a 2- to 3-cm intracranial dermoid. This extended intradurally but did not attach to brain. A second "arm" of the intranasal dermoid passed posteriorly toward the sphenoid bone.

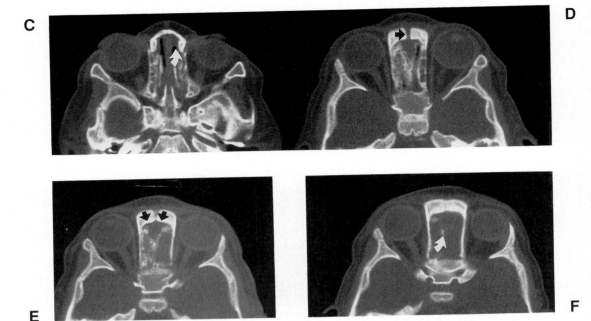

C D

E F

can wander extensively intra- and extracranially. In Bradley's review of 67 children with nasal dermoids, the lesion was confined to the skin in 61% and extended deeply to "invade" the nasal bones in 10%. The lesion extended into the septal cartilage in 10%, the nasal bones and cartilage in 6%, and the cribriform plate in 12%. Rare sinuses traverse the entire anteroposterior extent of the nasal septum to end at the basisphenoid, where they attach to the dura just anterior to the sella. The reported frequency of intracranial extension varies widely from 0 to 57% **(Option (C) is false).**

Intracranial extension can be associated with cysts and sinuses at any site. Sinuses at the base of the columella are least likely to extend intracranially. Thus, in Pensler's series, each of four sinuses situated at the base of the columella passed directly to the nasal spine of the maxilla, with no intracranial extension. However, Muhlbauer and Dittmar reported a similar sinus that ascended to end in the ethmoid air cells; it did not enter the cranial cavity.

True intracranial extension of (epi)dermoid usually affects the epidural space of the anterior fossa near the crista galli and may continue deeper, appearing between the two leaves of the falx as an interdural mass. Rarely, the lesions also extend into brain. An additional 31% of cases have intracranial extension of a fibrous cord devoid of (epi)dermal

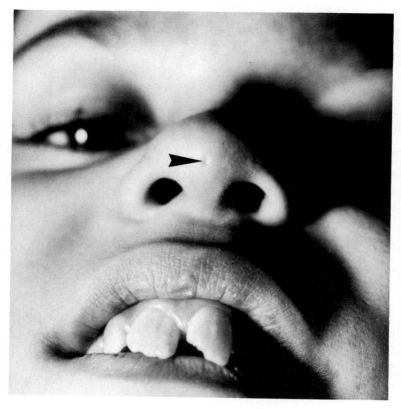

A

Figure 11-18. Nasal dermal sinus, intranasal dermoid, intracranial dermoid, and multilocular cerebral abscesses in a 10-year-old boy. (A) Patient photograph reveals a dermal sinus (arrowhead) at the nasal tip. (B to E) Serial axial CT scans demonstrate molding of the nasal bones by an intranasal mass (white arrow) and a bony canal (black arrows) through the nasal septum into the skull base. (F and G) Contrast-enhanced axial CT scans demonstrate the multilocular right frontal abscesses extending upward from the skull base. (H to K) At surgery, a probe was passed through the dissected dermal sinus tract (H, white arrow) into the extradural intracranial space (I, white arrow) between the dura (D) posteriorly and the cut end of the frontal bone (FB) anteriorly. The scalp (S) has been reflected forward over the frontal bone. Dissection downward along the falx (F) revealed the intradural dermoid (J, arrow), that was debrided to display the cyst wall (K, arrow).

elements (Figure 11-19). At present, intracranial extension of a fibrous cord is not considered significant and has not been associated with sequelae.

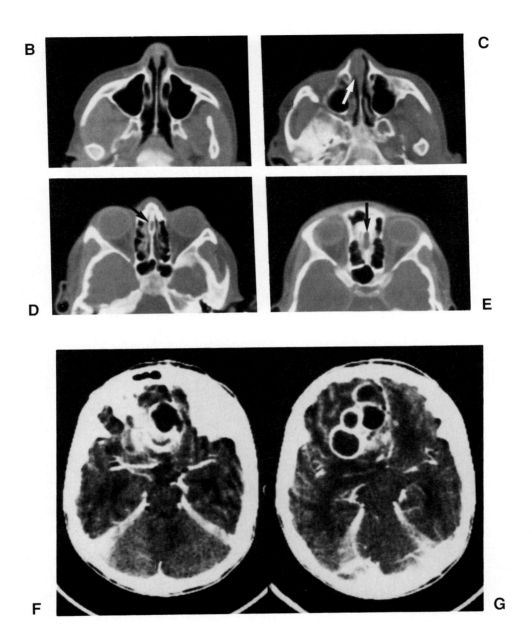

Nasal dermal sinuses are resected for cosmetic reasons, to avoid or treat the complications of local infection, and to prevent or treat secondary meningitis and cerebral abscess. Late development of squamous cell carcinoma is a theoretical rationale for resection, but such

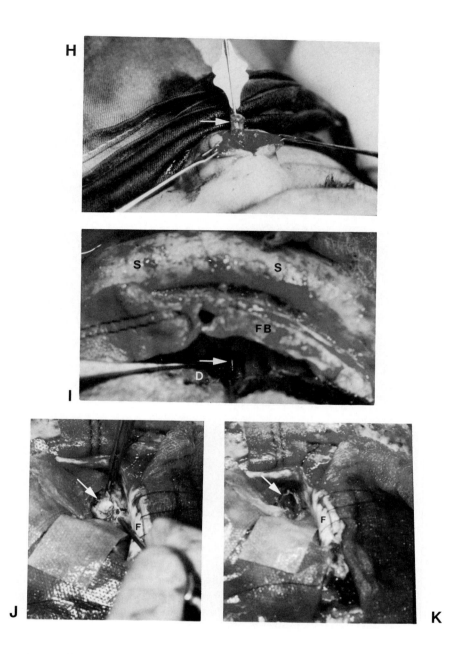

carcinoma has not yet been observed with nasal dermal sinuses **(Option (D) is false).**

In patients with dermal sinuses and cysts, CT successfully displays the course of the tract and any sequelae of infection. The ostium and tract usually appear as an isodense fibrous channel or as a lucent dermoid

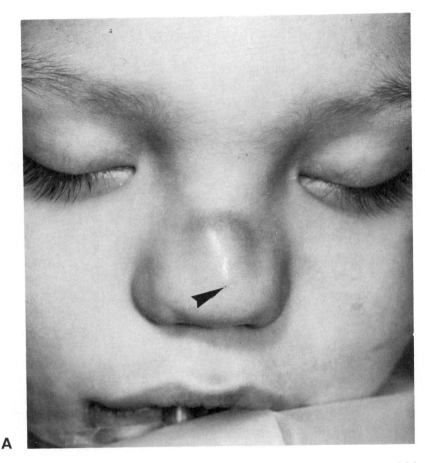

A

Figure 11-19. Nasal dermal sinus with fibrous cord in a 2-year-old boy.
(A) Photograph of the face demonstrates reddening and swelling of the
nasal bridge, just superior to a small sinus ostium (arrowhead). (B to E)
Direct coronal (B and C) and axial (D and E) CT scans demonstrate
asymmetric distortions of the crista and cribriform plate (arrowheads)
and widening of the upper nasal septum (arrowheads). At surgery, the
dermal elements and patent sinus stopped inferior to the skull base. The
wide foramen cecum and scalloped anterior border of the crista were
occupied by a fibrous cord that was continuous with the falx superiorly.
(Reprinted with permission from Naidich [5].)

channel that extends inward for a variable distance. Bony canals indicate
the course of the sinus through the nasal bones, ossified nasal septum,
and skull base. An uncomplicated dermoid cyst appears as a well-defined
lucency with an isodense capsule (Figure 11-20). Swelling and edema

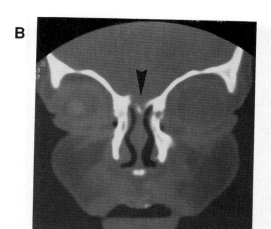

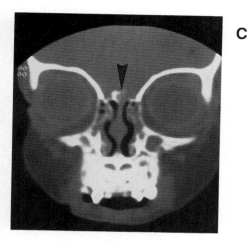

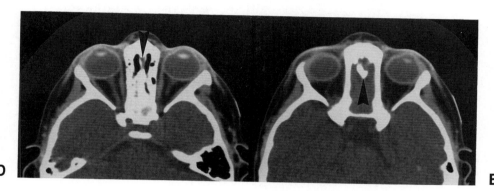

around the cyst suggest secondary inflammation (Figure 11-21). The intracranial ends of dermoid cysts typically lie in a hollowed-out gully along the anterior surface of a thickened enlarged crista. This hollow gives a false impression of a "bifid" crista. The intracranial portion of the dermoid may be lucent or dense.

Unfortunately, the only sure proof of intracranial extension is the actual demonstration of intracranial mass. CT demonstration of an enlarged foramen cecum and distorted crista galli is suggestive of intracranial extension but is not proof of such extension. Foraminal enlargement and distortion of the crista seem to form part of this malformation and may be present (i) with intracranial extension (Figures 11-17 and 11-18), (ii) without intracranial extension, or (iii) with intracranial extension of a fibrous cord rather than a dermoid (Figure 11-19) **(Option (E) is false).** To avoid unnecessary craniotomies, therefore, surgical studies suggest that the best approach is to dissect the

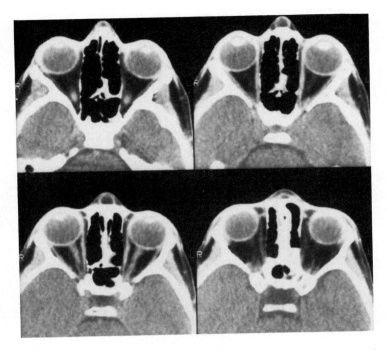

Figure 11-20. Axial noncontrast CT scans showing an extranasal epidermoid cyst with no infection in a 4-year-old boy. The well-defined isodense cyst wall and lucent center are clearly separable from the adjoining soft tissues. The nasal bones are flattened. No intracranial component is present.

extracranial portion of the tract along its entire length from the superficial ostium to the extracranial surface of the enlarged foramen cecum. The tract is then severed, and the severed end is sent for pathological examination. If the cephalic end has dermal elements, the dissection is then extended intracranially. If no dermal elements are found and if no mass was shown by CT, the procedure is concluded at that point.

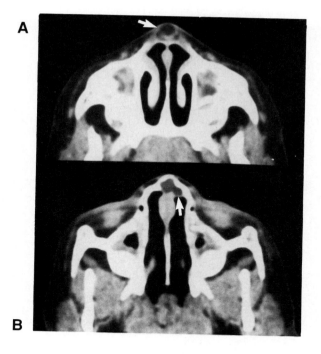

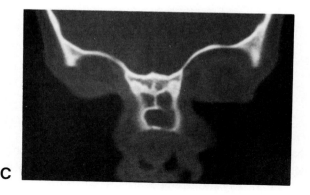

Figure 11-21. Mixed extranasal-intranasal dermoid with infection. (A and B) Axial noncontrast CT scans demonstrate extranasal (A) and intranasal (B) mass (white arrows), scalloped erosion of the nasal bones, and edema of the fat planes surrounding the cyst. Direct coronal (C) and reformatted sagittal contrast-enhanced CT scans (D and E) show the broadening and erosion of the nasal bridge and the relationship of the extranasal and intranasal portions of the dermoid cyst.

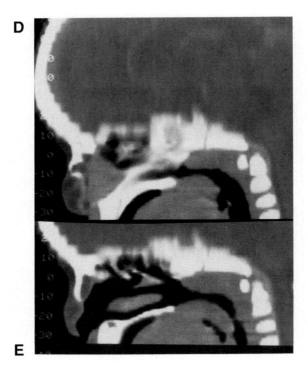

D

E

Question 52

Concerning nasal gliomas and cephaloceles,

    (A) an intranasal mass that is connected directly to the brain is a nasal cephalocele, not a nasal glioma

    (B) extranasal gliomas typically present as midline lesions at the nasal root

    (C) in infants, nasal gliomas are more common than inflammatory nasal polyps

    (D) nasal gliomas are very low-grade neoplasms

    (E) nasal gliomas are easily identified by their characteristically increased attenuation on computed tomography

Nasal "gliomas" are benign congenital masses of glial tissue that occur intranasally and/or extranasally at or near the root of the nose. They may be connected to the brain by a pedicle of glial tissue. By definition, they do not contain any cerebrospinal fluid (CSF)-filled space that is connected to either the ventricles or the subarachnoid space of the head.

Nasal gliomas and cephaloceles form a spectrum of related diseases. Characteristic cephaloceles contain ependyma-lined ventricles filled with

CSF. Prototypical nasal gliomas consist of solid masses of glial tissue that are entirely separate from the brain. Transitional forms include solid lesions with microscopic ependyma-lined canals, solid lesions intimately attached to the brain by glial pedicles with no ependyma-lined spaces, and solid lesions attached to the dura by fibrous bands with no glial pedicles. Analysis of cases reveals that the presence or absence of a pedicle and the presence or absence of thin ependyma-lined channels are not helpful in making surgically and radiologically useful distinctions among these lesions. Thus, the differential diagnosis between nasal gliomas and cephaloceles depends on the presence (cephalocele) or absence (nasal glioma) of communication between the intracranial CSF and any fluid spaces within or surrounding the mass **(Option (A) is false).** Indeed, nasal gliomas remain connected with intracranial structures in 15% of cases, usually through a defect in or near the cribriform plate.

Nasal gliomas are uncommon lesions, with perhaps 100 cases now reported. They occur sporadically, with no familial tendency and no sex predilection. They are rarely associated with other congenital malformations of the brain or body.

Nasal gliomas are subdivided into extranasal (60%), intranasal (30%), and mixed (10%) forms (Figure 11-22). The extranasal gliomas lie external to the nasal bones and nasal cavities. Most frequently, these gliomas occur at the bridge of the nose, to the left or right of the midline, but, curiously, not in the midline itself **(Option (B) is false).** Extranasal gliomas may also be found near the inner canthus, at the junction of the bony and cartilaginous portions of the nose, or between the frontal, nasal, ethmoid, and lacrimal bones.

Intranasal gliomas lie within the nasal or nasopharyngeal cavities, within the mouth, or, rarely, within the pterygopalatine fossa (Figure 11-23). In mixed nasal gliomas, the extranasal and intranasal components communicate via a defect in the nasal bones or around the lateral edges of the nasal bones (Figure 11-22). Rarely, the two portions communicate through defects in the orbital plate of the frontal bone or the frontal sinus. When extranasal gliomas lie to both sides of the nasal bridge, the two components communicate with each other via a defect in the nasal bones, constituting a mixed nasal glioma.

Clinically, extranasal gliomas usually present in early infancy or childhood as firm, slightly elastic, reddish to bluish, skin-covered masses. Capillary telangiectasias may cover the lesion. They exhibit no pulsations, do not increase in size with the Valsalva maneuver (crying), and do not pulsate or swell following compression of the ipsilateral jugular

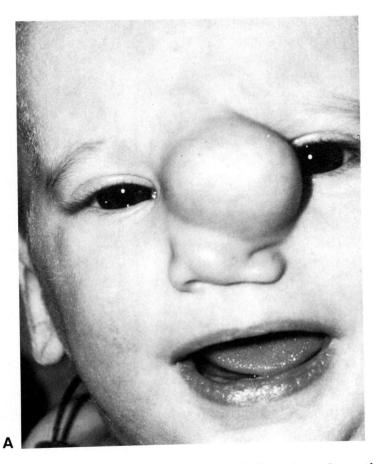

A

Figure 11-22.   Mixed extranasal-intranasal glioma in an 8-month-old boy
with a nasal mass that was present at birth and has grown in proportion
with the child. (A and B) Two views of the face demonstrate a 3-by-3-cm
firm left paramedian subcutaneous mass that displaces the septal and
alar cartilage, narrowing the nostril. The mass did not pulsate or change
size with crying. (C and D) At surgery, the mass was not bound to the
subcutaneous tissue. It lay nearly entirely external to the nasal bones,
to the left of midline. A narrow stalk (arrows) passed directly through the
left nasal bone and extended upward to the left cribriform plate. (E)
Bisecting the specimen revealed a homogeneous mass of smooth
grayish-white shiny tissue. Histologic examination revealed brain and
fibrous tissue consistent with nasal glioma.

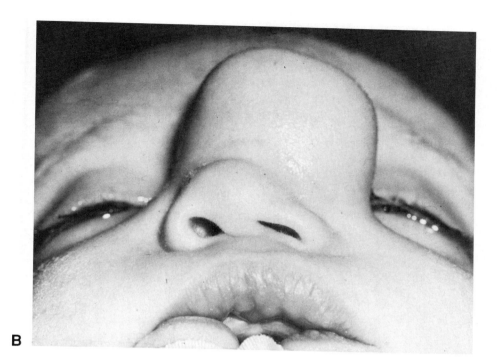

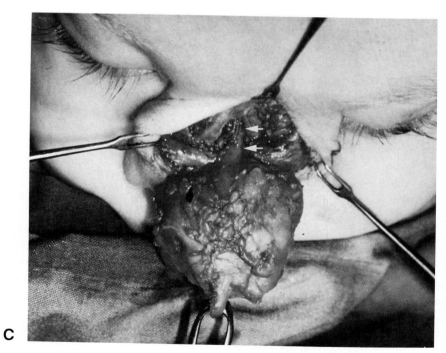

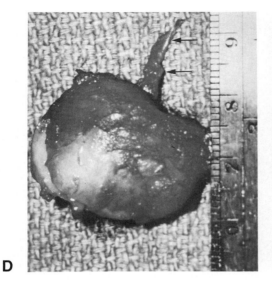
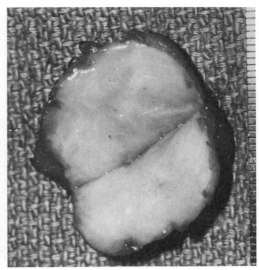

D   E

vein (negative Furstenburg sign). These lesions usually grow slowly in proportion to adjacent tissue but may grow more or less rapidly. They can cause severe deformity by displacing the nasal skeleton, the adjoining maxilla, and the orbital walls. Hypertelorism may result.

Intranasal gliomas usually present as large, firm, polypoid, submucosal masses that may extend inferiorly toward or nearly to the nostril. They usually attach to the turbinates and lie medial to the middle turbinate, between the middle turbinate and the nasal septum. Rarely, they attach to the septum itself. These intranasal masses expand the nasal fossa, widen the nasal bridge, and deviate the septum contralaterally. Obstruction of the nasal passage may lead to respiratory distress, especially in infants. Blockage of the nasolacrimal duct may cause epiphora on the affected side. CSF rhinorrhea, meningitis, and epistaxis may be the presenting complaints.

Intranasal gliomas are commonly confused with inflammatory polyps. However, nasal gliomas usually have a firmer consistency and appear to be less translucent than inflammatory polyps. Intranasal gliomas typically lie medial to the middle turbinate, whereas inflammatory polyps typically lie inferolateral to the middle turbinate. Only posterior ethmoid polyps project into the same space as the nasal glioma. Most important, nasal gliomas usually present in infancy, whereas ordinary nasal polyps are almost unheard of under 5 years of age **(Option (C) is true).**

Pathologically, nasal gliomas resemble reactive gliosis rather than neoplasia. No invasion of surrounding tissue has ever been observed; no

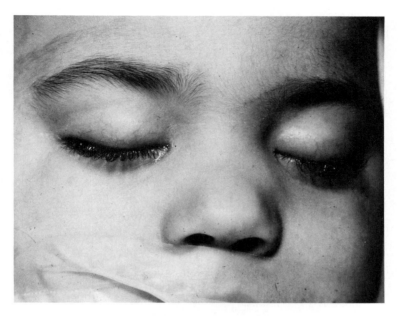

A

Figure 11-23. Intranasal glioma with intracranial attachments. (A) A photograph of the patient's face demonstrates widening of the nasal bridge and the left nostril (present prior to intubation). (B to D) Water-soluble positive-contrast cisternography. Axial (B), direct coronal (C), and reformatted sagittal (D) CT sections demonstrate a large left unilateral intranasal mass (arrowheads) that deviates the nasal septum rightward, bows the left nasal bone outward, and extends superiorly through a widened foramen cecum (black arrow) into the interdural space (white arrows) between the leaves of the falx. Opacified CSF outlines the intracranial portion of the mass but does not extend extracranially into or around the intranasal portion of the mass. (E and F) Frontal intraoperative photographs oriented like panels A and C. (E) The scalp (S) has been reflected over the orbits (O). Keyhole resection of the frontonasal junction exposes the frontal dura (D) and nasal cavity, bounded by remnant frontal bone (F) at the supraorbital ridges and remnant nasal bone (N) laterally. The frontal dura of each side is reflected inward in the midline (arrowheads) to form the falx. The interdural space (white arrows) is widened inferiorly. (F) Further dissection frees the interdural portion (between forceps) of the nasal glioma and proves that it is directly continuous with the intranasal portion (white arrows) of the mass.

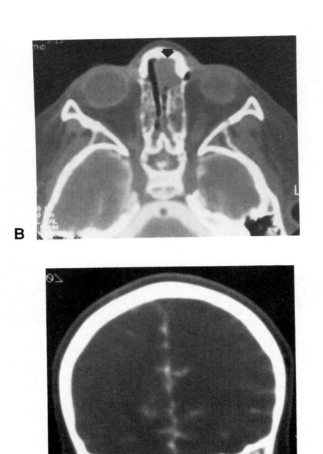

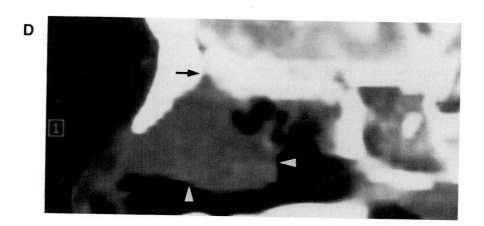

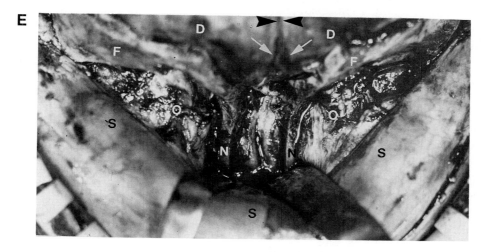

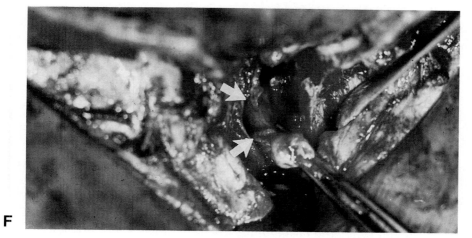

metastases have been reported. Thus, they are classified as heterotopias and not neoplasias **(Option (D) is false).**

Histologic studies show that the nasal glioma consists of small or large aggregates of fibrous or gemistocytic astrocytes. The cells may be multinuclear, but they exhibit no mitotic figures and no bizarre nuclear forms. Fibrous connective tissue enwraps the blood vessels and extends outward to form collagenous septa that partially subdivide the mass. Prominent zones of granulation tissue may be present. The lesion is usually not encapsulated. However, astrocytic processes, fibroblasts, and collagen may form a loose or dense connective tissue capsule. Extranasal gliomas are then surrounded by dermis with dermal appendages. Intranasal gliomas are surrounded by minor salivary glands, fibrovascular tissue, and nasal mucosa.

Only 10% of reported nasal gliomas contain neurons. This absence of neurons in 90% has been attributed to the insufficient supply of oxygen to support them or to the failure of neurons to differentiate from the embryonic neuroectoderm within the isolated glioma.

Imaging studies display the nasal glioma as an isodense soft tissue mass that deforms the nasal fossa **(Option (E) is false).** CT also demonstrates any bony evidence of extension through the glabella, nasal bones, cribriform plate, or foramen cecum (Figure 11-23). Calcification may be present in rare cases. Routine CT studies usually fail to differentiate between nasal glioma and encephalocele, unless the communicating CSF space is very large. It is often necessary to rule in or rule out CSF communication by positive-contrast CT cisternography in order to achieve the correct differential diagnosis (Figure 11-23).

Question 53

Concerning cephaloceles,

(A) the size of the fluid space within the sac determines patient prognosis
(B) sincipital cephaloceles are closely linked with other neural tube defects
(C) in nasofrontal cephaloceles, the ethmoid bone is displaced inferiorly

Cephaloceles are congenital herniations of intracranial contents through a cranial defect. When the herniation contains brain, it is a meningoencephalocele. If the herniation contains only meninges, it is a cranial meningocele. Cephaloceles are classified by the site of the cranial defect through which the brain and meninges protrude (Table 11-1). The

Table 11-1. Classification of cephaloceles*

1. Occipital cephaloceles
    Cervico-occipital (continuous with cervical
        rachischisis)
    Low occipital (involving foramen magnum)
    High occipital (above intact rim of foramen
        magnum)

2. Cephaloceles of the cranial vault
    Temporal
    Posterior fontanelle
    Interparietal
    Anterior fontanelle
    Interfrontal

3. Frontoethmoidal cephaloceles
    Nasofrontal
    Naso-ethmoidal
    Naso-orbital   } Sincipital cephaloceles

4. Basal cephaloceles
    Transethmoidal
    Sphenoethmoidal
    Transsphenoidal
    Frontosphenoidal

5. Cephaloceles associated with
        cranioschisis
    Cranial-upper facial cleft
    Basal-lower facial cleft
    Acrania and anencephaly

*Modified from Suwanwela and Suwanwela [27].

size of the fluid spaces does not determine patient prognosis **(Option (A) is false).**

Cephaloceles situated in the anterior part of the skull are often designated sincipital cephaloceles (Figure 11-24). These include the frontoethmoidal cephaloceles and the interfrontal subtype of cranial cephaloceles. Basal cephaloceles include intranasal, nasopharyngeal, and posterior orbital cephaloceles classified as transethmoidal, sphenoethmoidal, transsphenoidal, and frontosphenoidal cephaloceles. The fundamental difference between sincipital and basal cephaloceles is that sincipital cephaloceles always present as external masses along the nose, orbital margin, or forehead, whereas basal cephaloceles are not visible externally, unless they grow large enough to protrude from the nostril or mouth secondarily.

Cephaloceles are common lesions, with an incidence of 1 per 4,000 live births. Overall, occipital cephaloceles are the most frequent type (67 to 80%). Sincipital cephaloceles (15%) and basal cephaloceles (10%) are less common. The occipital and the sincipital cephaloceles appear to be distinctly different diseases. Occipital cephaloceles are linked with neural tube defects such as myelomeningocele; sincipital cephaloceles are not **(Option (B) is false).** Occipital cephaloceles are the most frequent type among people of European descent, while sincipital cephaloceles are the most frequent type among Malaysians and certain other Southeast Asian

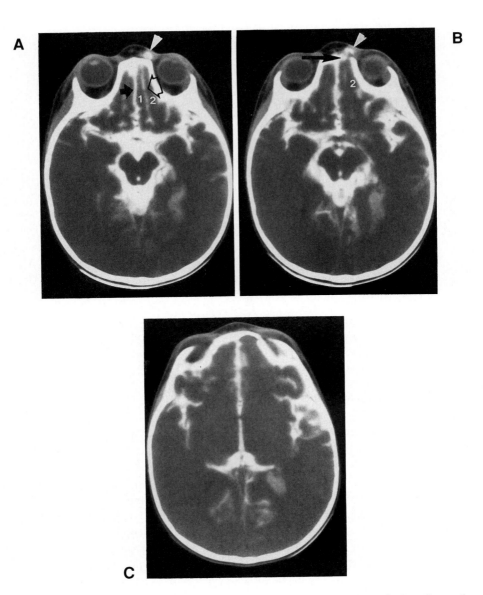

Figure 11-24. Sincipital cephalocele. Asymmetric left inferior frontal meningoencephalocele in a 17-month-old boy who had undergone partial resection of a "nasal glioma" at another institution. Axial (A to C) and direct coronal (D to F), water-soluble CT cisternograms reveal a left paramedian bone defect (black arrows) just superolateral to the nasofrontal suture (black arrowhead). The interhemispheric fissure (small black arrow), gyrus rectus (1) and olfactory sulcus (outline arrowhead) lie in normal position. The medial orbital gyrus (2) is directly related to the bone defect and is associated with scalloped erosion of the inner surface of the frontal bone. Contrast in the extracranial subarachnoid space (white arrowheads) outlines the herniated neural tissue and documents that this is an encephalocele and not a "glioma." At surgery the inferior surface of the frontal lobe protruded into the sac. Histologic examination of the resected specimen revealed brain tissue with disorganized neurons and fibroconnective tissue, a finding consistent with encephalocele.

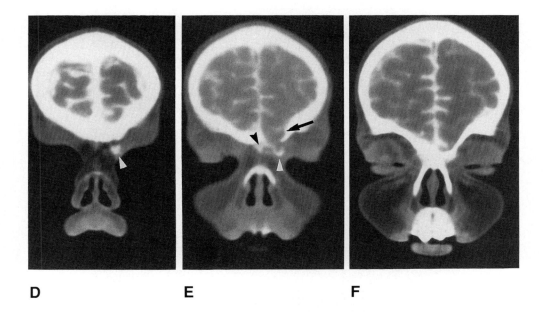

D   E   F

groups. Thus, among Australian aborigines nearly all cephaloceles are sincipital, whereas among Australians of European descent 67% are occipital and 2% are sincipital.

Frontoethmoidal cephaloceles are characterized by a cranial defect at the junction of the frontal and ethmoid bones. In 90%, the intracranial end of the defect is a single midline ostium that corresponds to the foramen cecum. In 10%, an intact midline bridge of bone divides the defect into bilateral paired ostia situated at the anterior ends of the cribriform plates.

The frontoethmoidal cephaloceles are subdivided into three types in accord with the position of the facial end of the cranial defect (Figure 11-25). In the nasofrontal form (50 to 61%), the facial end of the defect lies between the frontal and the nasal bones, and so the ostium presents at the nasion between deformed orbits (Figures 11-25 and 11-26). Specifically, in this type the frontal bones are displaced superiorly. The nasal bones, frontal processes of maxillae, and nasal cartilage are all displaced inferiorly, away from the frontal bone, but retain a normal relationship to each other. The ethmoid bone is displaced inferiorly, so that the midline portion of the anterior fossa is very deep and the crista projects into the defect from its inferior rim **(Option (C) is true).** The anterior portions of the medial orbital walls are displaced laterally. The

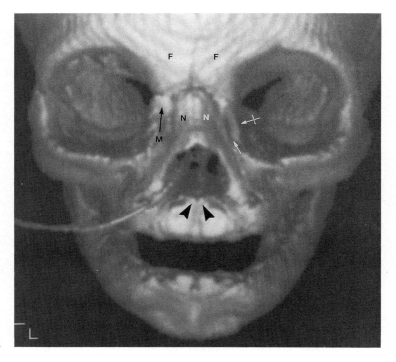

Figure 11-25. Pathways for the frontoethmoidal cephaloceles in a normal facial skeleton of a 5-month-old boy. (A to C) Reformatted three-dimensional CT images display the contours and relationships of the individual bones of the skull and face, plus the intervening sutures. E = ethmoid bone (lamina papyracea), F = frontal bone, L = lacrimal bone, M = frontal process of the maxilla, N = nasal bone. Note the interfrontal, internasal, frontonasal, and frontomaxillary sutures; the nasal spines (arrowheads) of the maxillae and the lacrimal sac fossa (arrow). The anterior crest of the lacrimal sac fossa is formed by the frontal process of maxilla; the posterior crest (crossed white arrow) is formed by the lacrimal bone. Cartilaginous structures are not displayed by this technique. (D) The sites through which the three subtypes of the frontoethmoidal cephaloceles protrude are indicated by the three numbered arrows. (1) Nasofrontal cephalocele. The facial end of the canal lies between the frontal and nasal bones. The frontal bones form the superior margin of the defect. The nasal bones, frontal processes of the maxillae, and nasal cartilage form the inferior margin of the defect. (2) Nasoethmoidal cephalocele. The facial end of the canal lies between the nasal bones and the nasal cartilage. The nasal bones and the frontal processes of the maxillae form the superior margin of the defect. The nasal cartilage and nasal septum form the inferior margin of the defect. (3) Naso-orbital cephalocele. The facial end of the canal lies in the medial wall of the orbit. The frontal process of maxilla forms the anterior margin of the defect. The lacrimal bone and lamina papyracea of the ethmoid form the posterior wall of the defect.

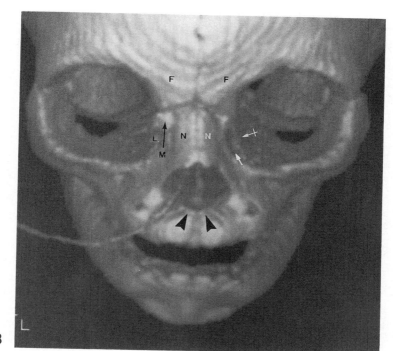

B

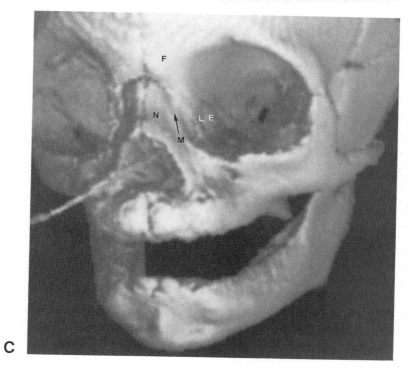

C

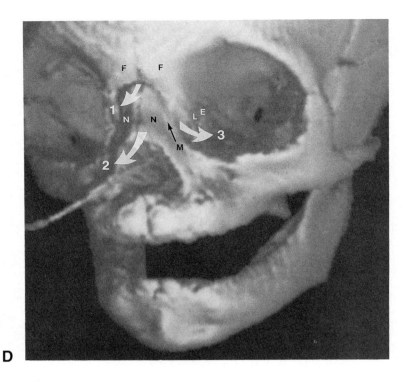

D

bone canal is short because the intracranial (frontoethmoidal) and the extracranial (nasofrontal) ends of the defect lie close together.

The associated soft tissue mass lies at the glabella or nasal root. The mass may be small (1 to 2 cm) or larger than the infant's head (Figure 11-26). Most of the nasofrontal cephaloceles are firm, solid masses and exhibit no transmitted pulsations. Some are cystic, compressible, and pulsatile and increase in size with the Valsalva maneuver (crying). The mass usually grows as the child grows. Cystic masses may increase in size disproportionately rapidly as CSF pools within the sac. The cephalocele may be covered by intact skin, thin skin that ruptures to leak CSF, or no skin at all, exposing brain to the environment. The falx frequently extends into the sac, partially subdividing it.

The herniated brain may be well preserved with recognizable gyri and sulci that converge toward the hernia ostium, or the herniated brain may be reduced to a mass of distorted gliotic tissue (Figure 11-27). Typically, the brain is not adherent to the base of the sac at the ostium, but may be adherent to the meninges at the dome of the sac (60%).

The tips of the frontal lobes usually protrude into the defect, symmetrically or asymmetrically. The olfactory bulbs may herniate with

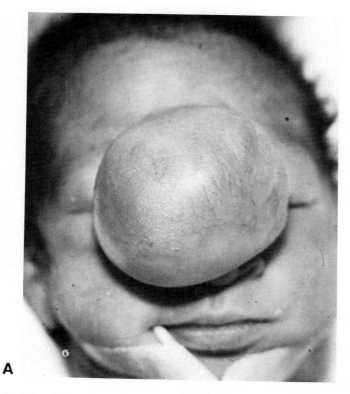

A

Figure 11-26. Nasofrontal form of frontoethmoidal cephalocele in a newborn girl. (A and B) Frontal and lateral views of the face. A large skin-covered midline mass protrudes between the two orbits, overlies the nasal bones and nasal cartilage, and compresses the nostrils. Arrow indicates the angle of observation for the surgical photographs. (C to F) Axial CT scans through the mass oriented as in the following surgical specimen (G). (C) Noncontrast CT scan and (D) contrast-enhanced CT scan obtained on different days. The mass is predominantly cystic. The inferior portions of both frontal lobes (arrows) protrude directly into the sac to different degrees and so appear multilobular. (E and F) The ostium of the cephalocele lies above the ethmoid (E) and nasal (N) bones but below the frontal (F) bones, and so the lesion is a frontonasal type of frontoethmoidal cephalocele. (G) Surgical photograph. View of the frontal bone (F) from above after reflection of the scalp (S) anteriorly and opening of the upper wall of the cephalocele to expose its contents. Most of the sac was filled with CSF. Portions of both frontal lobes (arrows) protrude into the sac, separated by the interhemispheric fissure. Multiple glial nodules (black arrowheads) stud the meninges that form the inner lining of the sac. White arrowheads indicate the ostium of the cephalocele.

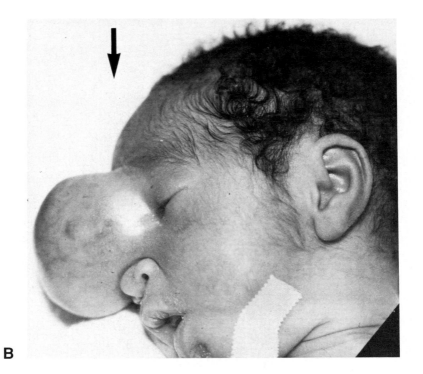

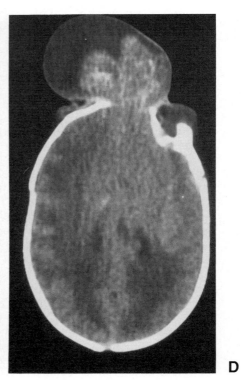

B

C

D

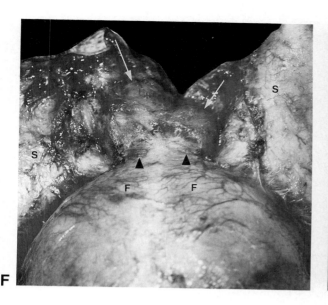

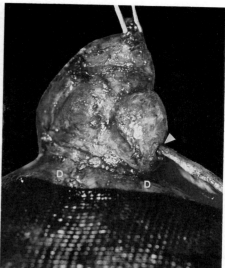

F

G

had concurrent agenesis of the corpus callosum with interhemispheric cyst.

Harverson et al. detailed the radiologic differences between the nasofrontal and nasoethmoidal cephaloceles. In the nasofrontal form the defect in the frontal bone is V-shaped. The superior aspects of the medial orbital walls are bowed and displaced laterally. The nasal bones remain attached to the cribriform plate at the lower margin of the ostium. Thus the cribriform plate and nasal bones lie unusually low between the orbits. There is a large gap between the frontal and ethmoidal bones. The soft tissue mass lies directly in front of the bone defect, usually in the midline, and is often spherical. Conversely, in the nasoethmoidal form the bone defect is usually circular and is situated between the orbits, causing increased interorbital distance. The nasal bones remain attached to the frontal bones along the upper margins of the ostium. The cribriform plate lies at a normal height with respect to the orbits. The soft tissue mass lies to one side of the midline, beside the nasal cartilage. It may be bilateral.

In the naso-orbital form of frontoethmoidal cephalocele (6 to 10%), the facial end of the defect lies at the medial wall of the orbit, so the ostium presents at the inner canthus and nasolabial folds. Specifically, the frontal process of maxilla is separated from the lacrimal and ethmoid bones. The abnormal frontal process of maxilla forms the anterior margin of the defect. The lacrimal bone and lamina papyracea of the ethmoid

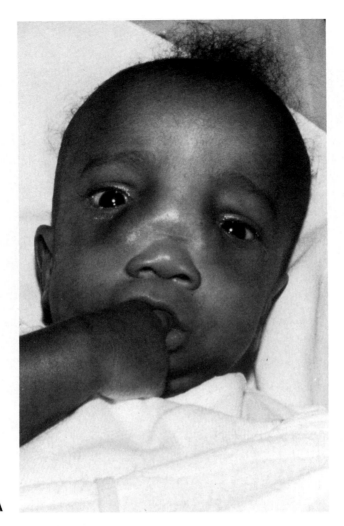

A

Figure 11-28. Nasoethmoidal form of frontoethmoidal cephalocele in a 5½-month-old boy with complete agenesis of the corpus callosum. (A) Patient photograph reveals hypertelorism, bulging at the glabella, and cystic swellings at the inner canthi and nasolabial folds bilaterally. (B to F) Water-soluble positive-contrast CT cisternograms. (B and C) Axial images demonstrate separation of the frontal (F) and ethmoidal (E) bones by the encephalocele. The lesion bulges into the left orbit, displacing the muscle cone and globe (G) laterally. A separate, tense cyst (C in panel B) lies anteromedial to the right globe. A = a large noncommunicating suprasellar arachnoid cyst. (D to F) Serial direct coronal CT scans demonstrate normal relationship of the frontal (F) and nasal (N) bones, ruling out the nasofrontal form of cephalocele. The facial end of the defect lies between the nasal bone and the nasal cartilage, and so this is a nasoethmoidal form of frontoethmoidal cephalocele. The left globe (G) is deviated and compressed by the cephalocele and associated cysts. The right cyst (C) lay anterior to maxilla, causing the visible swelling. The interhemispheric fissure (white arrowhead) deviates far to one side. At surgery the falx attached to the roof of the left orbit. The contralateral right frontal lobe extended into the midline and then herniated inferiorly.

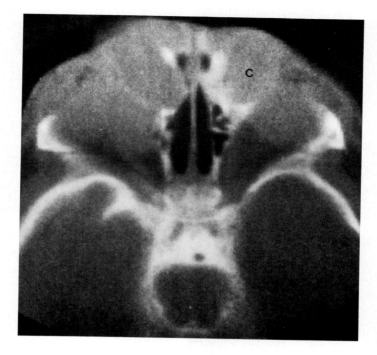

B

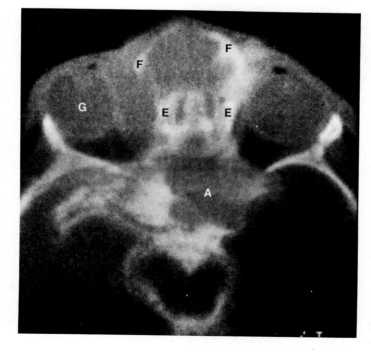

C

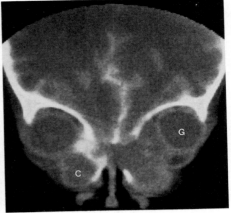

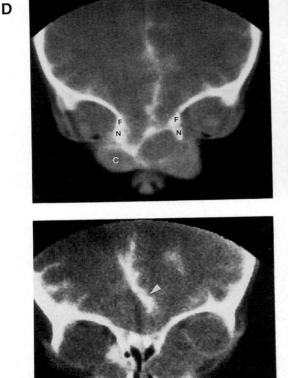

form the posterior edge of the defect. The frontal bones, nasal bones, and nasal cartilage retain their normal relationship to each other. In this type, the intracranial (frontoethmoid) and extracranial (medial orbital) ends of the defect are widely separated, so the canal is very long.

Patients with naso-orbital cephalocele may present with cystic soft tissue masses at the nasolabial folds between the nose and the lower eyelid. These folds contain nubbins of brain.

Suwanwela et al. reviewed the clinical findings in 25 patients with frontoethmoidal cephaloceles. Microcephaly was present in 24%, unilateral or bilateral microphthalmos was present in 16%, hydrocephalus was present in 12%, and seizures were present in 4%. Mental retardation was present in 43% of those old enough to test. CSF leakage and continuous bleeding from the exposed brain were major problems in those cephaloceles that lacked skin cover or in which the thin skin cover ruptured. Rappoport et al. found significant associated congenital anomalies, such as microphthalmos, mental retardation, and syndactyly with appendicular constriction bands in 33% of these patients. In one patient with a large frontoethmoidal cephalocele, an arachnoid cyst overlying the right frontal lobe communicated with the external sac.

Question 54

Concerning histiocytosis X,

(A) calvarial lesions are more commonly parietal than temporal
(B) involvement of the posterior pituitary gland most commonly accounts for concurrent diabetes insipidus
(C) calvarial lesions frequently erode the outer table to present as tender soft tissue masses
(D) calvarial lesions commonly erode through dura into the underlying cortex
(E) computed tomographic demonstration of a central density within the calvarial lesion rules out this diagnosis

Histiocytosis X designates a group of diseases that are characterized by the proliferation or infiltration of histiocytes in diverse tissues. The areas of involvement show predominant polygonal histiocytes with areas of necrosis and fibrosis and variable associated infiltrates of eosinophils, multinucleated giant cells, plasma cells, and lymphocytes. The etiology of this condition is unknown. The relationships among the different diseases in the group are obscure.

Originally, Hand (1893), Schüller (1915), and Christian (1919) described a triad of irregular defects of membranous bone, exophthalmos, and diabetes insipidus. Letterer (1924) and Siwe (1933) reported infants with fever, purulent otitis media, hepatosplenomegaly, generalized lymphadenopathy, and purpura. Lichtenstein and Jaffe (1940) and Otani and Ehrlich (1940) reported the solitary bone lesions termed eosinophilic granuloma. These were grouped together by Lichtenstein (1953) as histiocytosis X. In recent usage, the severe disseminated form, occurring in infants 0 to 2 years of age, is designated Letterer-Siwe disease. Multiple characteristic lesions evolving slowly in a child over 3 years of age are designated Hand-Schüller-Christian disease.

Histiocytosis X affects patients of any age, but it is most frequent in infants under 2 years of age. Boys predominate in a ratio of approximately

2:1. Most cases are sporadic, but families with histiocytosis X have been reported.

Histiocytosis X commonly affects the head and neck (up to 88% of patients). Lesions of the calvarium and the mandible predominate. Smith and Evans found skull lesions in 42% and mandibular lesions in 18% of 62 children with histiocytosis X. Surprisingly, Rawlings and Wilkins found that *calvarial* eosinophilic granuloma was usually an isolated lesion. No patient with multifocal eosinophilic granuloma had a calvarial lesion. No patient who presented with eosinophilic granuloma at a distant site later developed calvarial eosinophilic granuloma.

In the skull, the parietal bone is affected most commonly (42%), followed by the frontal bone (31%), temporal bone (12%), occipital bone (12%), and fronto-temporoparietal "bone" (4%) **(Option (A) is true).** The calvarial lesions of eosinophilic granuloma are usually located away from the sutures. Occasionally, a lesion may extend medially to overlie the midsagittal suture and sinus.

Characteristically, patients present with a painful enlarging skull mass. The mass is tender, firm, and fixed to the skull. Bone margins may be palpable (44%). Occasionally, the lesion is an asymptomatic incidental finding. Periorbital bone disease is often associated with proptosis and exophthalmos. Temporal bone disease is associated with vertigo and sensorineural hearing loss and can easily mimic mastoiditis, cholesteatoma, and malignant tumors such as rhabdomyosarcoma. Mandibular lesions are associated with periodontitis and with early eruption and displacement of teeth.

Dermatologic lesions are present in 42% of all cases of histiocytosis X and in 62% of affected infants. Tumefactions are commonly observed overlying the bone lesions. Seborrhea, mild eczema, or severe hemorrhagic eczema is observed in the scalp or along the hair line. Other common clinical findings in the head and neck include cervical lymphadenopathy (30%), aural lesions (21%) such as aural polyps and external otitis that are unresponsive to antibiotic therapy, and oral lesions (15%), especially oral ulcerations and tumefactions.

Intracranial involvement is common in patients with disseminated forms of histiocytosis X such as Hand-Schüller-Christian disease and Letterer-Siwe disease. The hypothalamus is affected most frequently, causing diabetes insipidus in one-half to one-third of cases **(Option (B) is false).** Growth hormone deficiency may also be present. Involvement of other areas is uncommon, but the optic chiasm, cerebellum, and spinal cord may be affected. Miller et al. used CT to demonstrate low-density suprasellar masses in five patients with histiocytosis X and diabetes insipidus. Associated hypothalamic mass was detected in three of the five (60%), and contrast enhancement was evident in three of the five (60%).

Skull radiographs are positive in 80% of those patients with diabetes insipidus, showing erosive changes about the sella in 60% and classic lesions of the skull and/or mandible in 60%. Surprisingly, bone destruction is associated with improved prognosis. In the series of Smith and Evans, 85% of survivors had bone lesions, whereas only 45% of fatal cases had bone lesions.

The typical calvarial lesion of eosinophilic granuloma is a sharply defined, lytic diploic lesion with no sclerotic rim and no periosteal reaction (Figure 11-29). It has a purely lucent matrix without the spoke-wheeling usually associated with hemangioma. A central density—termed button sequestrum—may remain within the center of the lesion. Eosinophilic granuloma usually erodes the inner and outer tables to differing degrees, giving the defect a sloping "beveled" wall. The calvarial lesions may be purely diploic. These lesions often present with pain alone. More frequently, the lesions erode through the outer table to present with a tender subgaleal soft tissue mass as well as pain **(Option (C) is true)**.

The lesion also commonly erodes through the inner table, displaces dura inward, and undermines the dura to form a small epidural mass around the circumference of the bone defect. Rarely, the lesion may invade through the dura into the cerebral cortex, causing seizures **(Option (D) is false)**.

On CT scans, calvarial eosinophilic granuloma appears as a lucent intradiploic lesion with sharply defined, irregular distribution of the inner and outer tables. Button sequestra appear as dense plates of bone within the lucent mass **(Option (E) is false)**. After contrast agent administration, the lesion usually shows moderately intense, inhomogeneous enhancement, with greatest density centrally or peripherally (Figures 11-29 and 11-30). The button sequestrum may enhance. Enhancing dura outlines the deep extent of the mass.

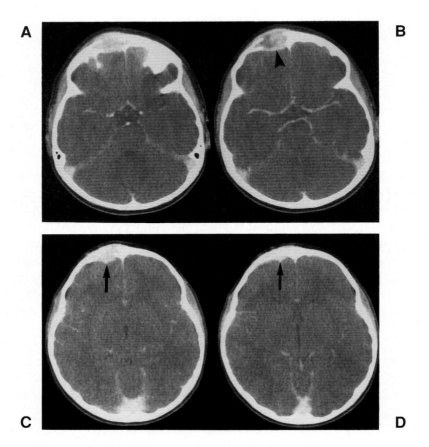

Figure 11-29. Eosinophilic granuloma of the frontal bone in a 3-year-old girl with a 3-week history of forehead swelling. Work-up revealed no other lesions. (A to D) Axial contrast-enhanced CT scans demonstrate a paramedian heterogeneously enhancing, frontal intradiploic soft tissue mass that erodes through the outer table to displace the scalp and through the inner table to displace dura (arrowhead) inward. The intracranial mass extends superiorly (arrow) deep to the margin of the bone defect. (E to H) Corresponding bone algorithm images demonstrate the expansion of the diploic space, mostly well-defined margins of the lesion and extension to the frontal midline. At surgery the external surface of the lesion was confined by pericranium. The tumor was delivered as an external "cap" followed by a soft center. The deep surface of the lesion extended into the dura but not deep to dura.

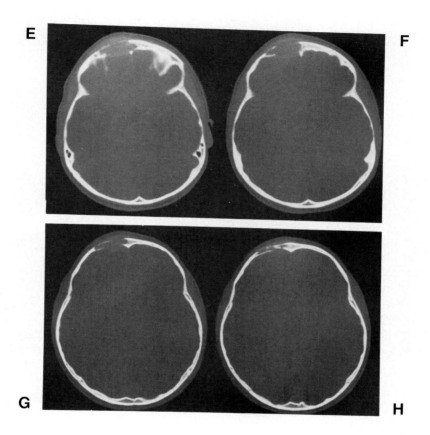

E   F

G   H

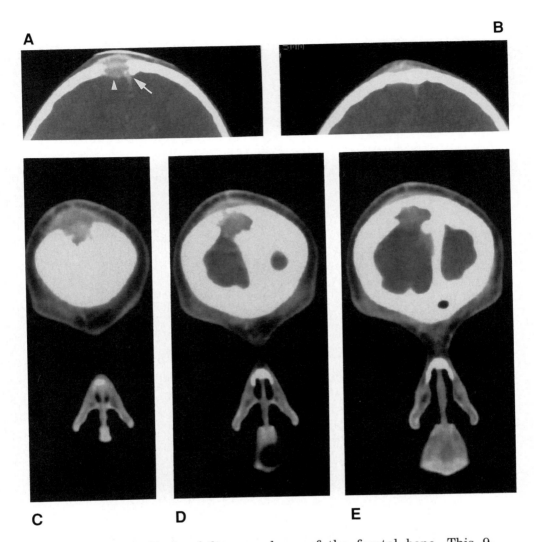

Figure 11-30. Eosinophilic granuloma of the frontal bone. This 9-year-old boy presented with frontal swelling. (A to E) Axial (A and B) and direct coronal (C to E) contrast-enhanced CT scans demonstrate a moderately well-defined intradiploic frontal bone lesion that erodes through the outer table to form a large subcutaneous mass and through the inner table to displace dura (white arrowhead) inward. The mass extends to the midline in relationship to the superior sagittal sinus (white arrow). The enhancement is inhomogeneous, with a central band of greater density. (F to J) Corresponding bone algorithm images display the slightly irregular scalloping of the lesion margins. At surgery the mass could not be separated from the dura.

F

G

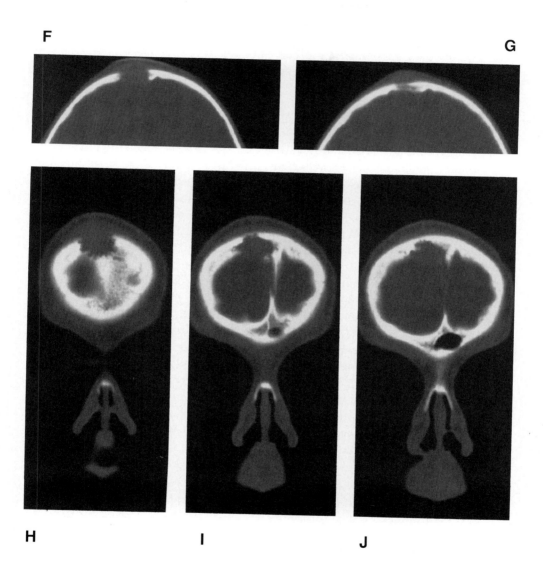

H

I

J

Question 55

Concerning sinus pericranii,

(A) it signifies chronic elevation of intracranial pressure
(B) it most commonly involves the frontal region
(C) it lies within 2 cm of the true midline, to either side of the superior sagittal sinus
(D) it is usually associated with well-defined calvarial defects
(E) it communicates with the dural venous sinuses via emissary and diploic veins

Sinus pericranii is a collection of nonmuscular venous blood vessels or venous hemangiomas that adhere tightly to the outer surface of the skull and that communicate directly with an intracranial venous sinus by way of many diploic veins of various sizes. The lesion receives no direct blood supply from either the internal or external carotid artery. Rather, the sinus fills with blood from the intracranial venous sinuses and drains back to those sinuses. The etiology of the condition is unknown, but relationships to trauma are postulated as one potential cause.

Patients with sinus pericranii typically present with a round, slowly enlarging scalp mass that is fluctuant but not pulsatile. The mass enlarges with increased intracranial pressure from crying, dependent position, or jugular compression (Figure 11-31). However, there is no evidence that the lesion results from an acute or chronic elevation of intracranial pressure **(Option (A) is false).** It diminishes in size with head elevation and disappears entirely upon prolonged digital compression. The subjacent bone is scalloped or fenestrated. The mass is fixed to the calvarium, but the overlying skin is usually normal. Neurologic examination is characteristically normal, although the patient may complain of headache, vague fullness, nausea, or vertigo. Sinus pericranii may first be detected at any age from birth onward. Males are affected more commonly than females (65 vs. 35%).

Sinus pericranii is usually frontal in location (40%). Parietal (34%), occipital (23%), and temporal (4%) sites are less common **(Option (B) is true).** The lesion often lies near the superior sagittal sinus, especially the central and posterior thirds of the sinus. However, the lesion itself need not be midline. It may lie far lateral, even over the mastoid bone **(Option (C) is false).**

The sinus clearly lies deep to the galeal aponeurosis. Its exact relationship to the periosteum is controversial, because the periosteum is difficult to define, even by histologic examination. Some lesions appear to be subperiosteal, others appear to be intraperiosteal, and still others appear to be extraperiosteal but subgaleal.

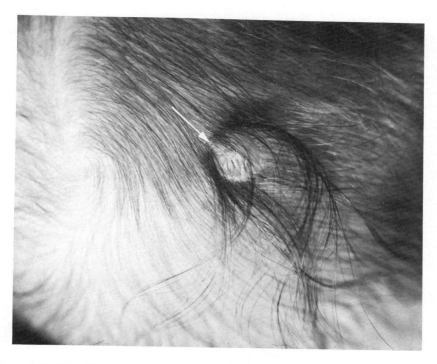

A

Figure 11-31. Sinus pericranii in a 4-month-old boy with a scalp lesion since birth. (A) Photograph of the top of the patient's head reveals a right posterior parietal paramedian zone of atrophic skin (white arrow) surrounded by a ring of abnormal hair. The atrophic zone bulged outward with crying. The lesion and the surrounding hair have increased in size disproportionately rapidly. (B to E) Direct coronal contrast-enhanced CT scans displayed from posterior (B) to anterior (E) reveal an enhancing cutaneous and subcutaneous lesion (white arrowhead in panel A) that communicates with the superior sagittal sinus via a large, obliquely oriented paramedian channel (white arrows). (F and G) Intraoperative photographs. (F) At surgery, the lesion (arrow) was seen to extend through the skin to the parietal bone (P), where it entered an oblique osseous canal. D = dura. (G) Exposure of the subjacent dura disclosed a dural defect (white arrow) through which the lesion (white arrowhead) continued anteromedially to join with the superior sagittal sinus.

Skull radiographs usually reveal a well-defined bone defect that may extend partially or completely through the calvarium **(Option (D) is true).** The edges of the defect are usually sharply marginated, but they may have irregular crevices or vascular honeycombing. Noncontrast CT scans are usually negative, except for the bone defect. Calcifications are

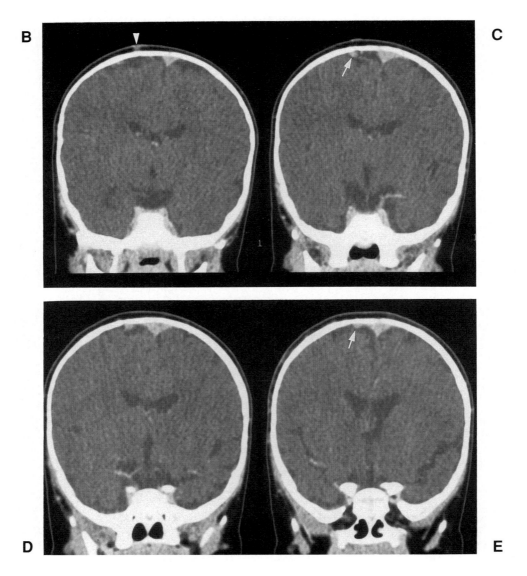

B

C

D

E

not a feature of this condition. Contrast-enhanced CT scans may show the transosseous communications and enlarged size of the subjacent veins or sinuses (Figure 11-31). Internal carotid, external carotid, and vertebral arteriograms are typically negative. Direct puncture of the lesion yields large volumes of venous blood. Injection of a contrast agent through that needle opacifies the sinus and documents the transosseous passage of contrast material through multiple enlarged diploic and epidural veins

Notes

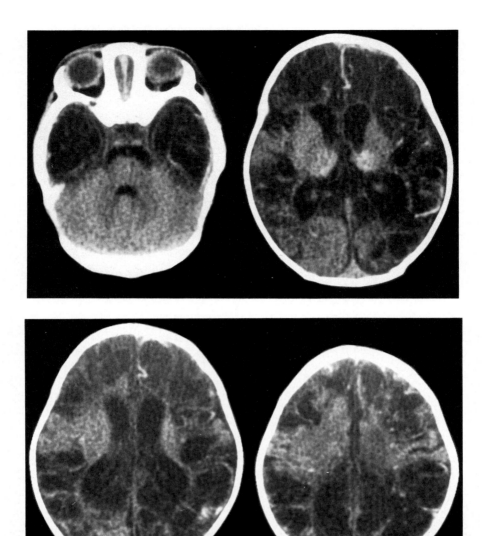

Figure 12-1. This full-term infant girl was born with the umbilical cord wound once about the neck and had Apgar scores of 9 and 9 at 1 and 5 minutes, respectively. On day 13 she developed cyanosis, apnea, and seizures. Gram stain and cultures and titers of virus in blood and in cerebrospinal fluid were all negative. Physical examination showed a lethargic girl with weak grasp, increased extensor tone, posturing, and weakly up-going toes bilaterally. You are shown four sections of a noncontrast computed tomographic (CT) scan obtained at 8 weeks of age.

Case 12: Multicystic Encephalomalacia

Question 56

Which *one* of the following is the MOST likely diagnosis?

(A) Multicystic encephalomalacia
(B) Porencephaly
(C) Schizencephaly
(D) Hydranencephaly
(E) Middle cerebral artery emboli

The test images (Figure 12-1) display modest ventricular enlargement; intact septum pellucidum; intact corpus callosum; well-defined, thickened ventricular walls; and replacement of most of the brain parenchyma by multiple bilateral cysts of diverse sizes and shapes (see Figure 12-2). Multiple intervening strands or septa of variable length, thickness, and orientation separate the cysts into multilocular cavities. These features of a "Swiss cheese" brain are typical of multicystic encephalomalacia (also called multilocular cystic encephalopathy, polyporencephaly, multiple encephalomalacia of infancy, and progressive degenerative encephalopathy, among other terms) **(Option (A) is correct).** The diagnosis of this acquired lesion is further supported by the progression of brain rarefaction in this patient from a nearly normal appearance at 14 days (Figure 12-3) to severe cystic change at 8 weeks (Figures 12-1 and 12-2).

Porencephaly (Option (B)) is unlikely because it is typically associated with unilocular smooth-walled cysts. Properly used, the term porencephaly designates a lesion that arises *in utero*, either as a genetic defect or as an injury (insult) acquired *in utero*. Porencephaly is not multicystic and does not show the multiple septations that are seen in this patient.

Schizencephaly (Option (C)) is discounted because the lesions of schizencephaly are characterized by unilateral or bilateral columns of heterotopic gray matter that extend through the full thickness of the cerebral wall, from the ependymal to the pial surfaces. These columns line a cerebral cleft. Multicystic lesions do not form part of the spectrum of

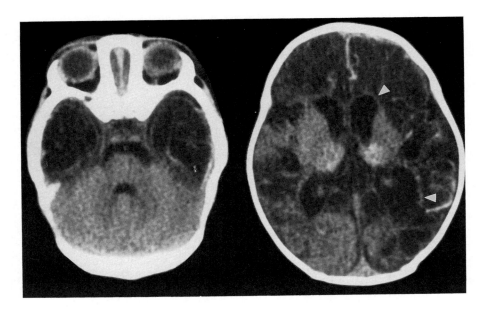

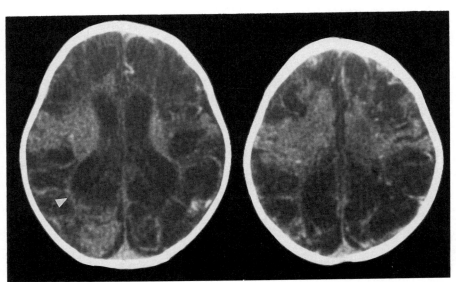

Figure 12-2 (Same as *Figure 12-1*). Noncontrast axial computed tomograms at 8 weeks (the test images) reveal enlargement of both lateral ventricles with slack contours of the ventricular walls, flat callosal angle, and no particular prominence of the temporal horns. These findings indicate ventriculomegaly secondary to atrophy. The major portions of both cerebral hemispheres have been replaced by multiple cortical and subcortical cysts of various sizes and shapes with intervening trabeculae of variable thickness. In many places, this cystic replacement extends from the pial surface of the hemisphere to the ependymal surface of the ventricle. The walls of the ventricles (white arrowheads) remain well defined, appear thickened, and clearly separate the ventricles from the parenchymal lesions. Serpiginous zones of increased density along the cortex may represent hemorrhage into the residual cortex or thrombosed surface vessels. The cerebellum is nearly unaffected. The corpus callosum and septum pellucidum are intact. The changes are those of multicystic encephalomalacia.

308

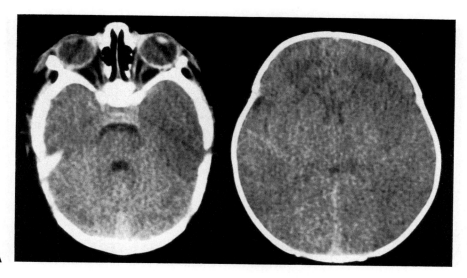

A   B

Figure 12-3. Same patient as in Figures 12-1 and 12-2. Multicystic encephalomalacia from presumed viral encephalitis. (A to D) Noncontrast axial computed tomograms at age 14 days, 1 day after her episode of apnea and seizures, reveal slightly reduced attenuation of the parenchyma diffusely, focally more prominent lucency in the right temporoparietal region (white arrow), loss of definition of the gray-white interface at that region, ventricles of normal size, lack of midline shift, and no evidence of pre-existing congenital malformation of brain structure. These changes are consistent with encephalitis or with hypoxic-ischemic damage. (E and F) Noncontrast axial computed tomograms at age 22 days reveal interval increase in ventricular size with no sign of hydrocephalus, diffuse reduction in the attenuation value of the parenchyma, greater prominence of the right temporoparietal lesion (white arrow), and loss of the gray-white junction at additional sites, such as the left frontal convexity. These changes are consistent with interval evolution of an inflammatory or ischemic process but fail to differentiate between the two. The overall clinical picture in this infant was thought to be most consistent with a viral encephalitis that progressed to multicystic encephalomalacia.

schizencephaly, and so the features illustrated here cannot be due to schizencephaly.

Hydranencephaly (Option (D)) is characterized by massive destruction of the cerebral hemispheres, reducing the cerebral walls to thin membranes over much or all of the brain. Consequently, there is massive dilatation of the remaining CSF space, with extremely large ventricles, the so-called "bubble brain." Hydranencephalic cavities are usually

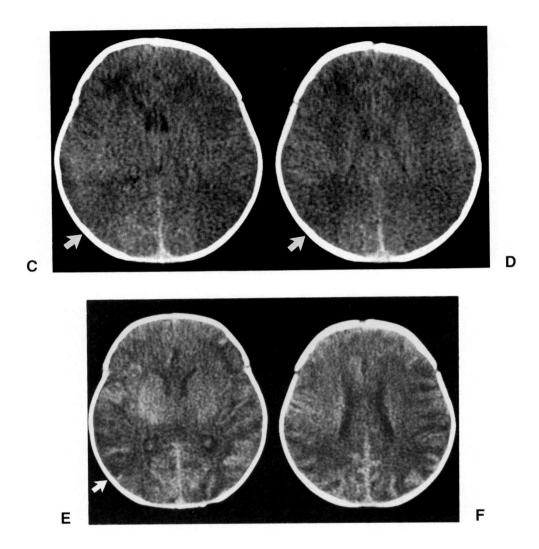

C   D

E   F

unilocular, but they may be bilocular, with one cavity in each hemisphere. They are not multicystic, and thus hydranencephaly is not likely.

Middle cerebral artery emboli (Option (E)) are not a likely cause for the findings in this patient. The lesions observed in the test images are widespread through anterior, middle, and posterior cerebral artery territories and are roughly symmetrical. With emboli, one usually observes a more patchy, asymmetric distribution and varying severity of infarction.

A variety of different insults may act on the developing central nervous system (CNS) to cause cystic replacement of the brain parenchyma. Such insults include hemorrhage, multifocal arterial and venous thromboses, diffuse anoxia, and infection. The results of such insults appear to depend less on the specific nature of the insult than on the precise stage in development at which the insult occurred. Therefore, the differing features of these lesions can be appreciated most easily when one understands how the developing brain responds to injuries at different times during gestation (see below).

Question 57

Features characteristic of multicystic encephalomalacia include:

(A) origin of cysts prior to the third month of gestation
(B) bilateral involvement
(C) direct continuity between the lesion cavities and the ventricles
(D) uniform size of individual cysts
(E) smooth lesion walls

The immature CNS of the fetus responds to an insult very differently from the more mature CNS of a full-term infant. Experimental data from animals indicate that the immature fetal CNS responds to an insult by (1) very rapid liquefaction and dissolution of necrotic tissue; (2) very rapid, complete clearance of necrotic material by macrophages, which then disappear rapidly from the lesion; and (3) very little or no proliferation of any glial scar.

For these reasons, and especially because there is no scarring, the lesions that affect the immature CNS create substantial, unilocular, smooth-walled cavities. The walls of the cavities consist of a thin layer of glial tissue deficient in neurons. There is no actual scarring.

Characteristically, these early insults affect the full thickness of the cerebral mantle, including the ependymal/subependymal zone, such that the parenchymal cavities appear to be confluent with the ventricle; no intervening ventricular wall can be discerned (Figure 12-4). In most cases, the superficial surface of the lesion is formed by a thin membrane that encloses the cavity and that lies just under the inner table. Alternatively, this tissue may be deficient, leading to communication with the surface. Extracerebral collections, such as subdural hygromas, may displace the superficial membrane medially.

Because these changes occur in the developing fetus, they may influence the course of subsequent development. This creates secondary distortions that could not arise had the insult occurred after development was complete. Thus, gray matter heterotopias, callosal agenesis, and septal agenesis may occur with insult to the fetus but not with insult to the full-term infant.

Conversely, the more mature CNS responds to an insult with less rapid and less complete dissolution of tissue, less rapid and less complete clearance of necrotic debris, and significant glial scarring. For those reasons, lesions developing toward the end of gestation and in the full-term infant typically take the form of a Swiss cheese brain, with multilocular, scarred, "shaggy-walled" cavities of different sizes and shapes (Figure 12-5). The cavities are separated by septa of different lengths, thicknesses, and orientations. Characteristically, the ventricular walls are preserved and appear thickened because of subependymal gliosis, as noted in the test images. When the destruction preferentially involves the cortical and subcortical layers of the brain, the thick "subependymal" layer also includes the better preserved subependymal brain parenchyma.

Since damage to the fetal brain and to the infantile brain results in such different, distinguishable pathological changes, it is worthwhile to provide separate names to designate each type of pathology. In keeping with Friede, the term porencephaly should be reserved solely to describe damage *in utero*, before the brain is able to make a significant glial scar. Typically, this porencephalic lesion will then appear as a circumscribed, unilocular, smooth-walled cavity; usually one cavity appears within each hemisphere.

The term encephalomalacia should be reserved for damage occurring intrapartum or postpartum (and on into adulthood), after the brain is able to make a significant glial scar. Typically, the severe encephalomalacic lesion will appear as multilocular cysts with intervening trabeculae— the Swiss cheese brain.

The precise time of transition from porencephaly to encephalomalacia is not known. During the last weeks of gestation, the brain begins to be able to elaborate a glial scar; the pathological appearance undergoes evolution and is difficult to classify. No specific neuroanatomical or neuropathological event marks the moment of birth; thus, it may be impossible to view a lesion and state unequivocally that this lesion occurred during birth, 2 weeks prior to birth, or 2 months after birth. However, one can often look at the brain and discern that the lesion clearly developed *in utero* (porencephaly) or that it was, at least, a late

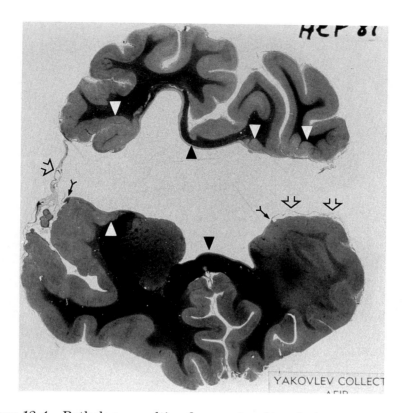

Figure 12-4. Pathology resulting from an insult early in gestation. Case HCP-81-59, coronal section 580, through the frontal lobes (reprinted with permission from the Yakovlev collection at the Armed Forces Institute of Pathology [AFIP]). On each side, unilocular, smooth-walled cavities communicate freely with the ventricle. Columns of heterotopic gray matter (white arrowheads) line the cavities. No discernible wall separates cavity from ventricle. These features indicate damage to the brain early in embryogenesis. The smooth walls and unilocularity indicate that the lesion occurred before the brain could make a glial scar. The columns of heterotopic gray matter indicate that the lesion occurred before the normal cortex was formed. The specific anomaly illustrated is designated agenetic porencephaly—schizencephaly with open lips. In this condition, symmetrical defects extend through the full thickness of the cerebral mantle. Microgyric gray matter (white arrowheads) lines the walls of the defects, and a pial-ependymal "roofing" membrane (open black arrows) originates from elevated pial-ependymal ridges (fishtail black arrows) to enclose the CSF. The pial-ependymal membrane is often most visible when the pial-ependymal ridge is displaced inward by an adjacent gyrus. This membrane is believed to represent the agenetic zone of the mantle that has become stretched and displaced outward by the dilated ventricle. The cavity within the brain parenchyma is the lateral diverticulum of the ventricle on each side. The septum pellucidum is frequently absent. The corpus callosum (black arrowheads) may be thin or absent.

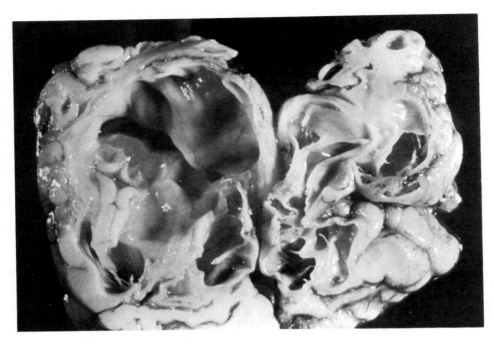

Figure 12-5. Severe multicystic encephalomalacia. Pathological specimen. Coronal section through the parieto-occipital lobes shows severe destruction of the brain parenchyma with formation of multiple cystic spaces separated by thin strands of residual gliotic brain parenchyma. The ventricles do not communicate with the cyst cavities. (Reprinted with permission from Raybaud [12].)

gestational or perinatal event (encephalomalacia), as in this case **(Option (A) is false).**

Pathological examination of brains from individuals with multicystic encephalomalacia reveals reduced brain size and brain weight. Typically, multiple cavities form within the greater parts of both cerebral hemispheres (Figures 12-5 to 12-7) **(Option (B) is true).** Such cavities may lie within the outer layers of the white matter and/or within the inner layers of the cortex. Often, they replace nearly all of the cerebral hemispheres. The cysts may be distributed randomly, but most cavities lie within the general territory of the anterior and middle cerebral arteries.

Portions of the brain are usually spared in a nearly characteristic pattern. The walls of the ventricles persist as thickened layers of tissue. This is an important distinguishing criterion of multicystic encephalomalacia **(Option (C) is false).** The portions of the temporal lobes below the superior temporal gyri, the basal ganglia, the brain stem, and the cerebellum are *relatively* preserved (Figure 12-6). The septum pellucidum and the corpus callosum are usually intact.

The multiple cysts vary widely in size and shape **(Option (D) is false).** The cavities are separated by gliotic tissue of various thicknesses. Many of the cavities are traversed by fine trabeculae. These septations may give the cavity a "shaggy," scarred wall **(Option (E) is false).** As described by Friede, microscopic examination of these lesions shows "infarction with organization or incomplete necrosis of brain parenchyma... . Organizing cavities are filled with fat-laden macrophages that also scatter through the adjacent glial scar...." The scar contains reactive astrocytes.

The major cerebral blood vessels and the carotid arteries appear to be patent. The mechanism of multicystic encephalomalacia may be acute elevation of intracranial pressure from any cause, e.g., brain edema following anoxia-ischemia. The peripheral tissue becomes necrotic, because the peripheral arteries and veins are contained in narrow sulci adjacent to unyielding bone and dura; these vessels are narrowed by the pressure. The central, periventricular, and basal tissues are preserved, because the vessels that supply these regions are buffered against compression by the fluid-filled ventricles and by the large inferior cisterns. The brain stem and cerebellum would be similarly preserved, because the relatively large basal cisterns of the infant buffer the pressure.

Patients with multicystic encephalomalacia usually have one of two histories: (1) abnormal birth with prolonged labor, often with fetal distress, followed by cyanosis, resuscitation, and then seizures starting hours to days postnatally, or (2) suspected meningitis with lethargy, hypotonia, and seizures but with inconclusive to negative bacterial cultures and negative antiviral antibody titers. In some cases, specific organisms, such as *Hemophilus influenzae*, are implicated. There is an increased incidence of multicystic encephalomalacia in twin pregnancies. One twin may be a macerated fetus, suggesting that the other, viable twin may develop multicystic encephalomalacia as a result of twin-to-twin transfusion or disseminated intravascular coagulation. A suggested but unproved factor is maternal fever. Experimentally, placement of pregnant ewes in elevated ambient temperatures for 9 hours daily during the third trimester has been shown to cause subcortical cavities in the brains of the newborn lambs.

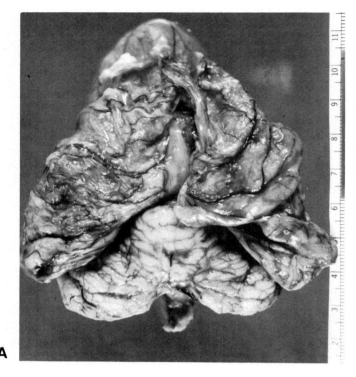

A

Figure 12-6. Severe multicystic encephalomalacia. This premature boy (34 weeks' gestation) presented with irregular respiration, apnea requiring intubation, and seizures at age 3 weeks. Cultures and titers of antibodies were all negative. Physical examination at 1 year of age revealed microcephaly, poor suck, no grasp, no gag, no spontaneous movements of the extremities, and seizures that progressed despite therapy. (A and B) Whole brain at necropsy at age 25 months viewed from above (A) and below (B) reveals marked reduction in brain size and weight, collapse of the cerebral hemispheres after ventricular and cisternal fluid leaked out, cerebral vessels coursing over the collapsed hemispheres, and relative sparing of the cerebellum and brain stem. (C and D) Coronal sections through the frontal horns (C) and the third ventricle (D) reveal enlarged frontal horns (F) and bodies (B) of the lateral ventricles, enlarged third ventricle (3), intact thickened ventricular walls (white arrowheads), relative sparing of the basal ganglia and thalami (T), and intact, thinned corpus callosum and septum pellucidum. C = caudate nucleus. Nearly all of the cerebrum has been replaced by multiple cysts of various sizes and shapes with intervening septa of variable thickness and length. (Reprinted with permission from Naidich and Chakera [5].)

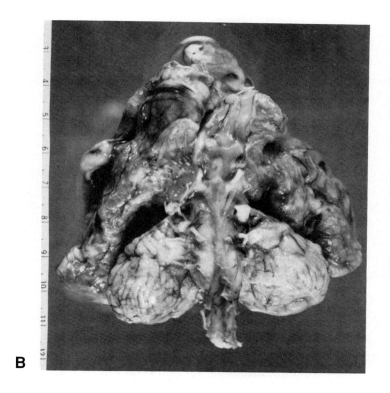

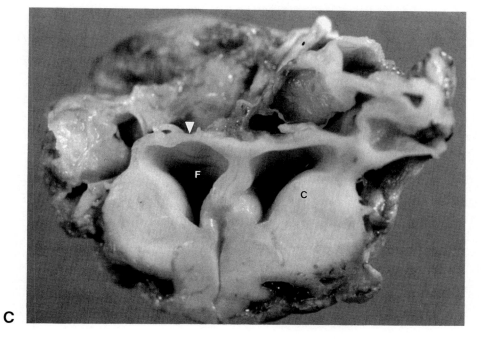

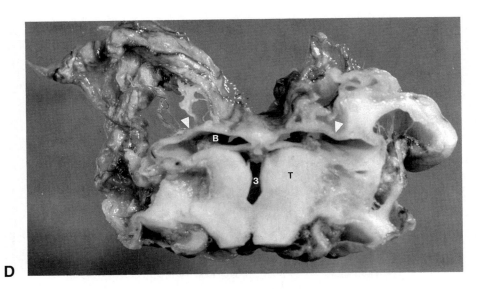

D

Imaging techniques demonstrate the pathological features expected for multicystic encephalomalacia (Figures 12-2, 12-8, and 12-9). CT scans typically display moderate ventriculomegaly, intact and thickened ventricular walls, and multiple bilateral supratentorial cysts. The septa between cysts may be resolved well or poorly, depending on their thickness and the resolution of the scanner. Certainly one sees only the largest cysts and the thickest septa under the best of circumstances. Nonetheless, it is easy to appreciate the multicystic nature of the pathology from the several large septa evident and from the mottled texture of the remainder of the parenchyma. The characteristic preservation of the walls of the ventricles, the *relative* sparing of the inferior temporal lobes and cerebellum, and the usual preservation of the septum pellucidum and corpus callosum are helpful in establishing the diagnosis. The cerebellum does show atrophic change in many cases; however, it is much less damaged than are the cerebral hemispheres. Similarly, the basal ganglia are relatively spared, but many cases demonstrate reduced size, reduced attenuation, and cystic replacement of the claustrum, the lateral portions of the caudate nucleus, and sometimes the lateral portions of the putamen. This is appreciated best by comparison with the normal brain (Figure 12-10).

It must be stressed that the examples illustrated in this section were specifically chosen to represent multicystic encephalomalacia that occurred rather late after birth. This was done to illustrate the evolution of the changes and document that the process did not occur *in utero* as a

318 / *Neuroradiology*

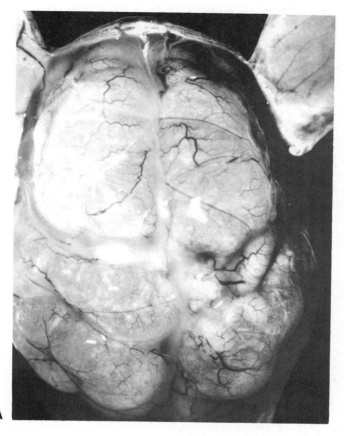

A

Figure 12-7. Severe multicystic encephalomalacia. Pathological specimens. (A to C) Whole brain viewed from above (A), from below (B), and
from the left side (C). (D) Coronal section through the temporal and
parietal lobes of the left hemisphere after impregnation of the cysts with
gelatin. This premature girl (32 to 34 weeks' gestation) presented with
respiratory distress at 24 hours, and seizures commenced on day 2 of life.
Cultures and titers of antibody were all negative. Sonography demonstrated a small Grade I subependymal bleed along the left frontal horn
on day 3. There is diffuse, approximately symmetrical replacement of the
cerebrum by multiple cysts with partial preservation of the anterior-
inferior surfaces of the frontal (F) and temporal (T) lobes and nearly
complete sparing of the brain stem (S) and cerebellum (C). Attenuated
cerebral vessels course over the outer surface of the multiple cysts. The
coronal section (panel D) demonstrates the multiple loculated cysts which
extend through the full thickness of the cerebral mantle from the
thickened gliotic, subependymal surface (black arrowheads) medially to
the pial surface laterally (arrow). Note the trabeculae that separate the
cysts and additional trabeculae (white arrowhead) visible through the
cysts. (Reprinted with permission from Naidich and Chakera [5].)

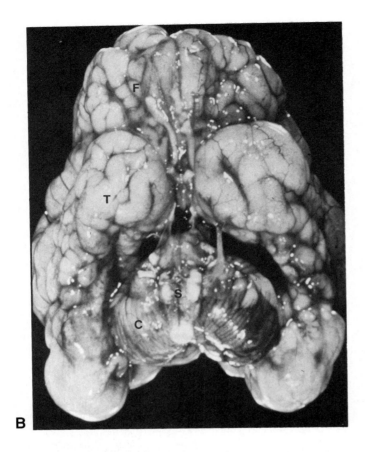

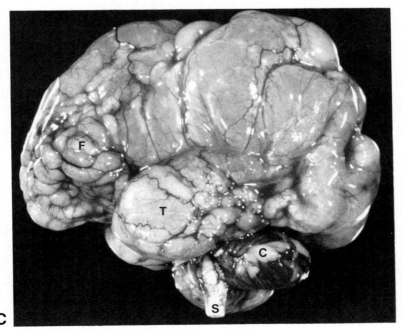

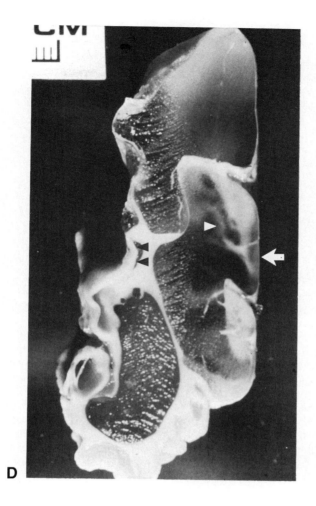

D

congenital malformation. Most cases of multicystic encephalomalacia have a history of birth asphyxia and show the full-blown picture of multicystic encephalomalacia on the CT scans obtained after birth.

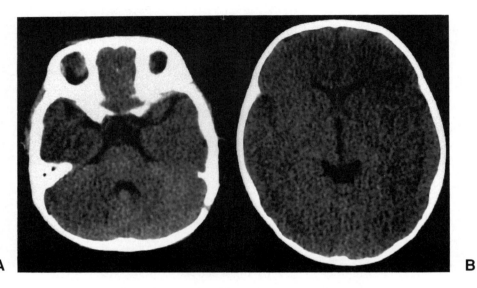

A   B

Figure 12-8.   Multicystic encephalomalacia. This full-term infant girl
was well until age 3 months, when she was found to be lethargic, limp,
breathing shallowly, and choking on sputum. Her rectal temperature at
admission was 42.2°C. Blood glucose was 25 mg/dL. Blood gases showed
a pH of 6.9, a pCO_2 of 60 mm Hg, and a pO_2 of 80 mm Hg. The patient
exhibited tonic-clonic seizures of all extremities and ceased spontaneous
respiration. Cultures and antibody titers were all negative. (A to D)
Noncontrast axial CT the day following admission reveals no definite
pathology. (E to H) Noncontrast axial CT 7 days later shows increased
size of the lateral ventricles, marked reduction in attenuation of most of
the cerebral hemispheres, loss of the gray-white interface in the affected
areas, reduced attenuation in the thalami (T) and medial basal ganglia,
and normal to increased attenuation in the corpus striatum (arrows)
bilaterally, consistent with hyperemia. The cerebellum, brain stem, and
patchy zones of frontal and occipital cortex are relatively spared. (I to L)
Noncontrast axial CT 18 days later (26 days after admission) shows
marked multicystic encephalomalacia. The ventricles are enlarged, with
slack contours and flat callosal angles consistent with atrophy. The
ventricular walls (large white arrowheads) are well defined and
thickened. Most of the cerebral parenchyma exhibits markedly reduced
attenuation with multiple faint trabeculae defining cysts of various sizes.
The lateral caudate nucleus (small white arrowhead), the regions of the
claustrum (crossed white arrow), and the lateral putamen are affected.
The thalami (T), medial lenticular nuclei (G), corpus callosum (white
arrow), septum pellucidum (open white arrow), and cerebellum appear
damaged but are relatively better preserved.

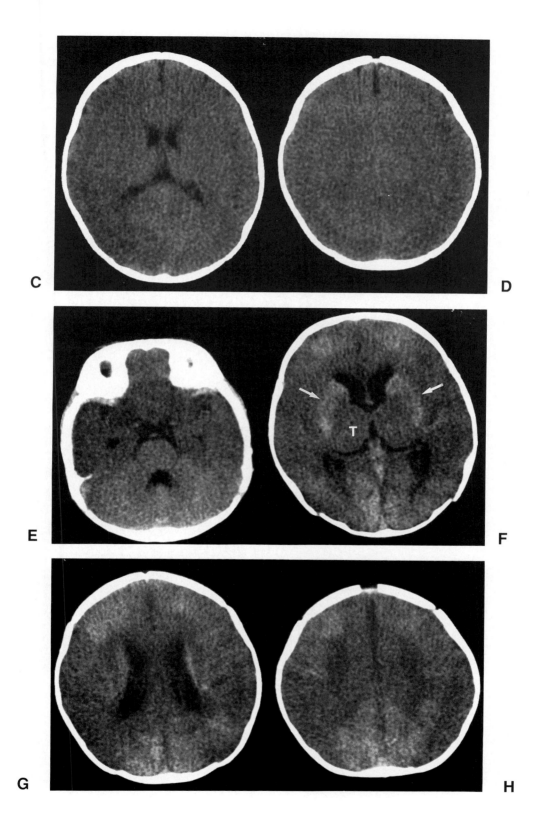

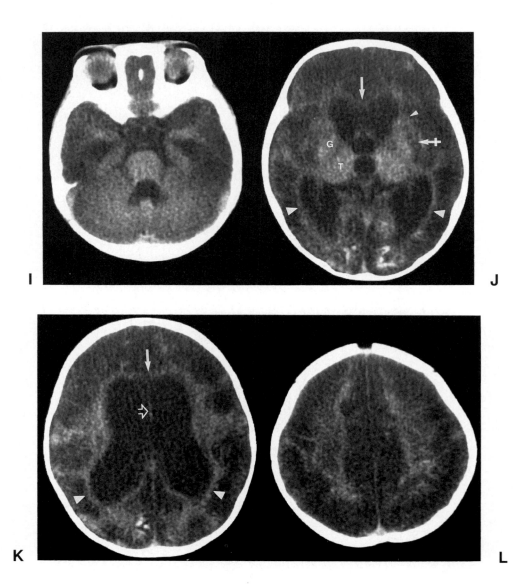

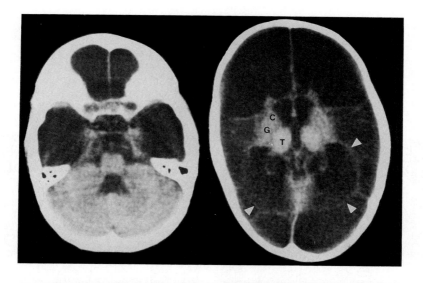

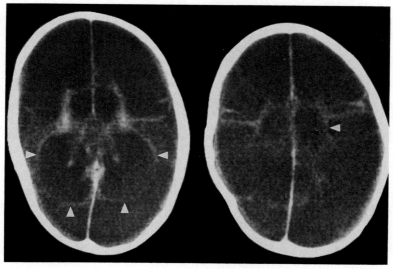

Figure 12-9. Multicystic encephalomalacia. This 4½-year-old boy had been a full-term infant born of monochorionic diamnionic twin pregnancy. Pregnancy was complicated by preeclampsia, death of one twin hours before delivery, failure of vaginal delivery, passage of meconium, and need for caesarean section. The dead twin was delivered as a slightly macerated fetus of normal weight (2.9 kg). The live twin weighed 3.2 kg. Apgar scores were 1 and 3 at 1 and 5 minutes. Despite intubation and suctioning of meconium from the tracheobronchial tree, the child suffered profound asphyxia with spastic quadriplegia, mental retardation, and seizures. Noncontrast axial CT reveals dilated lateral ventricles, well-defined thickened ventricular walls (white arrowheads), and replacement of the cerebral hemispheres by multiple cysts of various sizes and shapes, separated by septa of variable thickness and length. The lateral portions of the basal ganglia are also affected. There is relative sparing of cerebellum, brain stem, corpus callosum, septum pellucidum, thalami (T), and the medial portions of the caudate (C) and lenticular (G) nuclei.

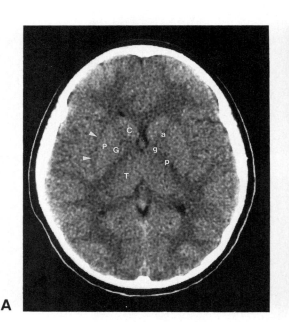 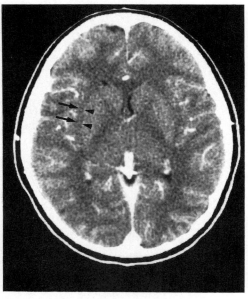

Figure 12-10. Normal noncontrast (A) and contrast-enhanced (B) axial CT through the basal ganglia of a 12-year-old girl. Note the positions and the proportions of the head of the caudate nucleus (C), putamen (P), globus pallidus (G), thalamus (T), and claustrum (the thin gray stripe indicated by the white arrowheads). The lenticular nucleus is composed of the putamen and the globus pallidus. The corpus striatum is composed of the caudate nucleus and the putamen. The anterior limb (a), genu (g), and posterior limb (p) of the internal capsule separate the lenticular nucleus laterally from the caudate nucleus and the thalamus medially. The external capsule (black arrowheads) separates the lenticular nucleus from the claustrum. The extreme capsule (black arrows) separates the claustrum from the insula. Following contrast enhancement, opacified vessels highlight the surface of the insula and indicate the thickness of the insular cortex between the vessels and the extreme capsule.

Question 58

Features characteristic of porencephaly include:

(A) postnatal onset of the pathology
(B) smooth lesion walls
(C) bilateral involvement
(D) multiloculated cysts
(E) continuity between lesions and ventricles

In 1859 Heschl coined the term porencephaly to designate circum-scribed defects which "have this in common, that in one or several places the cerebral substance is lacking through the entire thickness of the brain and so, if one disregards the purely membranous parts (which fill the defect), there is a canal through the brain which begins on the outer surface of the brain and ends in the cerebral ventricles." Although the term porencephaly is commonly used, loosely, to designate any hole in the brain, in the present discussion porencephaly will be used in the proper, restricted sense to describe circumscribed, smooth-walled defects that arise *in utero*.

Porencephaly signifies prenatal origin of the lesion, prior to develop-ment of the ability to form a glial scar **(Option (A) is false).** Depending on how early the insult occurs, two different forms of porencephaly can be discerned: agenetic porencephaly and encephaloclastic porencephaly.

Agenetic porencephaly results from an insult *in utero* prior to or during the formation of the cerebral cortex. As a result, the cavities of agenetic porencephaly are routinely associated with cortical malformations such as agyria, pachygyria, polymicrogyria, and gray matter heterotopias. Detection of cortical malformations in a patient with porencephaly signifies insult early in gestation (Figure 12-4). Because the corpus callosum and septum pellucidum form at about the same time as the cortex, agenetic porencephaly is also commonly (but not always) associated with septal and callosal dysgenesis. The characteristic example of agenetic porencephaly is schizencephaly (see discussion of Question 59).

Encephaloclastic (destructive) porencephaly results from necrotic softening and destruction of the previously formed cerebral wall. The insult occurs *in utero* after the cerebral cortex has formed. As a result, the cavities of encephaloclastic porencephaly characteristically are not associated with cortical malformations. Portions of the cortex are destroyed; adjacent cortex may be distorted secondarily. The convolutions bordering the lesion may be small because of atrophy and sclerosis, but true malformations of the adjacent cortex are usually absent. Infrequently, foci of pachygyria and polymicrogyria are observed in patients with encephaloclastic porencephaly. These foci may indicate repetitive insults to the brain both early and late in gestation. The septum pellucidum and corpus callosum may be present, absent, or partially destroyed in patients with encephaloclastic porencephaly. The characteristic example of encephaloclastic porencephaly is hydranencephaly (see discussion of Question 60).

Brains from infants with porencephaly usually disclose smooth-walled cavities that are oriented along the major fissures of the cerebral hemispheres, especially the central sulci and Sylvian fissures (Figure 12-11) **(Option (B) is true).** The defects are commonly bilateral **(Option (C) is true).** The cavities are unilocular on each side, resembling single cysts **(Option (D) is false).** The size of the cavity varies widely from patient to patient. The lateral wall of the lateral ventricle is focally deficient along the cavity on each affected side. The ventricles are directly continuous with the cavities through these defects; thus, the cavities contain clear CSF. Indeed, the cavities may properly be regarded as diverticular outpouchings of the ventricles **(Option (E) is true).**

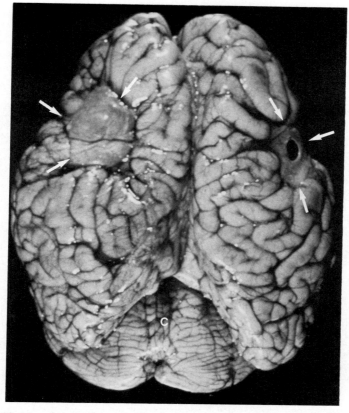

A

Figure 12-11. Agenetic porencephaly. Pathological specimen of schizen-cephaly with open lips. (A) View from above. Symmetrical membrane-covered defects (arrows) are present in the central regions of the two hemispheres. The cortex appears microgyric. The sulci converge toward the defects. On the left, a vessel courses across the membrane toward the distal cortex. On the right, the membrane exhibits an artifactual perforation. The cerebellum (C) appears normal. (B) Coronal section through the lateral ventricles and the anterior third ventricle (3). The corpus callosum (white arrowhead) is thin but present. Septum pellucidum is absent. The two lateral ventricles form a single cavity that extends laterally through the full thickness of each mantle, all the way to the "roofing" membrane (white arrows) that is formed by the pia-ependyma. No ventricular wall is visible medial to the membrane. Thus, the defects in the hemispheres are filled with freely communicating CSF and may be regarded as diverticula of the lateral ventricles. The walls of the defect are lined by columns of heterotopic gray matter (black arrowheads) that form a continuous sheet from the site of the original subependymal germinal matrix to the adjacent cortex. If these gray matter linings are regarded as the lips, then this is schizencephaly with open lips. (C) Coronal section through the posterior third ventricle (3) just behind the left defect. At this level, the lips of the left defect fuse together into a column (large black arrowheads) of gray matter that reaches from the lateral cortical surface toward (and, in other sections, to) the surface of the ventricle. The pia mater lining each bank of the sulcus (small black arrowheads) extends down into this column and, within it, merges with ependyma to form the pial-ependymal seam. Demonstration that the lips of the cerebral defect are lined by gray matter and that the lips merge together into a transcerebral column of gray matter at the edges of the defect confirms the diagnosis of schizencephaly. Islands of heterotopic gray matter (H) are found in both hemispheres lateral to the basal ganglia. (Reprinted with permission from Raybaud [12].)

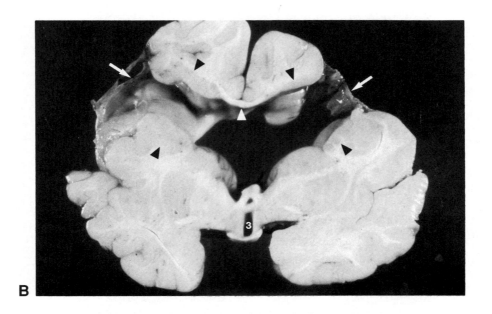

B

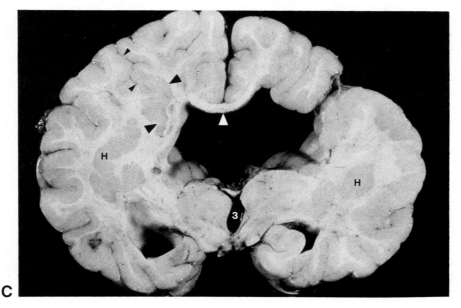

C

Question 59

Features characteristic of schizencephaly include:

(A) heterotopias of gray matter
(B) concurrent zones of polymicrogyria
(C) thrombosis of multiple middle cerebral artery branches
(D) absence of the interhemispheric fissure
(E) bilateral, paramedian hemorrhages

In 1946, Yakovlev and Wadsworth described schizencephaly and pre-sented evidence that it is a form of agenetic porencephaly dating to the second month of gestation. They clearly distinguished schizencephaly from the encephaloclastic porencephalies.

Schizencephaly is characterized by focal defects in the cerebral mantle (Figure 12-11). These defects are often bilateral but may be unilateral. They tend to occur along the major cerebral fissures, especially the Sylvian and central fissures. Several pairs of symmetrical defects may be present in a single brain.

Schizencephaly is routinely associated with disordered migration of subependymal neuroblasts; thus, the brain surrounding the defects exhibits subependymal masses of heterotopic gray matter and polymi-crogyria. Indeed, when schizencephaly appears to be unilateral, hetero-topias and foci of polymicrogyria are often found at the symmetrical site of the contralateral "normal" hemisphere. The subependymal gray matter and the polymicrogyric cortex form a continuous sheet of gray matter that appears to line the defect in the cerebral wall (Figures 12-4, 12-11, and 12-12) **(Options (A) and (B) are true).** There is no evidence of any glial or connective tissue scar along the defect. Secondary features include hypoplasia or aplasia of the white matter tracts, including corpus callosum, internal capsule, external capsule, cerebral peduncles, and the pyramids of the medulla. The lateral mass of each thalamus may be reduced in size.

In patients with schizencephaly, the ventricles are enlarged for one of two reasons. In some patients, there is persistent fetal ventriculomegaly with no true hydrocephalus. This moderate ventriculomegaly is desig-nated colpocephaly. In other patients, there is true hydrocephalus with very large ventricles.

The extent of the cerebral defect and the presence or absence of true hydrocephalus determine two different forms of schizencephaly. The layer of cortex adjacent to each side of the defect is called a cortical "lip." If the defect is small and there is no true hydrocephalus, then the cortices

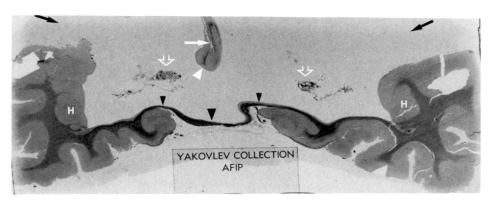

A

Figure 12-12. Agenetic porencephaly. Schizencephaly with open lips.
Coronal sections of the whole brain displayed from anterior to posterior.
(Case E.V. from the Yakovlov collection of the AFIP, with permission.)
(A) Section 1025. At the level of the choroid plexi (open white arrows),
the cerebral walls demonstrate large bilateral defects (black arrows) that
are lined by heterotopic gray matter (H). The corpus callosum is absent.
The dorsal hippocampus (white arrowhead) and interhemispheric fissure
(white arrow) occupy the midline superiorly. The commissure (large black
arrowhead) of the fornices (small black arrowheads) crosses the midline
inferiorly. The two lateral ventricles communicate freely from side to side
between the dorsal hippocampus and the commissure of the fornices. (B)
Section 1311. Just posterior to the right-sided defect, the gray matter
forms a continuous column (white arrowhead) from the brain surface
through the mantle to large masses of heterotopic subependymal gray
matter (H). The ventricle exhibits a slight outpouching or diverticle
(small black arrow) directed toward a line of union called the
pial-ependymal seam (small black arrowheads). Were these the sole
features present, this would be schizencephaly with closed lips. Patients
with schizencephaly with open lips characteristically exhibit these
changes at the edges of the open defects. Identification of these features
confirms that the open defect visible does represent schizencephaly and
not, for example, infarction. On the left, the cerebral defect (large black
arrow) is now smaller. At each edge of this defect the pia (crossed black
arrow) and ependyma (double-crossed black arrow) merge into a raised
pial-ependymal ridge (fishtail black arrow) that gives rise to the
pial-ependymal "roofing" membrane (open black arrows). This membrane
recurves outward toward the surface, so that the CSF-filled diverticulum
lies above the remnants of the brain. (C) Section 1396. Further
posteriorly, coronal sections demonstrate clearly the column of heterotopic gray matter (white arrowhead) and pial-ependymal seam (small
black arrowheads) on the right. On the left, the walls of the defect just
converge together, so that the two pial-ependymal ridges form a
pial-ependymal seam (small black arrowhead) between the cleft superficially and the diverticle (small black arrow) of the ventricle. Note that
the arachnoid and subarachnoid spaces pass deeply into the cleft to reach
the superficial surface of the seam. (D) Section 1551. Posterior to both
defects, the hemispheres are more nearly normal, but heterotopic gray
matter (H) still forms thick layers in the subependymal region and
scattered masses in the white matter.

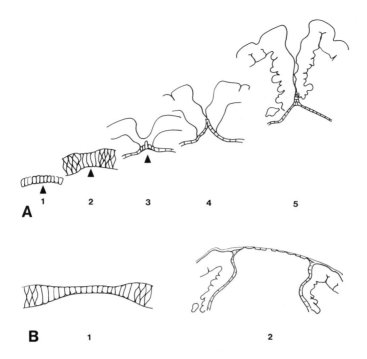

A

1   2   3   4   5

B   1   2

Figure 12-14. Morphogenesis of schizencephaly. Diagrams of the developing cerebral wall with the deep, ventricular surface toward the bottom and the superficial, cortical surface toward the top. The developing brain is growing outward toward the top. (A) Schizencephaly with closed lips. (1) The single layer of cells that forms the wall of the developing brain suffers an insult that damages a small zone (heavily inked cells, arrowhead). (2) This zone (arrowhead) fails to differentiate into the matrix, mantle, and marginal layers of His. (3) The affected region does not grow and thicken as much as the neighboring portions of the wall, and thus that portion (arrowhead) of the developing wall becomes dimpled on both the superficial (cortical) and deep (ventricular) surfaces. Because the wall did not differentiate into the three layers, gray matter forms throughout the full thickness of this zone. (4) With further growth, the cerebral wall becomes deeply furrowed. The adjacent cortices appear to roll inward to meet the diverticle of the ventricle. The pial and ependymal layers merge along the pial-ependymal seam. The gray matter forms a sleeve around the seam. (5) With further maturation, the zone assumes the configuration of schizencephaly with closed lips (see *Figure 12-13A).* (B) Schizencephaly with open lips. (1) The insult affects a wider area of the brain wall. (2) Developing hydrocephalus thins the affected segment and pushes it outward. As a result, the diverticle becomes a large ventricular outpouching between the adjacent columns of gray matter. The pial-ependymal seam is stretched out into the pial-ependymal membrane that forms the roof of this outpouching. All around the margin of the defect, the union of the pia and ependyma forms a thickened elevation called the pial-ependymal ridge.

or cleft that contains CSF and the usual cortical blood vessels. At first glance, this cleft appears to be an abnormally deep sulcus or fissure. Closer inspection, however, reveals that the deep fissure leads inward to a dysgenetic column of gray matter that reaches all the way to or nearly to the surface of the ventricle. At the bottom of the fissure, the layers of gray matter thicken, lose their normal layered architecture, and appear to merge into a solid cellular seam of gray matter. This seam is continuous with the disorganized gray matter of the dysgenetic zone and, through that, with the masses of subependymal gray matter (Figure 12-15). Blood vessels roll in with the cortex to reach the depth of the seam, where they become continuous with subependymal veins. The arachnoid extends into the cleft but does not appear to join in the formation of the seam. There is no evidence of vascular thrombosis or of glial or connective tissue scar **(Option (C) is false).** This situation is schizencephaly with closed lips. Some of these cases have been reported as septo-optic dysplasia with porencephaly or heterotopias.

If the dysgenetic zone is large and there is true hydrocephalus, then the ballooning ventricles push the dysgenetic zone outward as the brain thickens (Figure 12-14B). Thus, the margins of the adjacent cortex become widely separated, rather than rolled in. The separation may be narrow (Figure 12-16) or wide (Figure 12-17). The zone of separation typically takes the shape of an ovoid, with its long axis oriented along a major cerebral fissure. This is schizencephaly with open lips.

In schizencephaly with open lips, the edge of the dysgenetic zone is delimited by the margin of the surrounding cortex. At the margin, the gray matter of the cortex is still continuous with the heterotopic gray matter in the subependymal region. Indeed, at the poles of the ovoid defect, where the lips are least separated, one can still trace the cortical margins into a pial-ependymal seam identical to that seen in schizencephaly with closed lips (Figures 12-11, 12-12, and 12-17).

All along the cortical margin of the defect, the ependyma on the deep surface of the cortex and the pia mater on the outer surface of the cortex merge together to form an elevated, serrated thickening called the pial-ependymal ridge (Figures 12-11 and 12-12). This ridge gives rise to a thin, semitransparent membrane that arches over the opening between the lips (Figures 12-18 and 12-19). The membrane appears to correspond to the stretched dysgenetic zone. It is composed of two layers. The inner layer is ependyma that is continuous with the ependyma lining the entire ventricular system. The outer layer is pia mater continuous with the pia covering the cortex. These layers are fused together to form the pial-ependymal membrane. Outside this membrane is the arachnoid

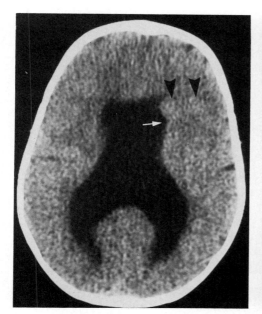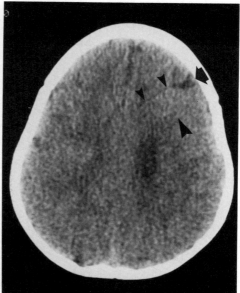

Figure 12-15. Agenetic porencephaly. Schizencephaly with closed lips. This 10-month-old boy presented with mild developmental delay, short stature, hypotonia, poor visual fixation, and hypoplastic optic nerves. Noncontrast axial CT demonstrates absent septum pellucidum, enlarged lateral ventricles, and a diverticular outpouching of the left frontal horn (white arrow). The diverticle is in direct line with a deep sulcus (black arrow) and a narrow lucency that may represent the deep continuation of the cleft (small black arrowheads). A column of heterotopic gray matter (large black arrowheads) extends across the expected position of the subcortical white matter and surrounds the lucent line. Note the resemblance of these findings to the pathological specimen illustrated in Figures 12-11C and 12-12B. Cases such as this one have also been reported in the literature as septo-optic dysplasia with heterotopic gray matter.

mater that is continuous with the arachnoid covering the adjacent cortex. The subarachnoid space is usually maintained between the arachnoid and the subjacent pial-ependymal membrane, but at points the arachnoid does fuse with the pia-ependyma. Normal patent blood vessels lie within the subarachnoid space and course over the pial-ependymal membrane, external to the defect, to supply the brain of the distal lip. Nodules of cerebral substance are commonly found in the subarachnoid space. Some of these nodules are free in the subarachnoid space. Others are attached

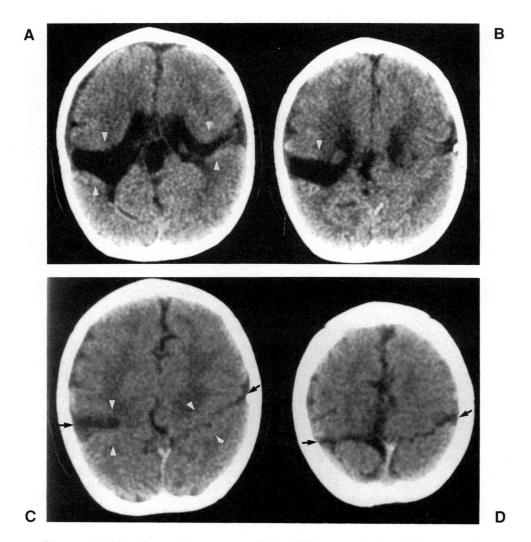

Figure 12-16. Agenetic porencephaly. Schizencephaly with narrowly open lips. This 22-month-old girl suffers from microcephaly, spastic quadraparesis (worse on the right side), and developmental delay. (A to D) Noncontrast CT demonstrates bilateral, slightly asymmetrical defects through the full thickness of the cerebral mantle. The defects are lined by gray matter (white arrowheads) and extend superiorly toward deep clefts and fissures (black arrows) in the mantle. These fissures represent the subarachnoid space situated between the adjacent banks of the in-rolled cortices (white arrowheads in panel C). Grossly, they resemble high continuations of the Sylvian fissures directed toward the vertex.

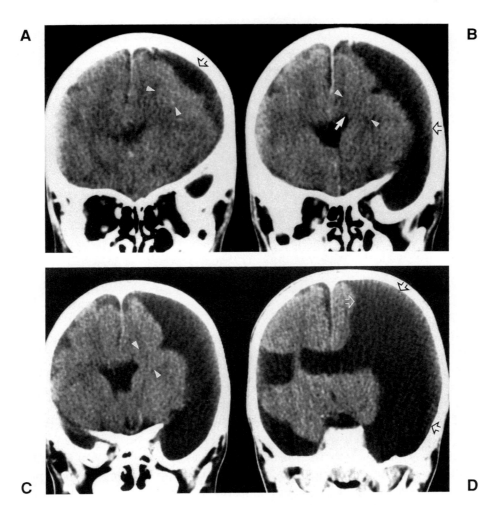

Figure 12-17. Agenetic porencephaly. Schizencephaly with open lips. This 13-month-old, premature boy (born at 30 to 32 weeks' gestation) was delivered by emergency caesarian section for *abruptio placentae.* He suffered bronchopulmonary dysplasia and had a single seizure shortly after birth. The child now manifests a developmental age of 5 months and hyperreflexia. Contrast-enhanced coronal CT scans displayed from anterior to posterior demonstrate the transition from the nearly normal brain with cortical thickening (white arrowheads) at the anterior edge of the defect (A) through the pial-ependymal seam and surrounding column of "gray matter" (between the white arrowheads) at the edge of the defect (B and C) to the full-thickness defect with marked outward expansion of the pial-ependymal roofing membrane (D to F) (open arrows). Note the small outpouching of the ventricle toward the seam (white arrow in panel B), the small transcerebral defect (black arrow in panel E), and a column of heterotopic gray matter (between black arrowheads in panel F) that closes the right defect posteriorly. The dilated left lateral ventricle causes asymmetric expansion of the left hemicranium. Such large ventricular diverticula may be mistaken for arachnoid cysts, unless the significance of the transcerebral defect and column of gray matter are appreciated.

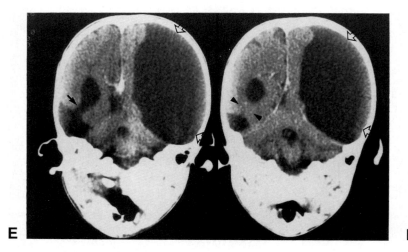

E   F

to the subjacent pia. These nodules may represent the disorganized gray matter that had been part of the seam and that now has been stretched and displaced outward with the membrane by the expanding ventricle. In accord with this concept, these nodules are found near the margins of the cortex rather than in the middle of the membrane.

The thin membrane that arches over the defect represents the pia and the ependymal lining of the ventricle. With hydrocephalus, therefore, the ventricle balloons into the cortical defect as a large, smooth-walled, laterally directed diverticulum. In schizencephaly with open lips, the "cavity" within the hemisphere is just the ventricle itself. No wall separates the cavity from the ventricle. In some cases, the membranous wall of the ventricle even bulges superficial to the cortex to form a large diverticulum that lies between the cortex and the inner table of the skull. Such diverticula should not be mistaken for arachnoid cysts (Figure 12-18).

In schizencephaly with open lips, the defects in the cortex are often very large. Nearly the entire frontal cortex, parietal cortex, and island of Reil may be absent, leaving only rudimentary occipital and temporal lobes posteroinferiorly. The medial surfaces of the hemispheres may also be deficient, leaving only a small rudiment of tissue at the base of the interhemispheric fissure. However, the interhemispheric fissure is still clearly identifiable **(Option (D) is false)**.

In some cases, the corpus callosum and the septum pellucidum are also deficient. In these cases, the rudiment of tissue found at the base of the interhemispheric fissure is the dorsal hippocampus, which would

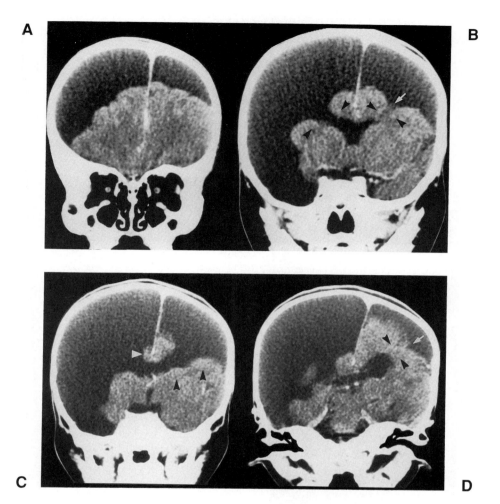

Figure 12-18. Agenetic porencephaly. Schizencephaly with open lips. This 2-year-old girl presented with severe developmental delay, microcephaly, spasticity, and contractures. (A to G) Contrast-enhanced coronal CT scans, displayed from anterior to posterior, demonstrate absent septum pellucidum, bilateral transcerebral defects that are lined by gray matter (black arrowheads in panels B and C), the column of gray matter (between black arrowheads in panel C) that surrounds the pial-ependymal seam and closes the left defect, a normal enhancing falx, shallow interhemispheric fissure, small midline remnant of dorsal hippocampus and adjacent cingulate gyrus (white arrowhead in panel C), just as in the pathological specimen (*Figure 12-12A*), and closing of the right cleft posteriorly (between white arrowheads in panels F and G), just as in the pathological specimen (*Figures 12-12B to 12-12D*). The brain surface appears notched (white arrows) where the cortical lips roll inward toward the defects. Marked expansion of the pial-ependymal "roofing" membrane forms a diverticulum of the ventricle that extends between the cortex and the inner table, mimicking an arachnoid cyst. (H to K) Axial CT scans obtained at the same time illustrate the appearance of these changes in the axial plane. Note the diverticle (small white arrow in panel I), the pial-ependymal and gray matter seams (between black arrowheads in panel I) at the inferior margin of the left defect, and the resemblance of the ventricular outpouchings to arachnoid cysts.

E 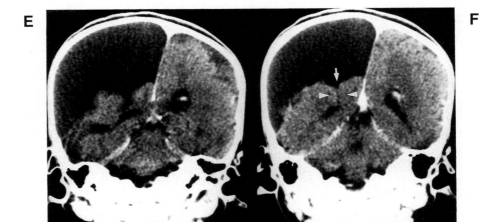 F

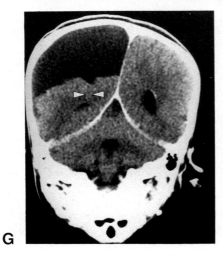
G

normally have lain atop the corpus callosum (Figure 12-11). The pial-ependymal membrane stretches from the residual temporal lobe (laterally and inferiorly) along the arc of the "convexity" to the midline, where it turns downward along the interhemispheric fissure to insert into the rudimentary dorsal hippocampus. The two lateral ventricles then communicate freely from side to side under the dorsal hippocampus (Figure 12-12A). The roof of the third ventricle is usually deficient, in whole or in part, and so the lateral and third ventricles form a widely communicating space.

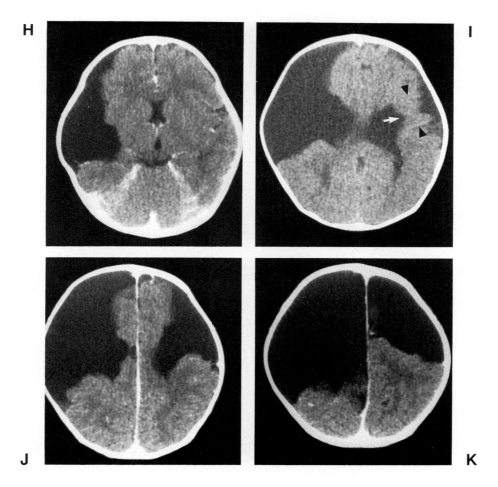

The bodies of the lateral ventricles are usually the largest part of the ventricular systems in patients with schizencephaly with open lips. The occipital horns are next most dilated and resemble posterior diverticular outpouchings of the ventricles. The temporal horns are usually very hypoplastic; the frontal horns may be entirely absent or very hypoplastic.

The angiographic features of schizencephaly are characteristic. These features include (1) in-curving of the cortical vessels along the rolled-in cortex at the margin of the defect, (2) continuity of these vessels with the subependymal veins, and (3) peripheral microgyria, visualized as small vessels forming characteristic reticular masses around the involved area. Hemorrhage is not a feature of schizencephaly **(Option (E) is false).**

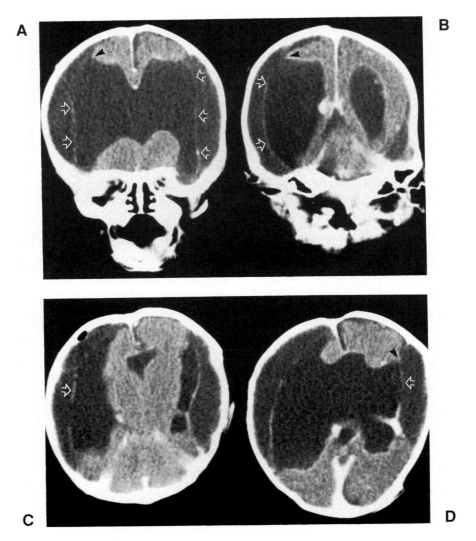

Figure 12-19. Agenetic porencephaly. Schizencephaly with open lips. This 1-month-old girl was a 4.4-kg full-term macrocephalic infant delivered by caesarian section for fetal distress. Apgar scores were 8 and 9 at 1 and 5 minutes, respectively. Following shunting, she developed Group D streptococcal meningitis. The neurological examination was normal for her age. Shown are contrast-enhanced coronal (A and B) and axial (C and D) CT scans. Shunt decompression of the ventricles has allowed the pial-ependymal "roofing" membrane (open white arrows) to collapse inward, revealing its course and its attachments at the pial-ependymal ridges (black arrowhead). The intense enhancement of the ventricular walls represents post-shunting ventriculitis. Note the resemblance to the pathological specimen illustrated in Figure 12-4.

Question 60

Features characteristic of hydranencephaly include:

(A) destruction of nearly all the solid portions of the cerebral hemispheres
(B) massively dilated lateral ventricles with thickened ependymal linings
(C) prominent zones of agyria and pachygyria
(D) occlusion of major portions of the circle of Willis
(E) likelihood of clinical recovery with nearly normal intellect, provided shunt therapy is instituted before age 2 months

Hydranencephaly signifies destruction of all or nearly all the solid cerebral tissue such that the cerebral hemispheres are replaced by thin-walled, membranous sacs that contain CSF (Figures 12-20 and 12-21) **(Option (A) is true).** The condition is rare, being found in 0.3% of autopsies in mentally defective children. Large hospitals see one to two such children annually.

Hydranencephaly was first described by Cruveilhier in 1835; the present term was coined by Kluge in 1902. Synonymous terms include hydrencephaly and "bubble brain." Although some authors refer to complete hemispheric necrosis in infants as "hydranencephaly of postnatal onset," such usage is confusing and should be avoided. In this discussion, hydranencephaly specifically refers to the severe form of encephaloclastic porencephaly that arises *in utero*.

On physical examination, the face of a patient with hydranencephaly is relatively normal. Eyes are present, indicating that the brain formed at some time during fetal life but was partially destroyed following development. Microphthalmia and chorioretinopathy are common.

The head may be of normal circumference or microcephalic at birth; it is rarely macrocephalic. During the next weeks of life, accumulation of fluid within the "ventricles" often causes progressive macrocephaly that may require shunt therapy (Figure 12-22). The cause of the ventricular distention is unknown. Some cases show obstruction of the foramina of Monro or aqueduct. Others show patent enlarged aqueducts and fourth ventricles. The choroid plexi are normal.

The dura is usually almost normal, but rarely it is pitted and deficient focally. The falx and tentorium are present but may be hypoplastic. The dural venous sinuses are intact. The leptomeninges (pia-arachnoid) are usually normal but may show evidence of hemorrhage.

The cerebral hemispheres are replaced by fluid-filled bubbles (Figures 12-20 through 12-22). The wall of the bubble is a thin, translucent membrane with no residual pattern of convolutions. The outer layer of

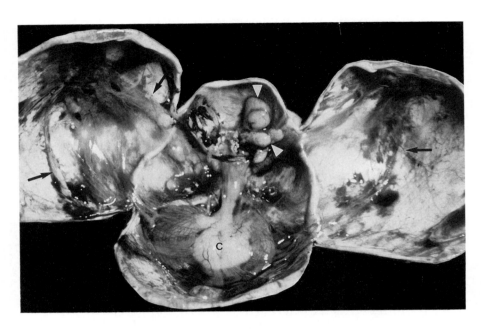

Figure 12-20. Severe encephaloclastic porencephaly. Hydranencephaly. This is a pathologic specimen of the brain, *in situ,* after opening the calvarium and spreading the bone plates laterally. This was a 2-day-old, 29-week-gestation premature girl with no spontaneous respiration at birth. Physical examination revealed macrocephaly, bilateral microphthalmia, malformed pinnae, absent external auditory canals, cleft soft palate, retroesophageal right subclavian artery, and hypoplastic adrenal glands. The major portions of both cerebral hemispheres are replaced by a thin gliotic translucent membrane (black arrows) that was attached to the dura of the skull base and vault and that separated from the calvarium when the skull was opened. The membrane enclosed choroid plexi and 630 mL of serosanguineous CSF. Remnants of gray matter (white arrowheads) persist along the orbital roof and at other scattered sites. The basal ganglia and thalamus were described by the pathologist as intact gross upon inspection but showed histological evidence of calcification and glial changes consistent with resolved intrauterine infection, possibly toxoplasmosis or cytomegalovirus. The cerebellum (C) appears grossly normal but exhibited abnormal lobation on histological examination. The brain stem was atrophic because of absence of the descending white matter tracts. The spinal cord lacked lateral columns.

the membrane abuts the dura of the convexities and the midline dura of the falx. The membrane may have light adhesions to the dura. The outer layer is formed by connective tissue that is continuous with the pia and arachnoid. It may show pigmentation, hemosiderin from old hemorrhage,

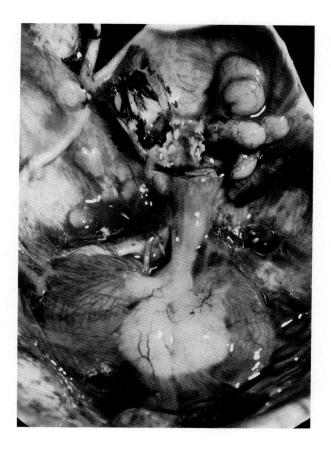

and fibrosis. The inner surface of the membrane is smooth, with an opaque layer of nervous tissue arranged in patches, in trabeculae, or as a thin continuous film. This nervous tissue consists mostly of astrocytes with a few residual neurons that may be mineralized. Ependyma is absent. No other remnant of the hemispheric wall is visible. Specifically, no tissue layer corresponding to the ventricular walls is present **(Option (B) is false)**. There is no thickened ependyma and no defined ventricular wall. Since the hydranencephalic membrane lies immediately subjacent to the inner table, it cannot be discerned unless subdural collections displace it inward (Figure 12-23).

The cerebral bubbles are filled with clear CSF. The septum pellucidum and corpus callosum are absent; thus, the two bubbles communicate freely across the midline.

The extent of cortical destruction varies but is always severe. Nearly always, both cerebral hemispheres are affected. Rarely, the process is

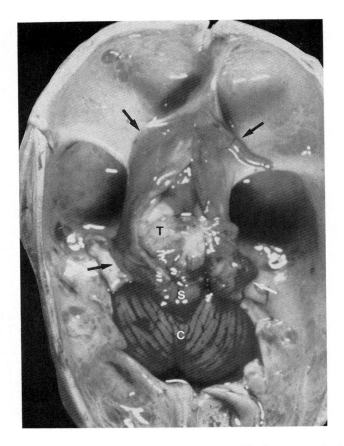

Figure 12-21. Encephaloclastic porencephaly. Hydranencephaly. Pathological specimen. This is a view of the hydranencephalic brain *in situ* after removal of the calvarium. Most of the brain has been reduced to a thin rim of gliotic tissue (arrows) that adheres closely to the meninges at the base of the skull and to the meninges attached to the calvarium. There is relative sparing of some portions of the inferior-medial surfaces of the frontal lobes, occipital lobes, and posterior temporal lobes. The deep gray nuclei, the thalami (T), the brain stem (S), and the cerebellum (C) are partially preserved. (Reprinted with permission from Raybaud [12].)

unilateral. The defect in the hemispheric walls typically corresponds to the territories supplied by the carotid arteries or to the anterior and middle cerebral arteries. When portions of the cerebral hemispheres are spared, rudimentary hippocampi and adjacent portions of the inferior temporal and occipital lobes are most nearly preserved. Typically, the hippocampal remnants show the most nearly normal lamination of

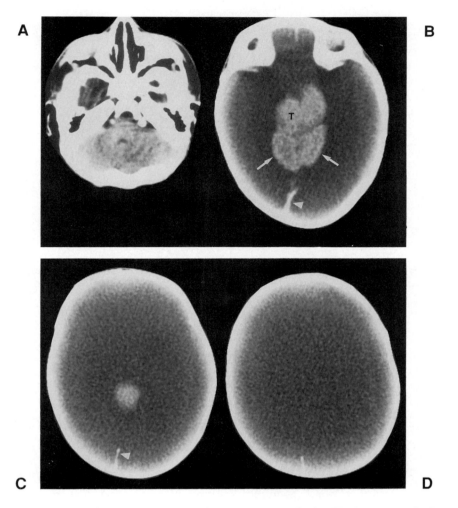

Figure 12-22. Severe encephaloclastic porencephaly. Hydranencephaly. This 8-day-old full-term boy was delivered by caesarean section for cephalopelvic disproportion. Physical examination revealed marked macrocephaly, pale right optic disk with no chorioretinitis, poor temperature control, and increased tone in all extremities. (A to D) Noncontrast axial CT scans demonstrate a relatively normal cerebellum (panel A), partial preservation of basal ganglia, thalamus (T), and posteromedial temporo-occipital lobes (arrows) (panel B), and replacement of the rest of the brain by bilateral fluid-filled sacs (bubble brain). The falx (white arrowheads) is hypoplastic but present. (E to H) Noncontrast coronal (panels E to G) and sagittal reformatted (H) CT images confirm the findings described above.

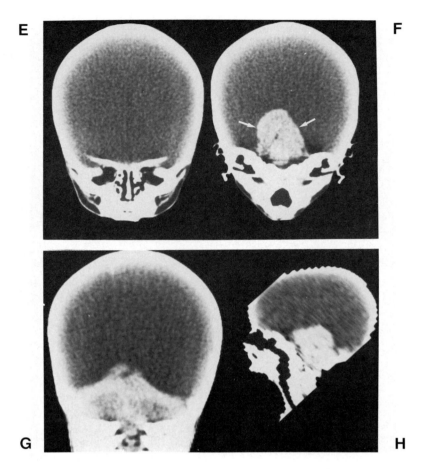

cortical layers. Other residual portions of brain may show foci of microgyria or pachygyria, but these are not characteristic features of hydranencephaly **(Option (C) is false).**

The basal ganglia form a characteristic hump overlying and anterior to the tentorial hiatus (Figure 12-22). The thalamus and corpus striatum are often rotated outward such that the internal capsule runs horizontally. The thalami are always atrophic, because the cortical projection nuclei and pulvinars are absent.

The cerebellum may be grossly normal or atrophic. Some cases show microfolia or cystic lesions. The cerebral peduncles and medullary pyramids are hypoplastic or absent, because the bubble brain gives rise to few descending corticospinal fibers.

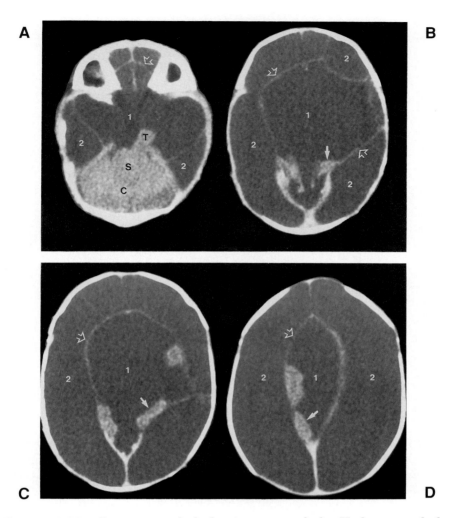

Figure 12-23. Severe encephaloclastic porencephaly. Hydranencephaly with bilateral subdural collections. This 3-day-old, full-term girl was born precipitously but had good Apgar scores of 8 and 9 at 1 and 5 minutes. She exhibited marked macrocephaly, lethargy, rigidity, and seizures. (A to D) Contrast-enhanced axial CT scans demonstrate replacement of most of the cerebrum by a fluid-filled sac (1). There is partial preservation of the cerebellum (C), brain stem (S), thalamus (T), and posteromedial temporo-occipital brain tissue (closed white arrows). In this case, large subdural collections (2) displace the hydranencephalic membrane inward (open white arrows), away from the calvarium, permitting it to be displayed by CT. (E) Following shunt therapy of the subdural collections, placement of positive contrast material through the catheter outlines the large, bilateral subdural spaces (2) and documents that these spaces do not communicate with the hydranencephalic cavity (1) (i.e., the "bubble").

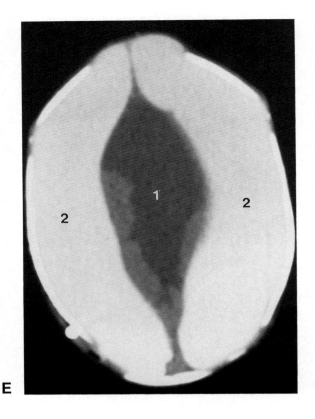

E

In patients with hydranencephaly, pathological examination nearly always shows an intact circle of Willis and intact major cerebral arteries **(Option (D) is false).** The sizes of the cerebral vessels are reduced in proportion to the small amount of residual tissue they need supply, but thromboses and obstructions are not a regular feature of hydranencephaly at postmortem. Absence of arteries occurs only in extreme cases in which even the diencephalon is destroyed. Rarely, vasculo-occlusive processes have been documented to cause unilateral hydranencephaly. This postmortem experience contrasts with the neuroradiologic, especially angiographic, experience *in vivo*.

In hydranencephaly, angiography demonstrates occlusion of the supraclinoid internal carotid arteries. In some cases, this occlusion is distal to the anterior choroidal arteries. In other cases, it includes these arteries. Fine collaterals form a vascular network that supplies the frontobasilar area and the basal ganglia. The basilar artery is normal and supplies any remnants of the temporal and occipital lobes through the posterior cerebral arteries.

At times, it may prove difficult to differentiate between severe hydrocephalus with massively dilated ventricles and severe forms of hydranencephaly. Partial restoration of the cerebral mantle after shunting indicates a diagnosis of hydrocephalus, not hydranencephaly (Figures 12-24 and 12-25). Angiography has been advocated for making the differential diagnosis prior to instituting therapy. Patients with hydrocephalus have a full complement of anterior and middle cerebral arteries. These arteries are very stretched but are always present no matter how thinned the mantle becomes. Hydranencephalic patients exhibit no filling of middle cerebral arteries.

Serious questions must be raised about the validity of either the angiographic and/or the postmortem criteria for a diagnosis of hydranencephaly, because the angiographic and postmortem experiences differ. Reports exist of patients with autopsy-proven hydranencephaly in whom a full complement of anterior, middle, and posterior cerebral arteries was documented by premortem Thorotrast angiography. Perhaps the angiographic criteria describe only the most severe cases of hydranencephaly. At present, angiography appears to be able to permit a diagnosis of hydranencephaly but cannot exclude hydranencephaly.

Clinically, two groups of hydranencephalic patients may be distinguished. The first group has greater loss of cerebral tissue and marked involvement of the basal ganglia and thalami. These patients are severely retarded, show poor autonomic regulation, and usually die before 1 month of age. The second group suffers less severe cerebral destruction; much of the basal ganglia are preserved. These infants seem normal for the first few months of life. Thereafter, they appear progressively more retarded, since they have no cerebral cortices to permit normal development. They are brought to medical attention several months after birth because of failure to thrive, seizures, hypotonia, or nonspecific complaints. They may exhibit a chronic decerebrate state. No therapy is known. These children do not develop normal intellect **(Option (E) is false).** Clinical recovery with nearly normal intellect after shunt therapy often occurs in children with severe hydrocephalus, but not in those with hydranencephaly.

The etiology of hydranencephaly remains obscure. It is generally agreed that hydranencephaly results from destruction and resorption of preformed solid cerebral tissue commencing before birth. However, it appears unlikely that the cause of the destruction is the same in all cases. Some cases may be due to toxoplasmosis, cytomegalovirus infection, or Venezuelan equine encephalitis. Others may represent bilateral carotid artery occlusion. Experimental studies in animals suggest that plugging

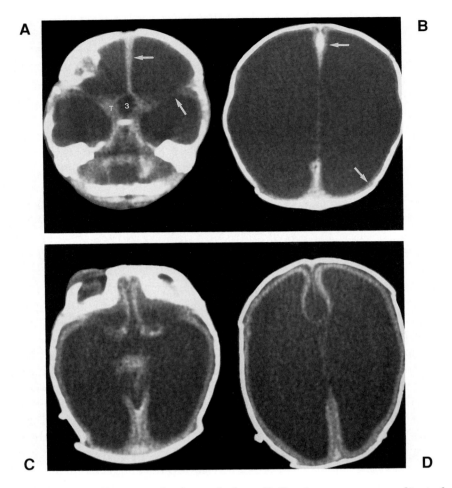

Figure 12-24. Extreme hydrocephalus. Following an uncomplicated pregnancy, this 1-week-old boy was delivered at term by use of forceps. Apgar scores were 3 and 5 at 1 and 5 minutes. Physical examination revealed macrocephaly and ambiguous genitalia. Poor respiratory effort required intubation shortly after birth. Increasing head circumference and bulging fontanelle required shunt diversion of CSF at age 1 week. (A and B) Prior to shunting, contrast-enhanced CT shows marked enlargement of both lateral ventricles with a paper-thin mantle, expansion of the third ventricle (3) so that the thalami (T) appear small, and preservation of the cerebellum. Although this appearance resembles hydranencephaly superficially, the presence of cerebral cortex (white arrows) in the midline, along the lateral convexities, and between the dilated frontal and temporal horns strongly suggests the correct diagnosis of severe hydrocephalus. (C and D) At 3 weeks after shunt therapy, the repeat computed tomogram reveals reduced head circumference, reduced ventricular size, and thickening of the cerebral mantle around the complete circumference of the ventricles. Widening of the inter-hemispheric fissure and slight inward collapse of the mantle permit CT display of the full thickness of the mantle. There are no focal defects to suggest agenetic porencephaly. The rapid interval thickening of the mantle rules out hydranencephaly.

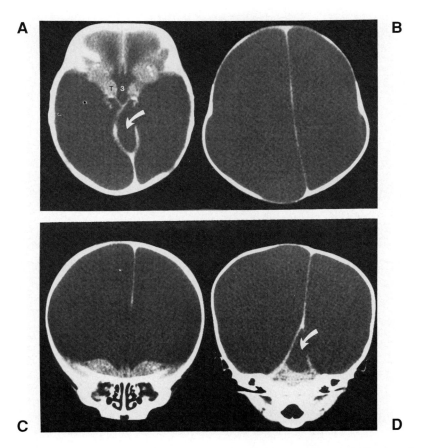

Figure 12-25. Extreme hydrocephalus. This 7-week-old full-term boy was born with macrocephaly. The parents were told that the child had "no brain tissue." A second opinion was sought. (A to D) Contrast-enhanced axial (A and B) and coronal (C and D) CT scans reveal marked asymmetric dilatation of both lateral ventricles, dilated third ventricle (3), extreme thinning of the cerebral mantle, anterior-inferior displacement of the basal ganglia and thalami (T), calcification of the ganglia, and a medial atrial diverticulum (curved white arrows) of the left lateral ventricle. The falx is present. No septum pellucidum is identifiable. (E to G) Noncontrast CT 2 months following shunting demonstrates the shunt tube, reduced ventricular size, thickened and collapsed but intact cerebral mantle (white arrows), and craniocerebral disproportion with large extracerebral collections of CSF. The parenchymal calcifications are more visible. Lucent lesions are present in both cerebellar hemispheres. It is not correct to diagnose hydranencephaly simply because imaging studies fail to demonstrate any cerebral mantle along the convexities.

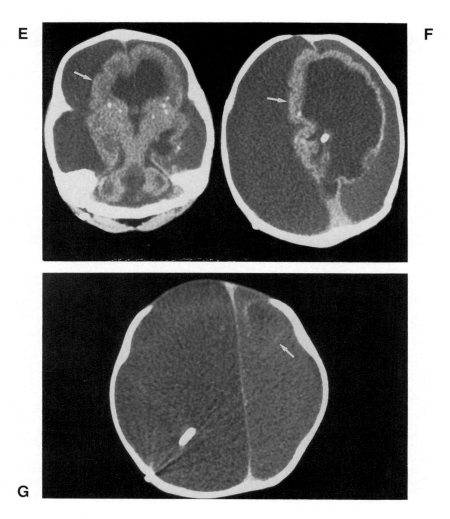

of the internal carotid artery may produce a condition similar to hydranencephaly. Hydranencephaly is classified as an encephaloclastic porencephaly, even though some cases exhibit foci of microgyria and pachygyria, which are migrational disorders more commonly found with agenetic porencephaly. Perhaps in these cases things begin to go wrong at an early stage and then deteriorate further later.

A "basket brain" is a form of destructive lesion that is intermediate in severity between schizencephaly and hydranencephaly. This condition involves large, bilateral hemispheric defects surrounded by residual brain (Figure 12-26). The residual basal portion of brain supplied by the two posterior cerebral arteries bears some resemblance to the bottom of a straw basket, while the residual midline strip of brain supplied by the anterior cerebral arteries resembles a high arched handle for the basket. The cingulate gyri and variable portions of adjoining cortex are spared and form sagittally oriented, parafalcine arches of tissue connecting the frontal and occipital portions of the brain. A similar lesion may be created by carotid artery ligation in monkeys.

Encephaloclastic porencephaly most frequently arises as a result of necrotic softening and destruction of the full thickness of the cerebral wall. When destruction is less severe, a thin, variably complete layer of cerebral substance may remain between the hole and the ventricle. Such defects may still be classified as encephaloclastic porencephaly if the cavities are unilocular and their walls are smooth (Figures 12-27 and 12-28). Such modest encephaloclastic cysts are most frequently unilateral. When bilateral, they are usually asymmetrical in position and extent. The convolutions bordering on the defect show various degrees of atrophy. The gyri may be small, but the small size represents ulegyria, not true microgyria. Concurrent anomalies in the organization of the mantle and true CNS malformations are rare.

The exact etiology of these mild forms of encephaloclastic porencephaly cannot be determined. Some lesions fall into no vascular territory. Other lesions are believed to represent arterial ischemic encephaloclastic porencephaly. These lesions can be diagnosed angiographically on the basis of the typical arterial-territory localization of the lesion and the persistence of a ventricular wall that depends for its vascularization on choroidal and striatal arteries (not on peripheral cortical branches). It is interesting to speculate on the similarities and differences between these less severe forms of encephaloclastic porencephaly and the periventricular leukomalacia observed in premature infants. Since we now keep alive very immature fetuses, perhaps we observe outside the uterus the same events that precipitate this milder form of encephaloclastic porencephaly *in utero*.

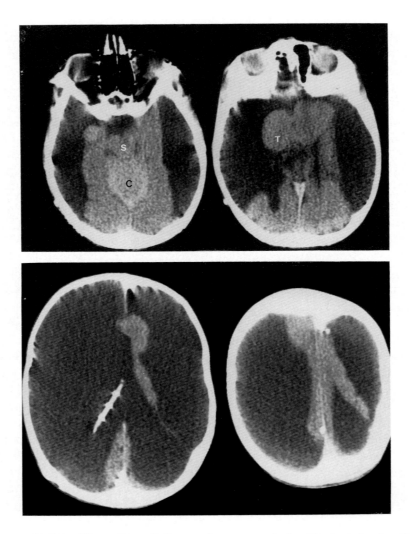

Figure 12-26. Transitional form of porencephaly. Basket brain. This 6-year-old boy with a normal birth history and progressive macrocephaly was shunted at age 1 year. He suffers severe retardation, frequent, prolonged seizures, and spasticity. Noncontrast CT demonstrates substantial defects in both cerebral mantles with preservation of relatively large portions of the medial temporal lobes, occipital lobes, and medial frontal and parietal lobes. The cerebellum (C), brain stem (S), and some of the deep gray nuclei (T) are also spared. Angiography revealed patent proximal middle cerebral arteries bilaterally but near absence of ascending opercular branches of the middle cerebral arteries on either side. Forms such as these are considered to be intermediate between schizencephaly and hydranencephaly. They are designated, generically, basket brain.

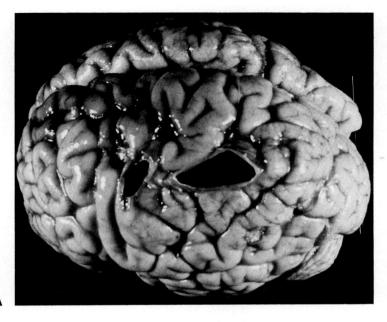

A

Figure 12-27. Less severe encephaloclastic porencephaly and hypoxic encephalopathy. This pathological specimen is from a 3-year-old boy, one of twins born septic at 6 months' gestation. The other twin died of sepsis at age 4 days. The 3-year-old twin suffered meningitis, seizures beginning at 9 months of age, and severe psychomotor retardation. (A) View of the dorsolateral surface. There is a double, (originally) membrane-covered defect in the left parietal region. The cortical pattern shows atrophy but no true polymicrogyria, even at the borders of the defect. (B) Coronal section through the foramina of Monro. The lateral and third (3) ventricles are of normal shape. The septum pellucidum is intact. The corpus callosum (double black arrowheads) is thin but present. There is a smooth-walled, left suprasylvian subcortical cavity (black arrow) affecting only the white matter. The ventricular wall (white arrowhead) is partially preserved. The basal ganglia are normal. (C) Coronal section through the posterior portion of the lateral ventricles. At this level, the defects are bilateral and affect the white matter and the cortex. On the left, the wall (white arrowhead) of the lateral ventricle appears paper thin. This cavity communicated with the ventricle further posteriorly. The right cavity (black arrow) did not communicate with the ventricle. Neither cavity exhibits a lining of heterotopic gray matter, rolled-in cortex, or associated polymicrogyria. Microscopic examination revealed patchy neuronal cell loss, astrocytic proliferation, hemosiderin-containing macrophages in the white matter adjacent to the cysts, preservation of most subcortical U-fibers near the cysts, extensive atrophy of the cerebrospinal tracts, and hypoxic damage to the hippocampi. (Reprinted with permission from Raybaud [12].)

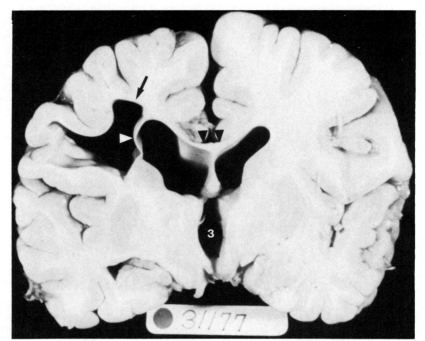

B

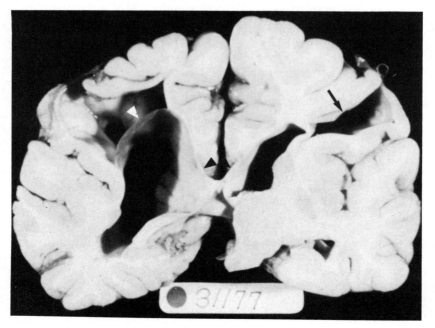

C

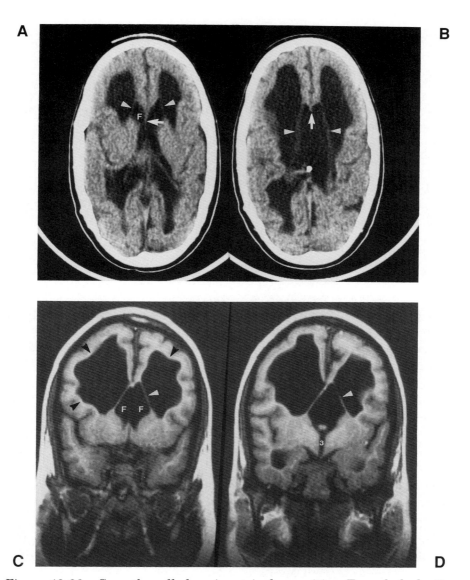

Figure 12-28. Smooth-walled periventricular cavities. Encephaloclastic porencephaly versus periventricular leukomalacia. This 9-year-old boy, formerly a 24-week-gestation premature infant, had developed respiratory distress syndrome and seizures at age 3 days. He had had open heart surgery for unknown heart disease and shunting for hydrocephalus with no shunt revision. Physical examination reveals severe retardation and spastic quadriplegia with contractures. (A and B) Noncontrast axial CT scans demonstrate shunted hydrocephalus with mild residual ventriculomegaly, slack ventricular contours, well-defined, thickened ventricular walls (white arrowheads), and bilateral, roughly symmetrical, smooth-walled, unilocular cavities lined by white matter. The septum pellucidum (white arrows) is partially preserved. There is no evidence of cortical defect or heterotopia. (C and D) Coronal spin-echo magnetic resonance images confirm the unilocular, smooth-walled nature of these defects, the lining of the defects by white, not gray, matter (black arrowheads), absence of heterotopias, near absence of the septum pellucidum, and preservation of thin walls (white arrowheads) of the lateral ventricles. F = frontal horn; 3 = third ventricle.

Question 61

In a neonate free from germinal matrix bleed and periventricular leukomalacia, cerebral infarction:

(A) is more often arterial than venous
(B) is more often thrombotic than embolic
(C) is commonly associated with sepsis and disseminated intravascular coagulation
(D) is more commonly unifocal in the premature infant but multifocal in the full-term infant
(E) occurs nearly twice as often in the right as in the left middle cerebral artery territory

Vasculo-occlusive disease occurring in early infancy can cause lesions that are superficially similar to those of schizencephaly, hydranencephaly, or multicystic encephalomalacia. Most often, however, the vasculo-occlusive diseases that develop during postnatal life are unilateral or asymmetrical and can be traced to a demonstrable occlusion in the vascular tree.

The precise incidence of thrombo-embolic occlusions of cerebral arteries in the neonate (0 to 28 days of age) remains unknown. Barmada et al. found cerebral infarctions in an arterial distribution in 32 of 592 neonates (5%) coming to postmortem examination. Venous infarctions were found in only 14 of these neonates (2%). In the neonatal period, therefore, arterial obstruction causes cerebral infarction more often than does venous obstruction **(Option (A) is true).** In older infants and small children, venous thrombosis is more frequent.

The most common cause of arterial obstruction and the most common cause of neonatal cerebral infarction appears to be embolism **(Option (B) is false).** Common sources of emboli include a recently thrombosed ductus arteriosus, thrombi from cardiac chambers, vegetations from heart valves, thrombi from placental and umbilical veins, and infarcted placental tissue. In neonates with sepsis, disseminated intravascular coagulation (DIC) plays a major role in causing cerebral infarction. In Barmada's study, autopsies of 11 infants with sepsis and arterial infarctions showed that the arterial occlusion was due to DIC in 9 (82%) and to arteritis from leptomeningitis in 2 (18%) **(Option (C) is true).** Occasionally, DIC of nonseptic origin also causes cerebral infarctions (Figure 12-29). The major cause of venous infarction appears to be stasis and thrombosis of the superior sagittal sinus from cardiac disease.

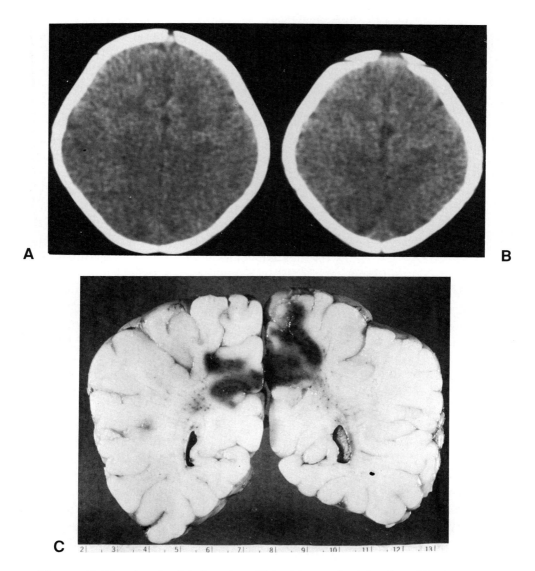

Figure 12-29. Cerebral infarction. This 11-month-old girl suddenly presented with fever, coma, purpura, scleral hemorrhages, and large, minimally reactive pupils. Work-up revealed no evidence of sepsis. Disseminated intravascular coagulation was treated by systemic heparinization. Repeated episodes of hypotension culminated in death the next day. (A and B) Noncontrast CT reveals loss of gray-white definition in the medial parietal lobes bilaterally, consistent with cerebral infarctions. (C) Coronal postmortem specimens demonstrate hemorrhagic necrosis of the cortex and subcortical white matter at the corresponding sites. Histologic sections revealed numerous thrombi in the small capillaries.

Specific analysis of neonates suggests that single large infarctions are predominant in full-term infants (Figure 12-30), whereas multiple small infarctions are predominant in premature infants. In Barmada's study, 8 of 14 full-term infants had single large infarctions and 6 had multiple small infarctions. Conversely, only 5 of 15 premature infants had single large infarctions, while 10 had multiple small infarctions, often adjacent to small thrombosed arteries or arterioles **(Option (D) is false).** Concurrent periventricular leukomalacia was found in 21% of the neonates with arterial infarctions; concurrent germinal matrix bleed was found in 17%. Cerebral infarctions occur in the distribution of the left middle cerebral artery more commonly than they do in that of the right middle cerebral artery (9:5). A twofold-greater incidence of left carotid artery infarction over right carotid artery infarction has also been observed in other series that include children of all ages (0 to 16 years) **(Option (E) is false).**

The gross and microscopic features of cerebral infarctions in neonates are very similar to those in adults, except that initially ischemic infarctions show a higher frequency of later hemorrhage in neonates. Advanced histopathologic changes in infants surviving only a few hours strongly suggest that infarction occurred *in utero* in some cases.

Clinically, neonates with cerebral infarctions most frequently show a generalized hypotonia. Most of these infants suddenly become lethargic and unresponsive, except to deep pain. Spontaneous movements and primitive reflexes become depressed. Autonomic instability is common. Most neonates with cerebral arterial infarction die rapidly. In Barmada's study, 50% had died by day 5 and 75% had died by day 10. One infant lived for 55 days.

Surprisingly, the risk of developing cerebral arterial infarctions seems more closely related to specific neonatal factors than to maternal problems. Maternal factors were implicated causally only when the infarction occurred a few days prior to birth or when labor was difficult and prolonged. Otherwise, the major risk factors seemed to be DIC associated with sepsis or respiratory distress syndrome (62%), prolonged cardiopulmonary arrest, sudden prolonged hypotension, and metabolic acidosis.

Cyanotic congenital heart disease is the condition that causes cerebrovascular occlusion most often if one considers children of all ages together, not neonates alone. Cerebrovascular thrombosis was observed in 3.8% of 1,875 patients with cyanotic congenital heart disease, especially tetralogy of Fallot; less often, transposition of the great vessels was observed. In 1973, Terplan found postmortem evidence of throm-

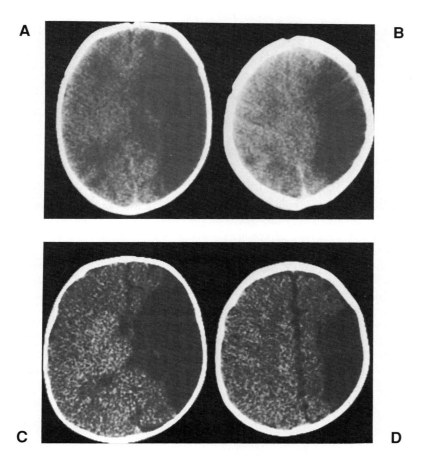

Figure 12-30. Middle cerebral artery infarction in a 39-week-gestation boy born to a 26-year-old diabetic mother. Apgar scores were 5 and 9 at 1 and 5 minutes. The right arm was ecchymotic, pulseless, and flaccid. Cardiac catheterization demonstrated complete occlusion of the right subclavian artery distal to the vertebral artery. The right arm was ultimately amputated. The final diagnosis was hypercoagulable state of unknown nature and middle cerebral artery infarction, probably secondary to internal carotid artery occlusion. (A and B) Day 5 of life. (C and D) Age 3 months. These images demonstrate evolution of a middle cerebral artery territory infarction from the acute state, with ill-defined margins and associated mass, to the chronic state, with sharply defined margins and ipsilateral hemiatrophy. (Case courtesy of R.A. Zimmerman, Philadelphia.)

boembolic cerebral infarctions in 17% of 500 patients with congenital heart defects. Such infarctions were four to five times more frequent in patients subjected to cardiac catheterization and/or surgery, suggesting an iatrogenic factor.

Thomas P. Naidich, M.D.

SUGGESTED READINGS

MULTICYSTIC ENCEPHALOMALACIA

1. Crome L. Multilocular cystic encephalopathy of infants. J Neurol Neurosurg Psychiatry 1958; 21:146–152
2. Crome L, Williams C. The problem of familial multilocular encephalomalacia. Acta Paediatr 1960; 49:175–184
3. Hartley WJ, Alexander G, Edwards MJ. Brain cavitation and micrencephaly in lambs exposed to prenatal hyperthermia. Teratology 1974; 9:299–304
4. Lindenburt R. Compression of brain arteries as pathogenetic factor for tissue necroses and their areas of predilection. J Neuropathol Exp Neurol 1955; 14:223–243
5. Naidich TP, Chakera TM. Multicystic encephalomalacia: CT appearance and pathological correlation. J Comput Assist Tomogr 1984; 8:631–636
6. Rorke LB. Pathology of perinatal brain injury. New York: Raven Press; 1982
7. Yoshioka H, Kadomoto Y, Mino M, Morikawa Y, Kasubuchi Y, Kusunoki T. Multicystic encephalomalacia in liveborn twin with a stillborn macerated co-twin. J Pediatr 1979; 95:798–800

PORENCEPHALY

8. Braun JP, Tournade A. Porencephaly. J Neuroradiol 1982; 9:161–178
9. Cohn R, Neumann MA. Porencephaly. A clinicopathologic study. J Neuropathol Exp Neurol 1946; 5:257–270
10. Dekaban AS. Large defects in cerebral hemispheres associated with cortical dysgenesis. J Neuropathol Exp Neurol 1965; 24:512–530
11. Friede FL. Porencephaly, hydranencephaly, multilocular cystic encephalopathy. In: Freide FL (ed), Developmental neuropathology. New York: Springer-Verlag; 1975:102–122
12. Raybaud C. Destructive lesions of the brain. Neuroradiology 1983; 25:265–291

SCHIZENCEPHALY

13. Aicardi J, Goutieres F. The syndrome of absence of the septum pellucidum with porencephalies and other developmental defects. Neuropediatrics 1981; 12:319–329
14. Barkovich AJ, Chuang SH, Norman D. MR of neuronal migration anomalies. AJR 1988; 150:179–187
15. Bird CR, Gilles FH. Type I schizencephaly: CT and neuropathologic findings. AJNR 1987; 8:451–454
16. DiPietro MA, Brody BA, Kuban K, Cole FS. Schizencephaly: rare cerebral malformation demonstrated by sonography. AJNR 1984; 5:196–198
17. Klingensmith WC III, Cioffi-Ragan DT. Schizencephaly: diagnosis and progression in utero. Radiology 1986; 159:617–618
18. Olson LD. Agenesis of the septum pellucidum associated with gray matter heterotopia. Minn Med 1985; 68:843–845
19. Yakovlev PI, Wadsworth RC. Schizencephalies. A study of the congenital clefts in the cerebral mantle. I. Clefts with fused lips. J Neuropathol Exp Neurol 1946; 5:116–130
20. Yakovlev PI, Wadsworth RC. Schizencephalies. A study of the congenital clefts in the cerebral mantle. II. Clefts with hydrocephalus and lips separated. J Neuropathol Exp Neurol 1946; 5:169–203

HYDRANENCEPHALY

21. Crome L. Hydrencephaly. Dev Med Child Neurol 1972; 14:224–226
22. Crome L, Sylvester PE. Hydranencephaly (hydrencephaly). Arch Dis Childhood 1958; 33:235–245
23. Dublin AB, French BN. Diagnostic image evaluation of hydranencephaly and pictorially similar entities, with emphasis on computed tomography. Radiology 1980; 137:81–91
24. Hamby WB, Krauss RF, Beswick WF. Hydranencephaly: clinical diagnosis. Presentation of seven cases. Pediatrics 1950; 6:371–383
25. Harwood-Nash DC, Fitz CR. Neuroradiology in infants and children, vol 3. St. Louis: CV Mosby; 1976
26. Moser RP, Seljeskog EL. Unilateral hydranencephaly: case report. Neurosurgery 1981; 9:703–705
27. Muir CS. Hydranencephaly and allied disorders. A study of cerebral defect in Chinese children. Arch Dis Child 1959; 34:231–246

INFARCTION

28. Banker BQ. Cerebral vascular disease in infancy and childhood. Part 1: occlusive vascular diseases. J Neuropathol Exp Neurol 1961; 20:127–140
29. Barmada MA, Moossy J, Shuman RM. Cerebral infarcts with arterial occlusion in neonates. Ann Neurol 1979; 6:495–502
30. Gold AP, Challenor YB, Gilles FH, et al. IX. Strokes in children (part 1) by Strokes in Children Study Group. Stroke 1973; 4:835–858

31. Golden GS. Stroke syndromes in childhood. Neurol Clin 1985; 3:59–75
32. Joint Committee for Stroke Facilities. IX. Strokes in children (part 1). Neuropathology of strokes in children. Stroke 1973; 4:860–870
33. Joint Committee for Stroke Facilities. IX. Strokes in children (part 1). Diagnosis and medical treatment of strokes in children. Stroke 1973; 4:872–894
34. Mannino FL, Trauner DA. Stroke in neonates. J Pediatr 1983; 102:605–610
35. Ment LR, Duncan CC, Ehrenkranz RA. Perinatal cerebral infarction. Ann Neurol 1984; 16:559–568
36. Raybaud CA, Livet MO, Jiddane M, Pinsard N. Radiology of ischemic strokes in children. In: Bories J (ed), Cerebral ischaemia. Berlin: Springer-Verlag; 1985:117–128
37. Terplan KL. Patterns of brain damage in infants and children with congenital heart disease. Association with catheterization and surgical procedures. Am J Dis Child 1973; 125:175–185

Notes

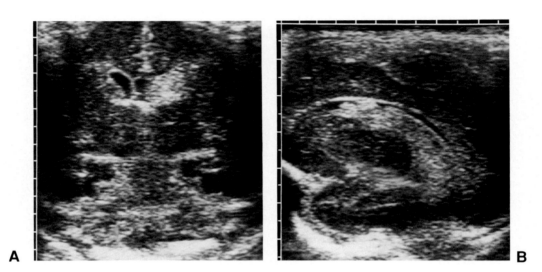

Figure 13-1. You are shown ultrasound images from a 28-week-gestation, premature infant. Figure 13-1A is a coronal scan through the body of the ventricles, and Figure 13-1B is a sagittal scan through the left lateral ventricle.

Case 13: Subependymal Hemorrhage

Question 62

Which *one* of the following is the MOST likely diagnosis?

(A) Subependymal hemorrhage
(B) Parenchymal hemorrhage
(C) Choroidal hemorrhage
(D) Periventricular leukomalacia
(E) Tuberous sclerosis

The most likely diagnosis in the test patient is subependymal hemorrhage (SEH) **(Option (A) is correct).** The coronal and sagittal ultrasound scans (Figure 13-1) of this premature infant display a focal area of increased echogenicity that lies immediately adjacent to the left lateral ventricle at the site of the subependymal germinal matrix. The lesion does not extend very far laterally, so it is highly likely to have remained confined to the subependymal germinal matrix (Figure 13-2, arrows). The lesion is very echogenic, so it is an acute SEH. Because of the exact site of the lesion, parenchymal hemorrhage (Option (B)) and choroidal hemorrhage (Option (C)) are less likely in this patient. Parenchymal hemorrhage is diagnosed when the zone of abnormal, increased echoes extends farther laterally than would be expected for a germinal matrix, even one that was expanded by a focal bleed. While this is admittedly a subjective judgement, most parenchymal hemorrhages do extend far enough laterally to be differentiated by "eye" alone. Choroidal hemorrhages typically expand the choroid plexus. They then either bulge into the ventricle, producing a bulbous zone of increased echoes confluent with the echogenic choroid plexus, or they rupture into the ventricle, causing both an expansion of the echogenic choroid plexus and echogenic intraventricular blood, perhaps with CSF-blood levels. Periventricular leukomalacia (Option (D)) is typically situated just slightly away from the margin of the ventricle, within the periventricular white matter. The lesion represents a coagulation necrosis in the watershed territory between two sets of arterial feeders: (1) the

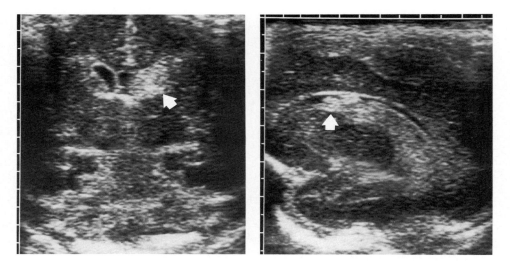

Figure 13-2 (Same as Figure 13-1). Subependymal hemorrhage. Arrows indicate focal areas of echogenicity confined to the subependymal germinal matrix.

paramedian set of "perforators" that penetrate upward from the base of the brain toward the lateral side of the ventricle and (2) the deep medullary perforators that arise from the convexity arteries and pass inward from the surface of the hemisphere toward the lateral margin of the ventricles. In premature newborns, the watershed usually lies in the periventricular white matter a few millimeters lateral to and superior to the outer angle of the ventricle. Thus, periventricular leukomalacia typically appears as a lesion centered further lateral to and slightly superficial to the lateral margin of the ventricle, not immediately adjacent to the edge of the ventricle and not immediately inferior to the floor of the ventricle as is true of SEH.

Tuberous sclerosis (Option (E)) can affect the subependymal tissue, can be echogenic, and can cause findings resembling those in the test images. However, tuberous sclerosis is an uncommon disease and, when present, does not usually produce such large lesions so early in life. Conversely, SEH is common in premature infants. In the absence of any other sonographic findings to suggest tuberous sclerosis (see Figure 13-29), the diagnosis of subependymal germinal matrix bleed is far more likely and more appropriate than would be a diagnosis of tuberous sclerosis.

Question 63

Concerning subependymal hemorrhage,

- (A) it occurs most frequently in full-term infants
- (B) when present, it nearly always manifests during the first 24 hours of life
- (C) subependymal hemorrhage alone is designated as Grade 0 hemorrhage
- (D) it occurs most commonly along the inferolateral border of the frontal horn
- (E) it is an uncommon, clinically insignificant finding in routine sonograms

SEH occurs primarily in preterm infants with a gestational age of less than 32 weeks **(Option (A) is false).** The likelihood of suffering a subependymal hemorrhage appears to correlate with the size of the germinal matrix at the time of actual birth. The germinal matrix is largest at 24 to 32 weeks' gestation; it then involutes so that it is virtually absent in the full-term, 40-week-gestation infant (Figure 13-3). Thus the incidence of SEH may be as high as 75% in premature infants of 26 weeks' gestation, becomes sharply reduced to about 35% in infants of 32 weeks' gestation, and is very low in full-term infants.

SEH typically occurs during the first week of life. Sonograms in preterm infants have shown that 86% of hemorrhages occur in the first 3 days of life (36% on day 1, 32% on day 2, and 18% on day 3). However, hemorrhages may first appear as late as 7 to 8 days of life **(Option (B) is false).**

Isolated SEH is designated Grade I, not Grade 0 **(Option (C) is false).** Since the severity of intracranial hemorrhage influences the prognosis of the patient, a number of grading systems have been proposed. The most widely used classification system is as follows: (i) Grade 0, normal (no hemorrhage); (ii) Grade I, SEH (Figures 13-1 and 13-4A left); (iii) Grade II, intraventricular hemorrhage with no ventricular dilatation (Figures 13-4A right and 13-5); (iv) Grade III, intraventricular hemorrhage with ventriculomegaly (Figures 13-4B and 13-6); and (v) Grade IV, intraparenchymal hemorrhage (Figures 13-4C and D and 13-7).

Several practical problems with the grading system must be noted. (1) A Grade I hemorrhage that may be inconsequential in one patient can evolve to a Grade IV hemorrhage in another patient, with catastrophic consequences. Therefore, the grade assigned to any intracranial hemorrhage must be modified by the findings of the serial ultrasound studies. The patient's prognosis must then be based upon the worst grade reached. (2) Three other forms of intracranial hemorrhage are not addressed by the grading system given above. These include parenchymal hemorrhages that do not represent extensions of SEH, choroidal hemorrhages,

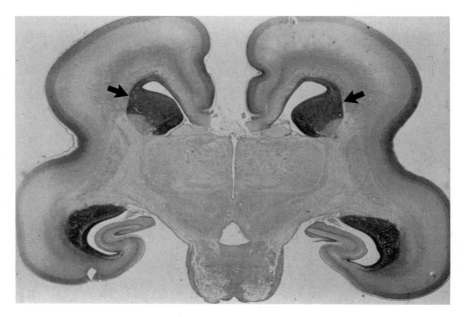

Figure 13-3. Coronal section from a 16-week-gestation fetus. The dark, highly cellular germinal matrix (arrows) lies in the subependymal position along the floor of the lateral ventricle. At this age it also sweeps around the ventricle to the roof of the temporal horn.

and cerebellar hemorrhages. It may be appropriate to consider the choroidal hemorrhage without ventriculomegaly as Grade II and to consider the choroidal hemorrhage with ventriculomegaly as Grade III.

The typical site of SEH is the germinal matrix that lies along the lateral portion of the floor of the frontal horn, and the lateral portion of the floor of the body of the lateral ventricle. The germinal matrix then sweeps posteriorly and inferiorly around the atrium into the roof of the temporal horn. When the germinal matrix involutes, it persists longest and remains largest in the region of the inferolateral wall of the frontal horn. This site, then, is the most common site of SEH **(Option (D) is true).** Anatomically, this portion of the germinal matrix (and associated bleeds) lies between the ependyma and the head of the caudate nucleus; that is, it lies superior to the caudate nucleus and anterior to the thalamus (Figure 13-3).

To understand the position and appearance of SEHs, it is first necessary to understand the anatomic relationships along the floor of the lateral ventricle (Figures 13-8 and 13-9). The floor of the lateral ventricle is made up of three structures: the caudate nucleus, the thalamus, and

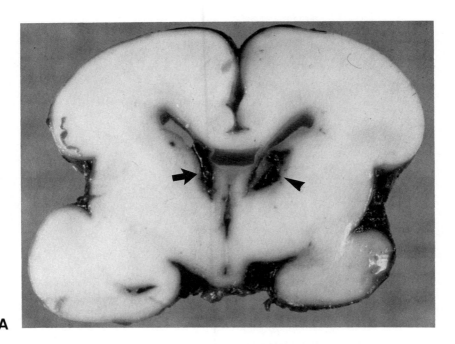

A

Figure 13-4. Grades of subependymal-intraventricular hemorrhage. Coronal anatomic specimens. (A) Grade II. On the left side, hemorrhage (arrowhead) is confined to the subependymal germinal matrix. Were this the only lesion, the hemorrhage would be categorized Grade I. However, the contralateral right hemorrhage (arrow) has broken into the ventricle and produced intraventricular hemorrhage with staining of the ventricular wall. There is no hydrocephalus. The patient must thus be categorized as having Grade II hemorrhage. Passage of blood outward has resulted in subarachnoid hemorrhage with staining of the external surface of the brain. (B) Grade III. Intraventricular hemorrhage forms blood casts of both lateral ventricles, including temporal horns. The ventricles are dilated. (C and D) Grade IV. Parenchymal hemorrhage with intraventricular hemorrhage and ventricular dilatation.

the fornix. The choroid plexus projects upward from the floor into the lateral ventricle. The precise interrelationships of these structures differ anterior to and posterior to the foramen of Monro (Table 13-1).

The portion of the lateral ventricle anterior to the foramen of Monro is called the frontal horn; that behind the foramen of Monro is called the body of the lateral ventricle. The floor of the lateral ventricle slopes downward and is higher laterally than medially. Because of this slope, the floor and the lateral wall are the same inferolateral surface.

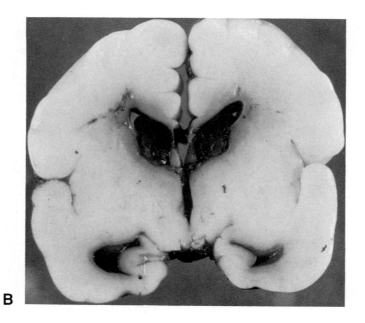

B

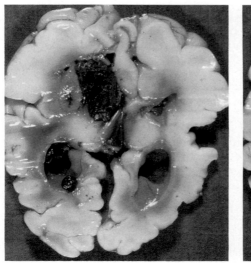

C

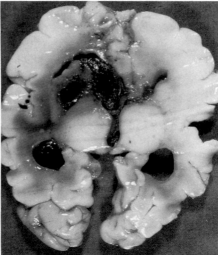

D

The portion of the caudate nucleus anterior to the foramen of Monro is designated the head of the caudate nucleus; the portion behind is designated the body. The thalamus lies entirely behind the foramen of Monro. The anterior end of the thalamus forms the posterior border of

378 / *Neuroradiology*

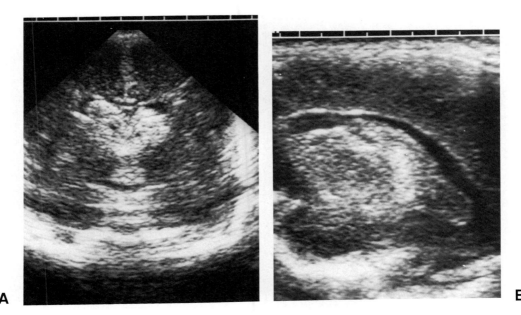

A   **B**

Figure 13-5. Coronal (A) and parasagittal (B) ultrasound images of a bilateral Grade II hemorrhage.

Table 13-1. Anatomic relationships along the floor of the lateral ventricle

Structure	Anterior to Foramen of Monro	Posterior to Foramen of Monro
Lateral ventricle	Frontal horn	Body
Caudate nucleus	Head	Body
Thalamus	None	Thalamus
Fornix	Anterior column	Body and crus
Choroid plexus	None	Choroid plexus

the foramen of Monro. The fornix lies on top of the thalamus near the midline and then separates from the thalamus to arc anteriorly, over the foramen of Monro. This arching anterior column of the fornix forms the anteromedial border of the foramen of Monro. The choroid plexus arises along the lateral border of the fornix and pushes up into the ventricle from the floor. It then curves medially and inferiorly through the foramen of Monro, along its posterior border, to merge with the choroid plexus of the third ventricle.

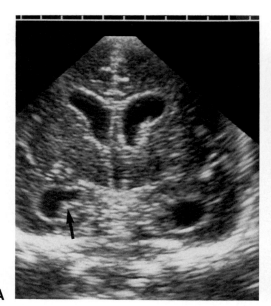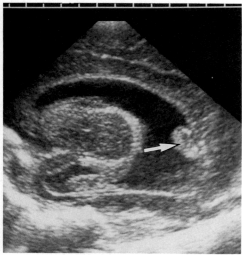

A

B

Figure 13-6. Coronal (A) and parasagittal (B) ultrasound scans of a Grade III hemorrhage (arrows) and ventricular enlargement.

In coronal sections anterior to the foramen of Monro, the floor of the frontal horn (i.e., inferolateral wall) is formed by the head of the caudate nucleus. There is no thalamus, fornix, or choroid plexus. The contour of the floor is convex upward as the bulbous head of caudate indents the ventricle (Figure 13-8A).

In coronal sections posterior to the foramen of Monro, the caudate nucleus becomes thinner and moves laterally, so that it forms only the small upper lateral margin of the floor of the ventricle. The thalamus forms the larger medial portion of the floor. The fornix sits on top of the medial portion of thalamus (Figures 13-8B and C). The choroid plexus enters the ventricle along the lateral edge of the fornix and—mushroom-like—overlaps the edge of fornix and the adjacent thalamus. A well-defined caudothalamic groove separates the caudate nucleus from the thalamus. This contains the thalamostriate vein.

In sagittal views (Figure 13-9), the caudate head projects anterior to the foramen of Monro and to the thalamus. The thalamus and the choroid plexus lie behind the foramen of Monro. The caudothalamic groove separates the caudate nucleus (anterosuperior to it) from the thalamus (posteroinferior to it). In the midline, one sees the frontal horn (or cavum

380 / *Neuroradiology*

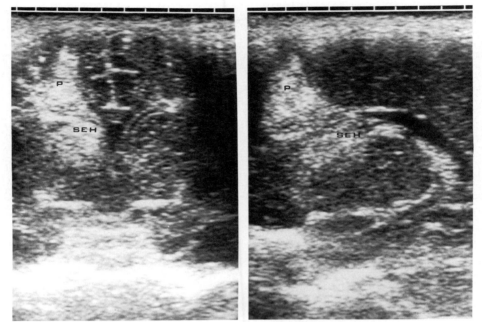

A   **B**

Figure 13-7. Coronal (A) and parasagittal (B) ultrasound images of a Grade IV hemorrhage. Hemorrhage has extended from the subependymal germinal matrix (SEH) into the brain parenchyma (P).

septi pellucidi), the foramen of Monro, and the choroid plexus of the roof of the third ventricle. Off midline one sees the frontal horn and the body of the lateral ventricle, the caudate nucleus, the thalamus, and the intervening caudothalamic groove. The choroid plexus lies medial and posterior to the caudothalamic groove.

In ultrasound images the caudothalamic groove (and contained vein) are echogenic (Figure 13-10). The choroid plexus is highly echogenic (Figure 13-11). The caudate nucleus and thalamus are less echogenic than either the choroid or the groove. In the normal infant then, the echogenic choroid plexus lies posterior to the foramen of Monro and to the caudothalamic groove. No echogenic structure normally lies anterior to the foramen of Monro or to the groove. Echogenic lesions seen anterior to the groove cannot be normal choroid plexi. In the right clinical context then, any echogenic focus seen to lie anterior to the caudothalamic groove is best interpreted as an acute echogenic hemorrhage (Figure 13-2).

In coronal views, SEH lies lateral to the caudothalamic groove. Echoes detected medial to the groove may represent normal choroid plexus,

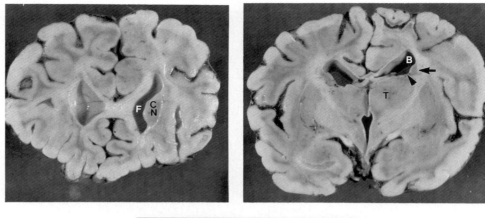

A

B

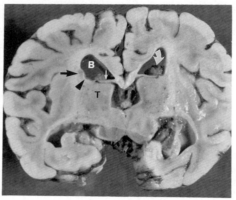

C

Figure 13-8. Anatomic relationships along the floor of the lateral ventricle. Coronal section specimens of a 7-month-old, *initially* 36-week-gestation, boy with transposition of the great vessels and cerebral atrophy. (A) Anterior to the foramen of Monro the head of the caudate nucleus (CN) indents the frontal horn (F) and forms the inferolateral wall of the ventricle. There is no choroid plexus in the frontal horn. (B and C) Posterior to the foramen of Monro the inferolateral wall of the body (B) of the lateral ventricle is formed by the caudate body (black arrow), the caudothalamic groove (arrowhead), the thalamus (T), and the fornix (white arrow) that sits atop the thalamus. The choroid plexus (curved white arrow) enters the ventricle along the lateral edge of the fornix and angles up into the CSF.

choroid plexus hemorrhage, or intraventricular clot adherent to the choroid plexus.

The caudothalamic groove should not be confused with the more echogenic choroid plexus in the roof of the third ventricle, which is visible

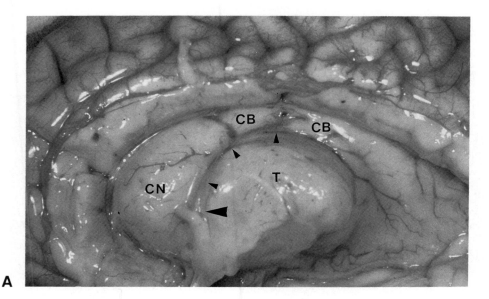

A

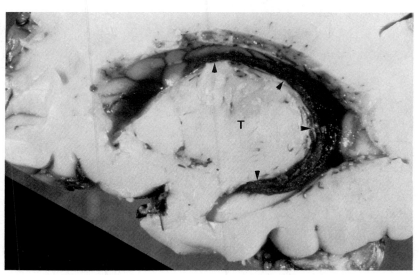

B

Figure 13-9. Anatomic relationships along the floor of the lateral ventricle. Sagittal specimens. (A) View of the lateral ventricle seen *from the midline* after stripping away the septum pellucidum, fornix, and choroid plexus. The large arrowhead marks the foramen of Monro. Note the bulbous head of the caudate nucleus (CN) that indents the frontal horn anterior to the foramen of Monro; the tapering body of the caudate nucleus (CB) that forms the lateral portion of the floor of the body of the ventricle behind the foramen of Monro; the thalamus (T) that forms most of the medial portion of the floor of the body of the lateral ventricle; and the caudothalamic groove (small arrowheads) that arcs anteriorly and medially to reach the foramen of Monro. (B) View of the lateral ventricle *from the lateral edge* of the ventricle showing the normal course of the choroid plexus (dark structure, arrowheads) around the thalamus (T) from the temporal horn inferiorly to the foramen of Monro superiorly. No choroid plexus enters the frontal horn.

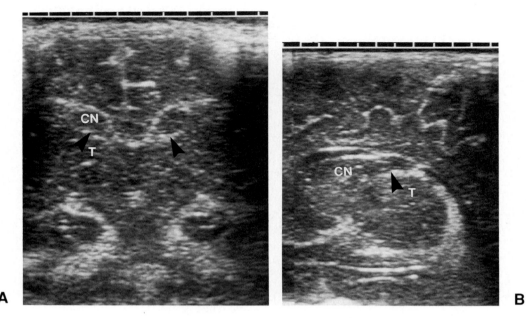

Figure 13-10. Coronal (A) and parasagittal (B) images of the caudotha-lamic groove (arrowheads) between the head of the caudate nucleus (CN) and the thalamus (T).

in more paramedian and midsagittal (midline) scans (Figure 13-12). The visibility of several midline structures, such as the cavum septi pellucidi, the cavum vergae, the third ventricle, the aqueduct of Sylvius or midline posterior fossa structures, should help one to avoid such a mistake.

SEH is frequently seen in routine sonograms of symptomatic and asymptomatic preterm infants. They are most common in those infants that are most immature (67% are seen at 28 weeks' gestation). Clinically, newborns with isolated SEH have a short-term outcome similar to that of preterm infants without SEH but with equivalent degrees of prematurity and respiratory distress. With time, the SEH either resolves completely or evolves into a small subependymal cyst of unknown significance (Figure 13-13). However, discovery of SEH must be considered a significant finding, because the SEH could extend and convert to intraventricular hemorrhage or intraparenchymal hemor-rhage. The prognosis of intraventricular hemorrhage and intraparenchy-mal hemorrhage is much less favorable. Therefore, initial detection of SEH mandates serial follow-up studies to monitor the course of the bleed and detect any unfavorable outcome **(Option (E) is false).**

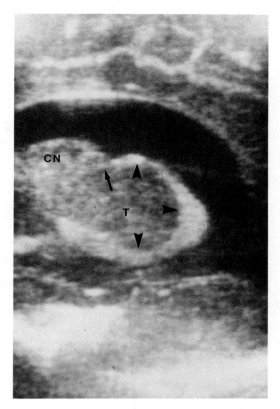

Figure 13-11. Parasagittal sonogram. Echogenic choroid plexus (arrow-heads) courses around the thalamus (T) toward the foramen of Monro. It does not extend anterior to the caudothalamic groove (arrow). CN = caudate nucleus.

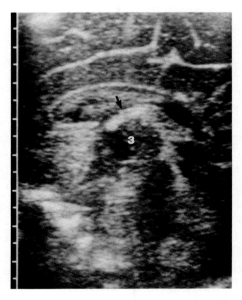

Figure 13-12. Nearly midline sagittal sonogram. The arrow indicates the echogenic choroid plexus in the roof of the third ventricle (3).

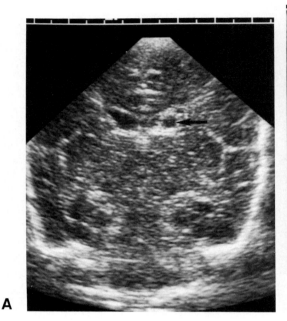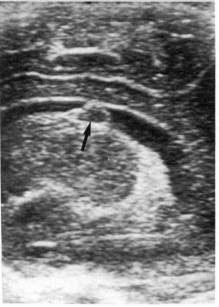

A   B

Figure 13-13. Coronal (A) and parasagittal (B) scans 3 weeks after an acute SEH demonstrate a small subependymal cyst (arrows).

Question 64

Concerning parenchymal hemorrhage in premature neonates,

    (A) both hypoxia and hypercapnia have been implicated in its pathogenesis
    (B) serial ultrasonography shows that it resolves in the same manner as subependymal hemorrhage
    (C) it most frequently affects the cerebellum
    (D) the morbidity directly related to it is very high
    (E) discovery of this condition mandates emergency arteriography

Most studies have shown a correlation between intraparenchymal hemorrhage, hypoxia, and hypercapnia **(Option (A) is true).** Many indices of possible hypoxia have been taken into consideration. These indices include fetal heart tones, Apgar scores, ventilator dependence, episodes of pneumothorax, and measurements of arterial blood gases. While the relative contributions of these factors have varied from one report to another, hypoxia and respiratory distress have invariably preceded the intracranial hemorrhage. Bolus intravascular injection and abrupt ligation of patent ductus arteriosus have also been shown to result in intracranial hemorrhage. In both settings, the fragile intracranial vessels are believed to distend suddenly and burst. Hypoxia and hypercapnia both lower the resistance of the intracranial vascular bed and, therefore, increase the cerebral blood flow. These are likewise believed to lead to distention and rupture of fragile capillaries or small vessels.

The sonographic appearance of parenchymal hemorrhage changes and passes through several phases over time. In phase I, acute parenchymal hemorrhage is highly echogenic and homogeneous, just like SEH (Figure 13-14A). The process of resolution of parenchymal hemorrhage is unlike that of the SEH, however **(Option (B) is false).** The parenchymal hemorrhage typically undergoes three additional phases. In phase 2, 1 to 2 weeks after the hemorrhage, the center of the parenchymal hematoma becomes hypoechoic. The periphery remains echogenic but becomes better demarcated from the surrounding brain (Figure 13-14B). In phase 3, by 2 to 4 weeks after the hemorrhage, the blood clot retracts and settles in a dependent position (Figure 13-14C). In phase 4, 2 to 3 months after the onset of the bleeding, necrosis and phagocytosis are complete, leaving an area of encephalomalacia that often communicates with the ipsilateral ventricle (Figure 13-14D). During this time, the ventricles become progressively dilated.

Parenchymal hemorrhages typically occur at different sites in the premature and the full-term neonate. In the premature neonate, parenchymal hemorrhages usually represent extensions of initial SEH into the brain substance of the frontal or parietal lobes. Less frequently the SEH extends into the occipital lobe. Thus, these sites are most frequent in the premature neonate **(Option (C) is false).**

Other conditions can cause artifactual or real parenchymal echogenicity that mimics the appearance of parenchymal hemorrhage. These include falx shadowing (Figure 13-15), cerebral edema (Figure 13-16), and cerebritis (Figure 13-17).

The frequency of cerebellar hemorrhage in living preterm infants is unknown. One autopsy study reported a frequency of 15 to 25% in preterm infants of less than 32 weeks' gestation. By common experience, however, cerebellar hemorrhage is very infrequent in premature neonates. Serial sonograms performed for monitoring of possible intracerebral hemorrhage rarely show cerebellar parenchymal bleeds. Perhaps these occur only with severe stress.

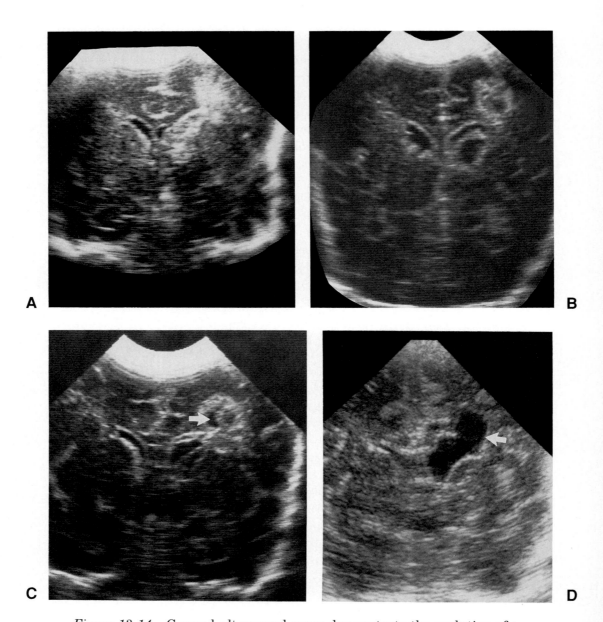

Figure 13-14. Coronal ultrasound scans demonstrate the evolution of a parenchymal hemorrhage. (A) Phase 1, acute Grade IV parenchymal hemorrhage is densely and homogeneously hyperechoic. (B) Phase 2, 1 to 2 weeks after the hemorrhage. There is now a hypoechoic center in the parenchymal hemorrhage. An ipsilateral subependymal cyst is also noted. (C) Phase 3, 2 to 4 weeks post-hemorrhage. Retraction of the blood clot leaves a crescent of anechoic fluid (arrow). (D) Phase 4, 2 to 3 months post-hemorrhage. The site of the bleed is now an area of encephalomalacia (arrow) that communicates with the ventricle.

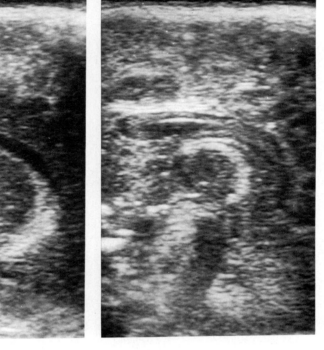

A

B

Figure 13-15. (A) Parasagittal sonogram illustrates the artifact of falx shadowing (arrow). (B) Midsagittal scan. Scanning in the midline directly through the falx maximizes the shadowing of the falx.

In full-term infants, SEH is rare. Consequently, parenchymal extension of SEH is also rare. In these circumstances, cerebellar parenchymal hemorrhage is far more common (Figure 13-18). In at least some cases, cerebellar hemorrhage in full-term infants has been associated with traumatic breech deliveries or mask ventilation. Cerebellar hemorrhages can be depicted best on transcranial sonograms by scanning in the coronal plane behind the ear (Figure 13-18) or by coronal scanning through the posterior fontanelle with the transducer angulated cephalad. Both methods show the anatomy of the occipital lobes, occipital horns (Figures 13-18B and 13-18C), and posterior fossa better than does scanning through the anterior fontanelle.

The morbidity directly related to parenchymal hemorrhages is very high **(Option (D) is true).** However, the mortality of greater than 50% quoted in the literature signifies only that high mortality is associated with, and not necessarily caused by, intraparenchymal hemorrhage.

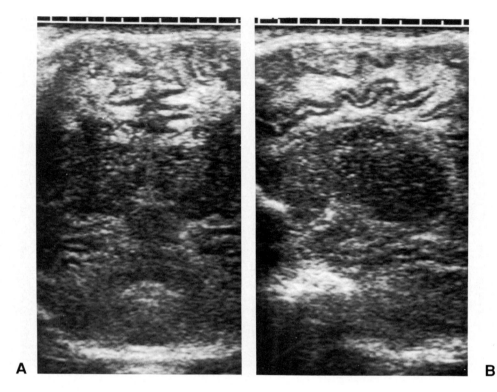

Figure 13-16. Coronal (A) and parasagittal (B) scans display the echogenic appearance of cerebral edema.

Preterm infants with intraparenchymal hemorrhage invariably, often simultaneously, suffer from many other life-threatening consequences of prematurity, such as acidosis, hypercapnia, congestive heart failure, necrotizing enterocolitis, etc.

Arteriography is rarely indicated for evaluation of intraparenchymal hemorrhage in the preterm neonate. Arteriovenous malformations are rarely the cause of the hemorrhage. Most of the bleeds occur as a result of hypoxia. Thus, it is unlikely that arteriography would disclose a remediable cause of hemorrhage. At the same time there is a risk of injury for little or no expected benefit **(Option (E) is false).** Ultrasonography is the modality of choice for initial detection of parenchymal hemorrhage in preterm infants; it often is the only test required for serial monitoring and management.

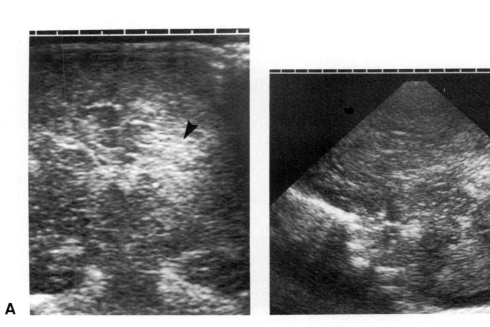

Figure 13-17. Coronal (A) and parasagittal (B) scans show the echogenic brain parenchyma in an infant with cerebritis. The single arrowhead in panel A indicates left parietal lobe involvement. The double arrowhead in panel B indicates right occipital lobe abnormality.

A

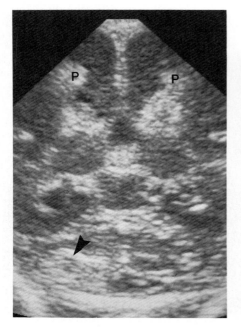

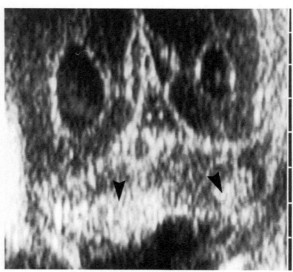

B

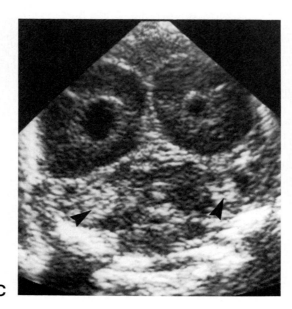

C

Figure 13-18. Coronal scan (A) through the anterior fontanelle shows bilateral parenchymal hemorrhages (P) and a single cerebellar hemorrhage (arrowhead). Transcranial coronal scan, with the transducer placed behind the ear (B), and coronal scan through the posterolateral fontanelle (C) show *bilateral* cerebellar hemorrhages (arrowheads) and asymmetrically dilated occipital horns.

Question 65

In the neonate, which *one* of the following is the MOST common etiology of choroidal hemorrhage?

(A) Prematurity
(B) Choroid plexus papilloma
(C) Arteriovenous malformation
(D) Forceps delivery
(E) Maternal diabetes

The most common cause of choroidal hemorrhage is prematurity **(Option (A) is correct).** The true frequency of choroidal hemorrhage is not known. Some authors believe that it accounts for only 3 to 7% of cases of intracranial hemorrhage, whereas others claim a frequency of 82%. Recent publications have suggested a frequency of about 60%. In premature infants, choroid plexus hemorrhage is not as easily diagnosed sonographically as are other forms of hemorrhage. The difficulty in diagnosing choroid plexus bleeds has three major causes. First, normal choroid plexus is so echogenic that isolated echogenic choroidal hemorrhage becomes difficult to diagnose (Figures 13-19 and 13-20). For example, on ultrasonography the choroid plexus on the affected side may appear only slightly larger and more echogenic than the normal side (Figure 13-21B). Second, technical problems such as asymmetrical, canted scans can display "different" sizes of two normal choroid plexi, leading to confusion (Figure 13-22). Although this confusion can be avoided by perfecting the scan, the possibility of technical error leads to undercalling asymmetric choroid plexi and possible choroid bleeds. Third, some groups of infants, such as those with myelomeningocele, have a prominent choroid plexus, especially in the region of the glomus. Thus, in 50% of myelomeningocele infants, the choroid plexus is pedunculated and hangs downward into the dependent portion of the ventricle. The bulbous glomus at the lowest end of the choroid plexus can be confused with choroidal hemorrhage or with an intraventricular clot attached to the choroid plexus. This compounds the difficulty of diagnosis.

If the ventricles are not dilated, isolated choroid plexus hemorrhage cannot be differentiated from intraventricular hemorrhage. A blood clot that is attached to the choroid plexus and extends posteriorly into a somewhat dilated occipital horn can be a useful clue for the diagnosis of choroid plexus hemorrhage (Figure 13-21A). A floating blood clot within the ventricle, not connecting with the choroid plexus, may be either a detached choroid plexus blood clot or an intraventricular hemorrhage

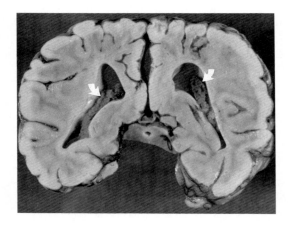

Figure 13-19. Same patient as in Figure 13-8. Coronal anatomic specimen of the choroid plexi (curved arrows) in the atria and posterior temporal horns.

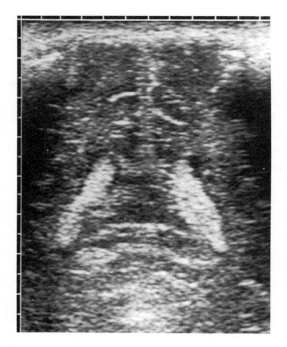

Figure 13-20. Coronal sonogram shows prominent but normal choroid plexi on both sides. This appearance should not be mistaken for choroidal hemorrhage.

A

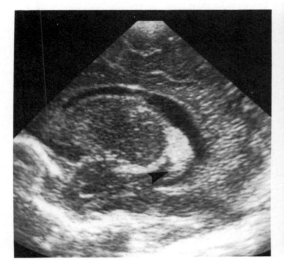

B

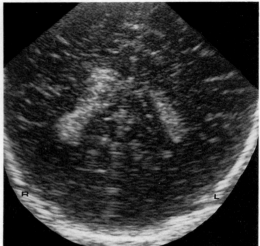

Figure 13-21. (A) Parasagittal scan demonstrates mild dilation of the lateral ventricle and a blood clot (arrowhead) attached to the choroid plexus. (B) Coronal sonogram shows an asymmetrically larger and more echogenic right choroid plexus in a baby with choroidal hemorrhage. This appearance is not remarkably different from that seen with normal variation (see Figure 13-20). (C) Nonenhanced CT of the head in the same baby showing the right choroid plexus (arrowhead) with a CT number much higher than that of the left choroid plexus. L = left, R = right.

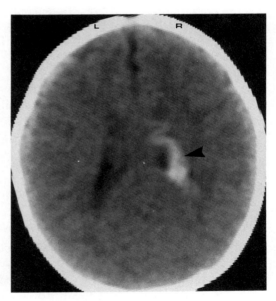

C

with intact choroid plexus. At present, it is believed that any intraventricular hemorrhage not associated with SEH probably originates from a choroid plexus hemorrhage.

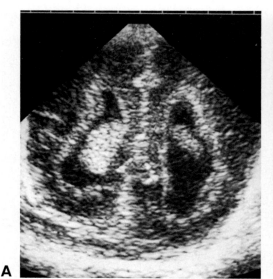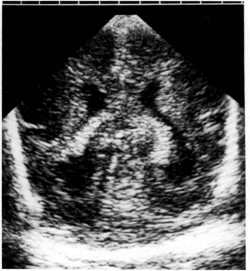

A   B

Figure 13-22. Infant sonogram. (A) Asymmetrical coronal scanning artifactually creates the impression that the right choroid plexus is larger and more echogenic than the left one. (B) When the scan is performed correctly, the choroid plexi are symmetrical.

CT documents choroidal hemorrhage more reliably than does ultrasonography. The noncontrast CT findings of choroidal bleed are frequently obvious because the affected choroid plexus has a much higher CT number than the contralateral choroid plexus (Figure 13-21C), even when the sonographic changes are subtle (Figure 13-21B).

Choroid plexus papillomas (Option (B)) are highly echogenic, appear as bulbous intraventricular masses, typically cause hydrocephalus, and may cause hemorrhage. When present, they are located primarily in the lateral ventricle(s) (Figure 13-23), specifically at the trigone. The ultrasonographic appearance can mimic an intraventricular hemorrhage, leading to misdiagnosis. However, the lesion is relatively rare, accounting for some 3 to 5% of brain tumors in children, and so it is not the most common cause of choroidal hemorrhage. One must always have a small awareness of the possibility of encountering a congenital choroid plexus papilloma while assessing an infant for possible intraventricular bleed. Absence of CSF-blood levels, absence of chemical signs of blood loss proportional to the age of infant observed, and, especially, any clear CSF from a ventricular tap should increase suspicion of possible papilloma.

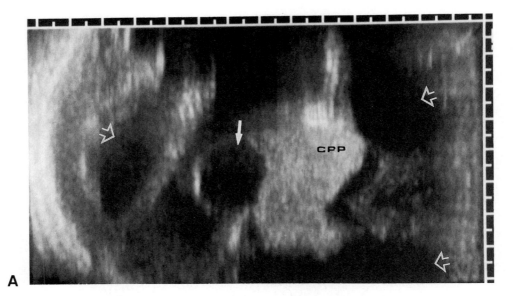

A

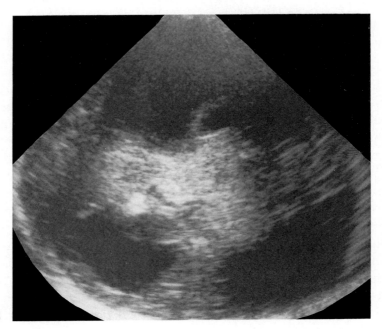

B

Figure 13-23. (A) Transcranial scanning in the "CT plane" shows a
choroid plexus papilloma (CPP), dilated lateral ventricles (open arrows),
and a large third ventricle (closed arrow). (B) Transcranial scanning
through the frontal bone shows the echogenic choroid plexus papilloma
and marked ventriculomegaly. (C) In another patient, coronal sonography
shows a choroid plexus papilloma (arrows) that hangs down from the
choroid plexus into the enlarged temporal horn.

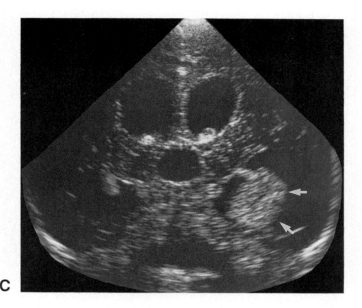

C

Doppler flow studies could be utilized to detect the increased flow associated with a hypervascular papilloma. In any doubtful case, CT with and without contrast enhancement or magnetic resonance imaging with and without contrast enhancement could clearly distinguish the nonhemorrhagic enhancing choroid plexus papilloma from the hemorrhagic nonenhancing clot. A hemorrhagic papilloma could remain indistinguishable from simple bleed, however.

Choroid plexus arteriovenous malformation (AVM) (Option (C)) could lead to choroidal and intraventricular hemorrhage. However, arteriovenous malformations are rare causes of choroidal hemorrhage. Small, so-called occult AVMs have been invoked to explain otherwise-mysterious choroidal bleeds. The frequency of these hypothecated lesions remains to be documented, especially those that are said to be undetectable because they "self-destruct" at the moment of hemorrhage. Large AVMs that incidentally affect the choroid plexus are more frequent and easily detected by ultrasonography, especially Doppler. These do not constitute a diagnostic problem.

Increased vascularity of choroid plexus due to either papilloma or arteriovenous malformation could be detected by Doppler flow studies, particularly in full-term babies. The Doppler flow studies in babies with choroidal hemorrhage are not expected to demonstrate high flow.

Choroidal hemorrhage (Option (D)) is observed in patients delivered both with and without forceps. There is no evidence that proper application and use of forceps predisposes to choroidal hemorrhage.

There is no evidence that maternal diabetes (Option (E)) directly results in choroidal hemorrhage. Babies born to diabetic mothers are nearly always full term and large in size. Thus, most are not at risk for hemorrhage. Nevertheless, 3% of neonates born to diabetic mothers are premature. A significant percentage of babies born to diabetic mothers may have severe respiratory distress. Thus, complications of respiratory distress could cause hypoxia and secondary intracranial hemorrhage. Nonetheless, prematurity remains the most common cause of choroidal hemorrhage.

Question 66

Periventricular leukomalacia refers to which *one* of the following?

(A) Transependymal migration of cerebrospinal fluid into the parenchyma in association with hydrocephalus
(B) Hemosiderin staining of the parenchyma following intraventricular hemorrhage
(C) Coagulation necrosis of the periventricular white matter
(D) Pathologic findings accompanying venous sinus thrombosis
(E) Failure of normal myelination comparable to that observed in metachromatic leukodystrophy

Periventricular leukomalacia (PVL) is an infarction of deep white matter, adjacent to the lateral angle of the lateral ventricles (Figure 13-24) **(Option (C) is correct).** This region of the brain is a watershed area that is fed by the end branches of the anterior, middle, and posterior cerebral arteries. PVL is believed to be the result of hypoxia and ischemia, which in turn lead to inadequate perfusion and nutrition of the watershed areas and development of coagulation necrosis of the white matter. The frequency of PVL is 7 to 22% in neonatal autopsy series. The frequency is 34% of preterm infants with birth weights of 1,501 g or less. Of those who died after being on assisted ventilation for more than 1 week, 59% had PVL. In one series, the autopsy frequency of PVL was 88% in 900-to 2,200-g preterm infants who lived for more than 6 days. Overall, PVL is the second most common lesion of the infant brain, the most common one being hemorrhage in the germinal matrix and ventricles.

In patients with PVL, the initial ultrasound scans may be normal. The first positive sonographic finding usually appears during the first week

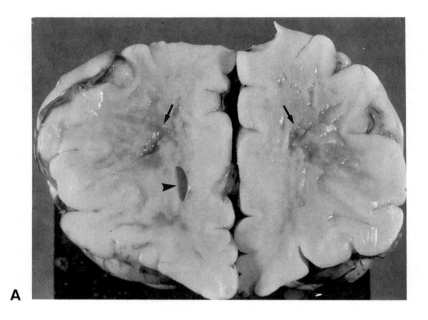

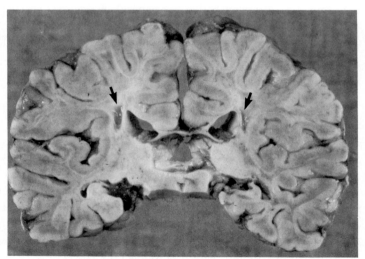

Figure 13-24. Anatomic specimens. (A) Acute periventricular leukomalacia. Coronal section at the anteriormost extent of the frontal horns
(arrowhead). Note the necrosis (arrows) of the white matter anteroposterior to the margins of the ventricle. (B) Chronic periventricular
leukomalacia. Coronal section shows dilated ventricles, cisterns and
fissures, and periventricular cavities (arrows).

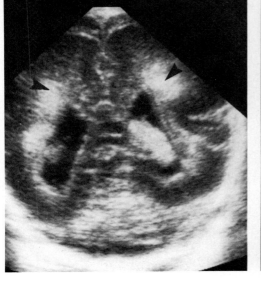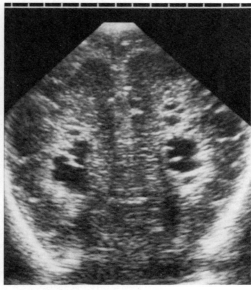

A   B

Figure 13-25. Coronal sonograms. (A) Periventricular white matter infarct (arrowheads). (B) Bilateral cystic encephalomalacia 3 weeks after the study shown in panel A.

of life as an intense periventricular echogenicity that probably represents white matter hemorrhage (Figure 13-25A). Some authors believe that nonhemorrhagic white matter infarct may be missed by ultrasonography, because infarct is often less echogenic than acute hemorrhage. Nearly 3 weeks later, cystic evolution of the lesion can be displayed by ultrasound imaging (Figure 13-25B). The cysts are multiple and variable in size. At this stage, significant ventriculomegaly is also evident on sonograms.

Not all lesions evolve to cavitation; those that do not may be overlooked by ultrasonography. In those that exhibit cavitation, the cysts may be very small (microcysts) or may have a greater diameter, in the range of 1 cm.

The exact timing of the onset of the lesions and their evolution may vary from one patient to another. Only serial studies in those who have hemorrhagic infarct can time the events accurately. Months after the baby leaves the nursery, severe motor, sensory, and mental retardation may become evident, followed later by spastic diplegia or quadriplegia, visual and auditory deficits, and convulsive disorders. Whether these unfavorable consequences are all secondary to PVL or whether some are due to concomitant or subsequent neuropathology is not known.

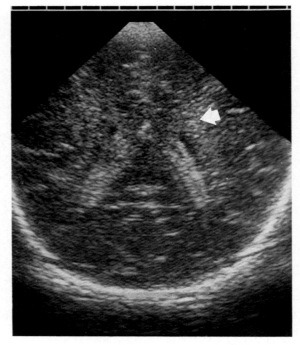

Figure 13-26. Normal peritrigonal blush (arrow).

The normal echogenicity of deep white matter, the "peritrigonal blush" (Figure 13-26), should not be misinterpreted as hemorrhagic infarct of deep white matter. Ninety-seven percent of newborns with a mean gestational age of 32 weeks demonstrate a normal peritrigonal (periventricular) echogenic blush. In full-term infants, the peritrigonal blush is not as prominent as that in preterm infants. This fine blush most likely represents both the white matter fibers and the penetrating medullary vessels that course radially from the cortex to the subependymal layer of the ventricle. This radial course is roughly perpendicular to the surface of the ventricle at each point along the changing curvature of the ventricle. From the anterior fontanelle such radial structures would provide multiple interfaces to the sonographic beam, especially at the frontal horns and atria.

Since the medullary vessels appear especially numerous and dilated in preterm infants, one normally observes linear echoes oriented roughly perpendicular to the margins of the ventricles that are more prominent in premature infants than in full-term infants. PVL should be suspected only if the periventricular blush is intense, coarse, and blotchy.

Cerebrospinal fluid (CSF) may migrate transependymally from dilated ventricles into the adjacent brain parenchyma (Option (A)). This fluid lies in the extracellular spaces of the periventricular white matter and is designated periventricular edema. In patients with periventricular edema, the sonographic image superficially resembles PVL. However, periventricular edema is not preceded by intensely echogenic white matter, as is PVL. Furthermore, the periventricular CSF edema does not result in formation of multiple periventricular cysts as PVL is known to do.

Not all patients with PVL have had intraventricular bleeding. Furthermore, if hemosiderin (Option (B)) stains the brain parenchyma, it would not manifest on sonograms as anechoic periventricular cysts.

The term periventricular leukomalacia has no specific relation to venous sinus thrombosis (Option (D)). Venous sinus thrombosis is extremely rare in preterm infants. Acute venous thrombosis may cause diffuse brain edema, concurrent venous hypertension, venular and capillary rupture, and intraparenchymal hemorrhage of the medial cerebral hemispheres, thalami, or basal ganglia. Chronic intracranial venous hypertension may cause ventriculomegaly without periventricular cysts.

PVL is an acquired central nervous system disorder seen mostly in hypoxemic preterm infants; it is not related to failure of normal myelination (Option (E)). Metachromatic leukodystrophy is a genetically determined metabolic disorder of sphingolipid metabolism in which cerebroside sulfate (sulfatide) accumulates excessively in many organs, especially brain and kidneys, because of deficient activity of a sulfuric acid esterase. Since neural cerebrosides and sulfatides are among the chief lipid components of myelin, all myelin-containing parts of the nervous system, both central and peripheral, are affected by this disease. The excessive accumulation of sulfatide in the nervous system leads to disintegration of myelin at all levels. Consequently, when stained with dyes such as toluidine blue and cresyl violet, the white matter stains purple, red, or even brown instead of the expected blue or violet—a phenomenon known as metachromasia. Therefore, the term metachromatic leukodystrophy means that the diseased cerebral white matter stains intensely and metachromatically because of the large amounts of phagocytosed sulfatide that accompany the breakdown of the myelin.

The sonographic appearance of metachromatic leukodystrophy is not known. On CT, the white matter has a very low attenuation value (Figure 13-27). The nature of the pathologic process and the CT appearance strongly suggest that, on ultrasonography, the white matter will be diffusely hypoechoic.

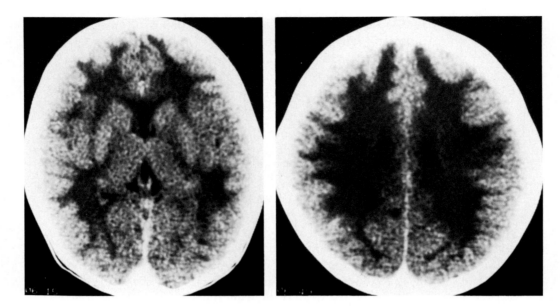

Figure 13-27. Noncontrast CT appearance of metachromatic leuko-dystrophy.

Question 67

Concerning neonates with tuberous sclerosis,

  (A) on CT, subependymal tumors are frequently seen to be calcified
  (B) subependymal tubers are highly echogenic
  (C) on CT, subependymal tubers are less frequently visible than are subcortical ones
  (D) detection of a large focus of increased echogenicity in the septum pellucidum strongly suggests the diagnosis of giant-cell astrocytoma
  (E) clinical stigmata are frequently absent

The literature indicates that children with tuberous sclerosis typically remain symptom-free during the neonatal period **(Option (E) is true).** Rarely, seizures commence as early as the first days of life. These children are more likely to be mentally retarded than are those who become symptomatic later in life. As the infant grows older, the disease is manifested as seizures, skin lesions, and mental retardation, not necessarily in that order. Some patients display only one or two

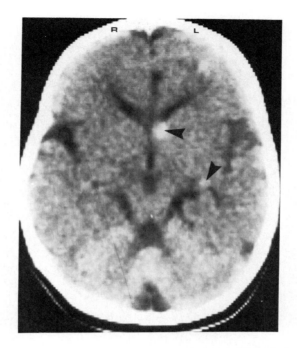

Figure 13-28. Tuberous sclerosis. Noncontrast CT of the head of an infant shows calcified subependymal tubers (arrowheads).

components of this classic clinical triad; a few remain asymptomatic for years. Girls are affected more often than boys.

Since most neonates remain asymptomatic, they are not often studied by CT or ultrasonography in the first 4 weeks of life, and thus the imaging features are not well characterized. In infants, however, it is true that (1) subependymal tumors are frequently seen to be calcified on CT studies (Figure 13-28), (2) subependymal tubers are highly echogenic (Figure 13-29), and (3) detection of a large focus of increased echogenicity in the septum pellucidum near the foramen of Monro strongly suggests the diagnosis of giant-cell astrocytoma **(Options (A), (B), and (D) are true).** Subependymal periventricular tubers are more frequently visible on CT than are subcortical tubers **(Option (C) is false).** The differential diagnosis includes toxoplasmosis, cytomegalic inclusion disease, Fahr's syndrome, and tuberculous meningitis.

David Yousefzadeh, M.D.
Thomas P. Naidich, M.D.

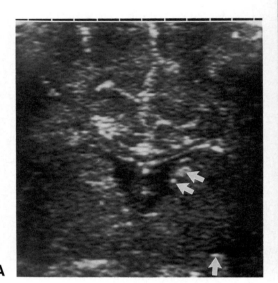
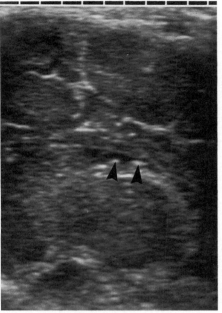

A

B

Figure 13-29. Tuberous sclerosis. Coronal (A) and parasagittal (B) ultrasound scans demonstrate highly echogenic subependymal tubers (arrows and arrowheads).

SUGGESTED READINGS

NEONATAL INTRACRANIAL HEMORRHAGE

1. Bowie JD, Kirks DR, Rosenberg ER, Clair MR. Caudothalamic groove: value in identification of germinal matrix hemorrhage by sonography in preterm neonates. AJR 1983; 141:1317–1320

2. Burstein J, Papile LA, Burstein R. Intraventricular hemorrhage and hydrocephalus in premature newborns: a prospective study with CT. AJR 1979; 132:631–635

3. Dykes F, Lazzara A, Ahmann P, Blumenstein B, Schwartz J, Brann AW. Intraventricular hemorrhage: a prospective evaluation of etiopathogenesis. Pediatrics 1980; 66:42–49

4. Emerson P, Fujimura M, Howat P, et al. Timing of intraventricular hemorrhage. Arch Dis Child 1977; 52:183–187

5. Grant EG, Kerner M, Schellinger D, et al. Evolution of porencephalic cysts from intraparenchymal hemorrhage in neonates: sonographic evidence. AJR 1982; 138:467–470

6. Johnson ML, Rumack CM, Mannes EJ, Appareti KE. Detection of neonatal intracranial hemorrhage utilizing real-time and static ultrasound. JCU 1981; 9:427–433

7. Larroche JC. Post-haemorrhagic hydrocephalus in infancy. Anatomical study. Biol Neonate 1972; 20:287–299

8. Norman MG. Perinatal brain damage. Perspect Pediatr Pathol 1978; 4:41–92

9. Pape KE, Wigglesworth JS. Hemorrhage, ischemia and the perinatal brain. London: Lavenham Press; 1979

10. Peterson CM, Smith WL, Franken EA. Neonatal intracerebellar hemorrhage: detection by real-time ultrasound. Radiology 1984; 150:391–392

11. Reeder JD, Kaude JV, Setzer ES. Choroid plexus hemorrhage in premature neonates: recognition by sonography. AJNR 1982; 3:619–622

12. Schellinger D, Grant EG, Manz HJ, Patronas NJ. Intraparenchymal hemorrhage in preterm neonates: a broadening spectrum. AJR 1988; 150:1109–1115

13. Shankaran S, Slovis TL, Bedard MP, Poland RL. Sonographic classification of intracranial hemorrhage. A prognostic indicator of mortality, morbidity, and short-term neurologic outcome. J Pediatr 1982; 469–475

14. Sherwood A, Hopp A, Smith JF. Cellular reactions to subependymal plate haemorrhage in the human neonate. Neuropathol Appl Neurobiol 1978; 4:245–261

15. Tsiantos A, Victorin L, Relier P, et al. Intracranial hemorrhage in the prematurely born infant. Timing of clots and evaluation of clinical signs and symptoms. J Pediatr 1974; 85:854–859

16. Volpe JJ. Neurology of the newborn, 2nd ed. Philadelphia: WB Saunders; 1987:311–361

17. Volpe JJ. Edward B. Neuhauser Lecture. Current concepts of brain injury in the premature infant. AJR 1989; 153:243–251

PERIVENTRICULAR LEUKOMALACIA

18. Bowerman RA, Donn SM, DiPietro MA, D'Amato CJ, Hicks SP. Periventricular leukomalacia in the pre-term newborn infant: sonographic and clinical features. Radiology 1984; 151:383–388

19. Chow PP, Horgan JG, Taylor KJW. Neonatal periventricular leukomalacia: real-time sonographic diagnosis with CT correlation. AJR 1985; 145:155–160

20. Flodmark O, Roland EH, Hill A, Whitfield MF. Periventricular leukomalacia: radiologic diagnosis. Radiology 1987; 162:119–124

TUBEROUS SCLEROSIS

21. Legge M, Sauerbrei E, MacDonald A. Intracranial tuberous sclerosis in infancy. Radiology 1984; 153:667–668

CHOROID PLEXUS PAPILLOMA

22. Chow PP, Horgan JG, Burns PN, Weltin G, Taylor KJ. Choroid plexus papilloma: detection by real-time and Doppler sonography. AJNR 1986; 7:168–170

CRANIAL ULTRASONOGRAPHY

23. DiPietro MA, Brody BA, Teele RL. The calcar avis: demonstration with cranial US. Radiology 1985; 156:363–364
24. DiPietro MA, Brody BA, Teele RL. Peritrigonal echogenic "blush" on cranial sonography: pathologic correlates. AJR 1986; 146:1067–1072
25. Mack LA, Rumack CM, Johnson ML. Ultrasound evaluation of cystic intracranial lesions in the neonate. Radiology 1980; 137:451–455
26. Netanyahu I, Grant EG. Prominent choroid plexus in meningomyelocele: sonographic findings. AJNR 1986; 7:317–321
27. Rumack CM, Johnson ML. Perinatal and infant brain imaging: role of ultrasound and computed tomography: Chicago: Yearbook Medical Publishers; 1984

Notes